Management of Peri-operative Complications

Guest Editors

LEWIS J. KAPLAN, MD
STANLEY H. ROSENBAUM, MD

SURGICAL CLINICS
OF NORTH AMERICA

www.surgical.theclinics.com

Consulting Editor
RONALD F. MARTIN, MD

April 2012 • Volume 92 • Number 2

SAUNDERS an imprint of ELSEVIER, Inc.

W.B. SAUNDERS COMPANY

A Division of Elsevier Inc.

1600 John F. Kennedy Blvd., Suite 1800, Philadelphia, PA 19103-2899

http://www.surgical.theclinics.com

SURGICAL CLINICS OF NORTH AMERICA Volume 92, Number 2
April 2012 ISSN 0039-6109, ISBN-13: 978-1-4557-3938-7

Editor: John Vassallo, j.vassallo@elsevier.com
Developmental Editor: Teia Stone

Surgical Clinics of North America (ISSN 0039–6109) is published bimonthly by Elsevier Inc., 360 Park Avenue South, New York, NY 10010-1710. Months of publication are February, April, June, August, October, and December. Business and Editorial Offices: 1600 John F. Kennedy Blvd., Suite 1800, Philadelphia, PA 19103-2899. Periodicals postage paid at New York, NY and additional mailing offices. Subscription prices are $339.00 per year for US individuals, $575.00 per year for US institutions, $166.00 per year for US students and residents, $415.00 per year for Canadian individuals, $714.00 per year for Canadian institutions, $468.00 for international individuals, $714.00 per year for international institutions and $229.00 per year for Canadian and foreign students/residents. To receive student/resident rate, orders must be accompanied by name of affiliated institution, date of term, and the *signature* of program/residency coordinator on institution letterhead. Orders will be billed at individual rate until proof of status is received. Foreign air speed delivery is included in all *Clinics* subscription prices. All prices are subject to change without notice. POSTMASTER: Send address changes to *Surgical Clinics*, Elsevier Health Sciences Division, Subscription Customer Service, 3251 Riverport Lane, Maryland Heights, MO 63043. **Customer Service (orders, claims, online, change of address): Telephone: 1-800-654-2452 (U.S. and Canada); 314-447-8871 (outside U.S. and Canada). Fax: 314-447-8029. E-mail: journalscustomerservice-usa@elsevier.com (for print support); journalsonlinesupport-usa@elsevier.com (for online support).**

Reprints. For copies of 100 or more, of articles in this publication, please contact the Commercial Reprints Department, Elsevier Inc., 360 Park Avenue South, New York, New York 10010-1710. Tel. (212) 633-3812, Fax: (212) 462-1935, e-mail: reprints@elsevier.com.

The Surgical Clinics of North America is also published in Spanish by McGraw-Hill Interamericana Editores S.A., P.O. Box 5-237 06500 Mexico D.F. Mexico; and in Portuguese by Interlivros Edicoes Ltda., Rua Comandante Coelho 1085, CEP 21250, Rio de Janeiro, Brazil; and in Greek by Paschalidis Medical Publications, Athens Greece.

The Surgical Clinics of North America is covered in *MEDLINE/PubMed (Index Medicus), EMBASE/Excerpta Medica, Current Contents/Clinical Medicine, Current Contents/Life Sciences, Science Citation Index,* and *ISI/BIOMED.*

Printed and bound by CPI Group (UK) Ltd, Croydon, CR0 4YY

Transferred to Digital Print 2012

Contributors

CONSULTING EDITOR

RONALD F. MARTIN, MD, FACS
Director, Surgical Education/Residency Program Director, Department of Surgery,
Marshfield Clinic and Saint Joseph's Hospital, Marshfield, Wisconsin; Clinical Associate
Professor, University of Wisconsin School of Medicine and Public Health, Madison,
Wisconsin; Colonel, Medical Corps, United States Army Reserve

GUEST EDITORS

LEWIS J. KAPLAN, MD, FACS, FCCM, FCCP
Associate Professor of Surgery, Section of Trauma, Surgical Critical Care and Surgical
Emergencies, Department of Surgery, Yale University School of Medicine, New Haven,
Connecticut

STANLEY H. ROSENBAUM, MD
Professor of Anesthesiology, Surgery and Internal Medicine, Department of
Anesthesiology, Yale University School of Medicine, New Haven, Connecticut

AUTHORS

STEVEN R. ALLEN, MD
Division of Traumatology, Surgical Critical Care and Emergency Surgery, University of
Pennsylvania, Philadelphia, Pennsylvania

KOEN AMELOOT, MD
Intensive Care Unit, Ziekenhuis Netwerk Antwerpen, Campus Stuivenberg/Erasmus,
Antwerpen, Belgium

PHILIP S. BARIE, MD, MBA, FIDSA, FCCM, FACS
Professor of Surgery and Public Health, Department of Surgery, Weill Cornell Medical
College; Chief, Preston A. (Pep) Wade Acute Care Surgery Service, New York-Presbyterian
Hospital-Weill Cornell Medical Center, New York, New York

THOMAS BUCHHEIT, MD
Associate Professor, Department of Anesthesiology, Duke University Medical Center,
Durham, North Carolina

CRAIG M. COOPERSMITH, MD
Professor of Surgery, Associate Director, Emory Center for Critical Care, Emory University
School of Medicine and Emory Healthcare, Atlanta, Georgia

H. GILL CRYER, MD
Professor of Surgery, Division of General Surgery, Chief of Trauma and Emergency
Surgery, UCLA Medical Center, University of California-Los Angeles, Los Angeles,
California

KIMBERLY A. DAVIS, MD, FACS, FCCM
Professor of Surgery, Vice Chairman of Clinical Affairs, Chief of the Section of Trauma, Surgical Critical Care and Surgical Emergencies, Department of Surgery, Yale University School of Medicine, New Haven, Connecticut

NELE DESIE, MD
Intensive Care Unit, Ziekenhuis Netwerk Antwerpen, Campus Stuivenberg/Erasmus, Antwerpen, Belgium

MICHAEL G. DOORLY, MD, MS
Clinical Instructor of Surgery and Colorectal Surgery Research Fellow, Keck School of Medicine, University of Southern California, Los Angeles, California

JOHN FILDES, MD
Chief, Division of Trauma & Critical Care, Vice Chair, Professor of Surgery, Department of Surgery, University of Nevada School of Medicine, Las Vegas, Nevada; Medical Director, American College of Surgeons Committee on Trauma, Chicago, Illinois

LTC (Ret.) LISA M. FLYNN, MD, RVT, FACS, USAR, MC
Assistant Professor of Surgery, Department of Surgery, Wayne State University, Detroit, Michigan

HEIDI L. FRANKEL, MD, FACS
Division of Trauma, Acute Care and Critical Care Surgery, Penn State Hershey Medical Center, Hershey, Pennsylvania; Division of Surgical Critical Care, University of Maryland R Adams Cowley Shock Trauma Center, Baltimore, Maryland

CARL GILLEBERT, MD
Intensive Care Unit, Ziekenhuis Netwerk Antwerpen, Campus Stuivenberg/Erasmus, Antwerpen, Belgium

SEON JONES, MD
Instructor of Surgery, Division of Trauma and Surgical Critical Care, Vanderbilt University Medical Center, Nashville, Tennessee

LEWIS J. KAPLAN, MD, FACS, FCCM, FCCP
Associate Professor of Surgery, Section of Trauma, Surgical Critical Care and Surgical Emergencies, Department of Surgery, Yale University School of Medicine, New Haven, Connecticut

MANU L.N.G. MALBRAIN, MD, PhD
Head of Department, Intensive Care Unit and High Care Burn Unit, Ziekenhuis Netwerk Antwerpen, Campus Stuivenberg/Erasmus, Antwerpen, Belgium

RONALD F. MARTIN, MD, FACS
Director, Surgical Education/Residency Program Director, Department of Surgery, Marshfield Clinic and Saint Joseph's Hospital, Marshfield, Wisconsin; Clinical Associate Professor of Surgery, University of Wisconsin School of Medicine and Public Health, Madison, Wisconsin; Colonel, Medical Corps, United States Army Reserve

ADRIAN A. MAUNG, MD, FACS
Assistant Professor of Surgery, Section of Trauma, Surgical Critical Care and Surgical Emergencies, Department of Surgery, Yale University School of Medicine, New Haven, Connecticut

ADDISON K. MAY, MD
Professor of Surgery and Anesthesiology, Division of Trauma and Surgical Critical Care; Director, Surgical Critical Care and Program Director, Surgical Critical Care and Acute Care Surgery Fellowship, Vanderbilt University Medical Center, Nashville, Tennessee

JOHN E. MAZUSKI, MD, PhD
Professor of Surgery, Section of Acute and Critical Care Surgery, Department of Surgery, Washington University School of Medicine, St Louis, Missouri

KEVIN W. MCCONNELL, MD
Assistant Professor of Surgery, Acute and Critical Care Surgery, Emory University School of Medicine, Atlanta, Georgia

LENA M. NAPOLITANO, MD, FACS, FCCP, FCCM
Division Chief, Division of Acute Care Surgery [Trauma, Burns, Surgical Critical Care, Emergency Surgery]; Professor of Surgery, Director, Trauma and Surgical Critical Care, Associate Chair, Department of Surgery, University of Michigan Health System, Ann Arbor, Michigan

AVERY B. NATHENS, MD, PhD
Division Head and Director of Trauma, Professor of Surgery, St. Michael's Hospital, University of Toronto, Toronto, Canada; Director, American College of Surgeons Trauma Quality Improvement Program, Chicago, Illinois

GRETA L. PIPER, MD
Assistant Professor of Surgery, Section of Trauma, Surgical Critical Care and Surgical Emergencies, Department of Surgery, Yale University School of Medicine, New Haven, Connecticut

SRINIVAS PYATI, MD
Assistant Professor, Department of Anesthesiology, Duke University Medical Center, Durham, North Carolina

JORDAN M. RAYMER, MD
Resident in General Surgery, Marshfield Clinic and Saint Joseph's Hospital, Marshfield, Wisconsin

MICHAEL F. ROTONDO, MD, FACS
Professor and Chairman of Surgery, Department of Surgery, The Brody School of Medicine, East Carolina University, Greenville, North Carolina

GAURAV SACHDEV, MD
Surgical Critical Care Fellow, Division of Acute Care Surgery [Trauma, Burns, Surgical Critical Care, Emergency Surgery], Department of Surgery, University of Michigan, Ann Arbor, Michigan

STEVEN J. SCHWULST, MD
Assistant Professor of Surgery, Division of Trauma and Critical Care, Department of Surgery, Northwestern University Feinberg School of Medicine, Chicago, Illinois

ANTHONY J. SENAGORE, MD, MS, MBA, FACS, FASCRS
Professor and Clinical Scholar, Division Chief of Colorectal Surgery, Charles W. and Carolyn Costello Chair for Colorectal Diseases, Keck School of Medicine, University of Southern California, Los Angeles, California

SAMUEL A. TISHERMAN, MD, FACS, FCCM
Professor, Departments of Critical Care Medicine and Surgery, University of Pittsburgh, Pittsburgh, Pennsylvania

BRETT H. WAIBEL, MD, FACS
Assistant Professor of Surgery, Department of Surgery, The Brody School of Medicine, East Carolina University, Greenville, North Carolina

Contents

For surgical patients, appropriate selection and administration of fluids can mitigate against organ failure, whereas improper dosing can exacerbate already injured systems. Fluid and electrolyte goals and deficiencies must be defined for individual patients to provide the appropriate combination of resuscitation and maintenance fluids. Specific electrolyte abnormalities should be anticipated, identified, and corrected to optimize organ functions. Using the strong-ion approach to acid-base assessment, delivered fluids that contain calculated amounts of electrolytes will interact with the patient's plasma charge and influence the patient's pH, allowing the clinician to achieve a more precise end point.

Cardiovascular dysfunction and failure are commonly encountered in patients with intra-abdominal hypertension or abdominal compartment syndrome. Accurate assessment and optimization of preload, afterload, and contractility are essential to restoring end-organ perfusion and maximizing patient survival. Application of a goal-directed resuscitation strategy, including abdominal decompression, when indicated, improves cardiac function, reverses end-organ failure, and minimizes intra-abdominal hypertension–related patient morbidity and mortality.

Hemorrhage remains a leading cause of morbidity and death in both civilian and military trauma. Restoration of effective end-organ perfusion by stopping hemorrhage and restoring intravascular volume in such a way as to minimize acidosis, hypothermia, and coagulopathy, almost always requires the use of blood and/or blood-component therapy. The best method to manage life-threatening hemorrhage is to avoid the circumstance that prompted it or to mitigate blood loss early in the injury cycle; otherwise, blood replacement must suffice. This article reviews current understanding of massive transfusion, along with its attendant unintended consequences, in the management of patients with profound hemorrhage.

Significant gastrointestinal (GI) bleeding in the postoperative period is an uncommon complication of surgery. The management of GI bleeding within the postoperative period is complex because of a larger differential for the source of bleeding and a more complex risk/benefit analysis. There is minimal published literature specific to the management of postoperative GI bleeding, and the infrequency, complexity, and variability of the clinical setting of this complication confound simplistic consideration of its cause and therapy. This article outlines a systematic evaluation of the patient, treatment options, and assessment of risk/benefit ratio for various treatment options.

With the success of damage-control surgery for the treatment of exsanguinating truncal trauma, it has been adapted to other surgical diseases associated with shock states, such as severe secondary peritonitis. The structured approach of damage control is easily adapted to and can incorporate the fundamental elements of the Surviving Sepsis Campaign. It is not meant to replace tried and true surgical principles, such as source control, but is a usable framework in managing the complicated circumstances seen with these patients.

Postoperative ileus is a preventable disease with surprising economic consequences. Understanding the triad of dysmotility in conjunction with an enhanced recovery program improves patient outcome, decreases length of stay in hospital, and lowers the cost. Alvimopan and other investigational promotility medications can help attain these goals. Surgeons should avoid labeling all postoperative abdominal distention as ileus, which not only prevents timely diagnosis and treatment of early postoperative small bowel obstruction or acute colonic pseudo-obstruction but also increases patient morbidity and mortality.

Nutritional support in surgical patients has evolved from simple provision of adequate calories to retard loss of lean body mass to the provision of specific nutrients in an attempt to manipulate metabolic and immune responses. Although still limited, the current understanding of this complex subject indicates that the type, route, amount, and composition of nutritional support provided to patients can affect their outcome. Further studies are, however, needed to better characterize the exact nutritional support that is most beneficial for a specific disease state and a specific patient.

Individual health care quality measures that have been shown to improve outcome can be combined together into what are called care bundles, with the expectation that this set of practices produces further improvements in outcome. Prevention of surgical site infection is the focus of several quality measures put forward by the Surgical Care Improvement Project; these can collectively be considered a bundle as well. Whether these process measures, which include several components related to the administration of antibiotic prophylaxis, are effective in decreasing rates of surgical site infection has come under considerable debate recently.

Postoperative organ failure is a challenging disease process that is better prevented than treated. Providers should use close observation and clinical judgment, and checklists of best practices to minimize the risk of organ failure in their patients. The treatment of multiorgan dysfunction syndrome (MODS) generally remains supportive, outside of rapid initiation of source control (when appropriate) and targeted antibiotic therapy. More specific treatments may be developed as the complex pathophysiology of MODS is better understood and more homogenous patient populations are selected for study.

Postoperative pulmonary complications (atelectasis, pneumonia, pulmonary edema, acute respiratory failure) are common, particularly after abdominal and thoracic surgery, pneumonia and atelectasis being the most common. Postoperative pneumonia is associated with increased morbidity, length of hospital stay, and costs. Few institutions have pneumonia prevention programs for surgical patients, and these should be strongly considered. Acute respiratory failure is a life-threatening pulmonary complication that requires institution of mechanical ventilation and admission to the intensive care unit, and is associated with increased risk for ventilator-associated pneumonia. This article discusses epidemiology, risk factors, diagnosis, treatment, and prevention of these pulmonary complications in surgical patients.

The increasing prevalence of multidrug-resistant (MDR) infections in clinical practice stems from clinical and veterinary antibiotic use, and animal husbandry. As resistance to antibiotics becomes more common, a vicious circle develops wherein increasingly broad-spectrum agents must be prescribed empirically to ensure that initial antibiotic therapy is adequate to the task, and new, ever more powerful agents are needed for the treatment of

MDR bacteria. Unfortunately, a dearth of new agents and drugs is in development. As clinicians we must learn to make do with what we have for the foreseeable future, according to the principles of antibiotic stewardship.

Although techniques for acute pain management have improved in recent years, a dramatic reduction in the incidence and severity of chronic pain following surgery has not occurred. Amputation and thoracotomy, although technically different, share the commonalities of unavoidable nerve injury and the frequent presence of persistent postsurgical neuropathic pain. The authors review the risk factors for the development of chronic pain following these surgeries and the current evidence that supports analgesic interventions. The inconclusive results from many preemptive analgesic studies may require us to reconceptualize the perioperative treatment period as a time of gradual neurologic remodeling.

Delirium is a common feature of the postoperative period, leading to increased morbidity and mortality and significant costs. Multiple factors predispose a patient to delirium in its hypoactive, hyperactive, or mixed forms. Tools have been validated for its quick and accurate identification to ensure timely and effective multidisciplinary intervention and treatment. A significant percentage of patients may require placement in skilled nursing facilities or similar care environments because of the long-lasting effects. The physician must be vigilant in the search for and identification of all forms of delirium and must effectively treat the underlying medical condition and symptoms.

In the perioperative period, patients may suffer complications leading to serious adverse events. Patient deterioration needs to be rapidly identified, and a rapid response system must be initiated. Additional personnel may also be needed. Rescue therapies, beyond the routine resuscitative efforts, may be needed in some cases. The types of complications that may be faced include a difficult airway, refractory hypoxemia, pulmonary embolism, myocardial infarction, cardiac arrest with restoration of pulse but ongoing coma, and stroke. Although perioperative complications can be catastrophic, rapid intervention, including rescue therapies when necessary, can improve outcomes.

The American College of Surgeons Trauma Quality Improvement Program (ACS TQIP) is a recent addition to the many quality improvement collaboratives that have been established in surgery. On the background of a well-established trauma center and its performance improvement activities, ACS TQIP offers the potential to advance trauma care and offers participating centers the opportunity to better understand their strengths and areas for improvement. The rationale for ACS TQIP's development, implementation challenges, and potential for advancing the quality of trauma care are described.

THE CLINICS ARE NOW AVAILABLE ONLINE!

Access your subscription at:
www.theclinics.com

Foreword

Management of Peri-operative Complications

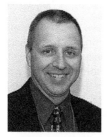

Ronald F. Martin, MD
Consulting Editor

Surgery is a humbling pursuit—or at least it should be. And there are few things as humbling to a surgeon as an operation that goes awry or worse.

There is great merit in knowing how to get out of trouble, whether it is in the operating room or on the wards. There is greater merit in knowing how not to get into trouble in the first place. The best surgeons with whom I have had the privilege to work have been masters at not only avoiding operative pitfalls but also being in the wrong place at the wrong time with the wrong resources to begin with. Certainly, the development of better technology for imaging and evaluation has been useful, but the people who routinely "make it look easy" are the ones who are expert preoperative assessors of patients because they understand the diseases they treat and the consequences to the patients who have them.

As in much of life, a gram of prevention is worth a kilogram of cure. In order to prevent peri-operative problems, one must first have a good working construct of what problems exist or can arise. This issue of the *Surgical Clinics of North America* provides an excellent review of challenging problems that present to us as well as those that we, sometimes, contribute to. In addition, a review of the strategies for mitigating these problems is provided as well as information on how to evaluate and track our success in our endeavors.

If we as a profession are going to make an impact on behalf of our patients, we will need to do some things better than we currently do. First, we need to measure more frequently and more accurately. As Lord Kelvin is attributed to stating, "If you cannot measure it, you cannot improve it." We are going to have to find the right metrics to meaningfully measure what we do. That will by necessity require that we develop quality metrics not just for outcomes but also for indications. Not all things are right for all people. One example a colleague of mine likes to cite is the proposed requirement to measure hemoglobin A1c on every primary care patient. Do we really feel compelled to track better or worse glucose control on someone with markedly

Surg Clin N Am 92 (2012) xiii–xiv
doi:10.1016/j.suc.2012.02.001
0039-6109/12/$ – see front matter

advanced cancer? As my colleague states, 100 percent compliance with some things just shows people aren't thinking. Furthermore, unless we plan to bankrupt the entire economy, we will need to assign value equations as part of our analysis. An uncomfortable part of this last suggestion is that we will need to seriously consider what the value of something is to individuals in light of other patient variables such as age and comorbid conditions. I know this smacks of *rationing health care*, but unless we believe that we can provide all care for all patients at all times under all circumstances, then we de facto already believe in some kind of rationing.

If we are going to assign value of treatments, then we have to have better data on the real costs and real benefits of the options that we are considering (some would argue that patient satisfaction as a different variable but I personally would submit that it is in the benefits). To get the kind of data we need to be more accurate, we will need mandatory reporting, information systems that interface better, and protections for participating that exceed the costs of participating, ie, tort reform. This may sound familiar, as we just reviewed patient safety in our last issue of the *Clinics* and some of the issues well overlap.

Personally, I have always found it emotionally easier to recognize or take care of a complication in one of my partner's patients or a patient who has been transferred to us from a referring facility than to do the same for one my own patients. I'd like to think that my intellect overrides my emotion in such situations and for the most part perhaps it does. Thankfully, I have the benefit of great partners and a stellar resident staff that wouldn't let me labor in a self-delusional state for very long should my attempts at self-deception start to prevail.

It takes a special kind of confidence to agree to operate on someone in the hopes of improving his or her lot in life. I like to think that confidence stems from years of practice and rigorous training in our subject matter, and sometimes it does, although the confidence some of us display is unjustified because either we don't know what we don't know or we just are not as capable of the introspection necessary to do this well. Improved knowledge of what can go wrong is always the best place to start when trying to avoid trouble. Judgment, however, is what prevails in the end. As it is said, good judgment comes from experience and experience comes from bad judgment. It is always preferable to gain experience from another's marginal judgment when possible.

I am indebted to Drs Kaplan and Rosenbaum for assembling this collection of thoughtful articles that demonstrate both the experience and the judgment accrued by so many over the years.

Ronald F. Martin, MD
Department of Surgery
Marshfield Clinic
1000 North Oak Avenue
Marshfield, WI 54449, USA

E-mail address:
martin.ronald@marshfield.org

Preface

Management of Peri-operative Complications

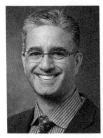 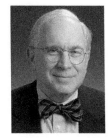

Lewis J. Kaplan, MD   Stanley H. Rosenbaum, MD
Guest Editors

This edition of *Surgical Clinics of North America* is devoted to the management of peri-operative complications, with a focus on patients with critical illness. We would like to thank all of our authors for their time and dedication in generating high-quality works within their respective areas of expertise. This text carries the reader through the universal therapies of fluids and electrolytes and then through specific complications, organ failure, rescue therapies, preventive measures, and the benchmarking of current and best practices. It is our hope that the information contained herein will enable our colleagues to provide optimal care better in and out of the ICU throughout all phases of peri-operative management.

Lewis J. Kaplan, MD
Department of Surgery
Section of Trauma
Surgical Critical Care and Surgical Emergencies
Yale University School of Medicine
330 Cedar Street, BB-310
New Haven, CT 06520, USA

Stanley H. Rosenbaum, MD
Department of Anesthesiology
Yale University School of Medicine
PO Box 208051
333 Cedar Street, TMP 3
New Haven, CT 06520-8051, USA

E-mail addresses:
lewis.kaplan@yale.edu (L.J. Kaplan)
Stanley.rosenbaum@yale.edu (S.H. Rosenbaum)

Surg Clin N Am 92 (2012) xv
doi:10.1016/j.suc.2012.01.016
0039-6109/12/$ – see front matter © 2012 Elsevier Inc. All rights reserved.

Fluid and Electrolyte Management for the Surgical Patient

Greta L. Piper, MD[a], Lewis J. Kaplan, MD[b],*

KEYWORDS

- Fluid balance • Electrolyte balance • Acid-base assessment
- Plasma volume • Hyperchloremic metabolic acidosis

Human cells consist of 65% to 90% water. Water and solutes pass through cell membranes both actively and passively. Specific fluid and electrolyte concentrations are necessary in order for cell metabolism to occur, and these balances are affected by different stresses including trauma, surgery, and critical illness. While fluid loss, both measurable and insensible, occurs with these stressors, replacement and maintenance fluids are commonly administered without consideration of specific patient needs. Protocols and order sets allow for one-size-fits-all fluid management that, though time efficient, may not optimize patient recovery and may be detrimental.

A patient's fluid and electrolyte status affects all organ systems. Appropriate selection and administration of fluids can mitigate against organ failure; improper dosing can exacerbate already injured systems. The human body in a state of wellness has a remarkable capacity to make small and large adjustments in fluid and electrolyte intake and mobilization for specific needs. In a state of illness these compensatory mechanisms are disrupted, and recovery is dependent on restoration of an appropriate balance.

In this era of ongoing identification and analysis of medical errors, fluid and electrolyte management has trailed behind the medical decisions that have immediate obvious adverse consequences, perhaps because the effects of fluid mismanagement appear as multiple organ system failings that are attributed instead to progression of the underlying disease in the patient. This predicament may also reflect a lack of understanding of the importance of considering individual volume and electrolyte abnormalities as a separate variable that can significantly alter a patient's course and outcome.

[a] Section of Trauma, Surgical Critical Care and Surgical Emergencies, Department of Surgery, Yale University School of Medicine, New Haven, CT, USA
[b] Section of Trauma, Surgical Critical Care and Surgical Emergencies, Department of Surgery, Yale University School of Medicine, 330 Cedar Street, BB-310, New Haven, CT 06520, USA
* Corresponding author.
E-mail address: Lewis.Kaplan@yale.edu

Surg Clin N Am 92 (2012) 189–205
doi:10.1016/j.suc.2012.01.004
0039-6109/12/$ – see front matter

FLUIDS AND GOALS

Patients are managed during their hospitalization with different types of fluids, including those designed to address the management of hypovolemia and those designed to address daily fluid and salt requirements. In general, each specific fluid prescription should address a distinct therapeutic goal to be achieved. To this end, each fluid type is individually discussed here, beginning with resuscitation fluids, as patients presenting to the emergency department (ED) or operating room (OR) commonly require management of hypovolemia from external fluid or blood losses, or internal losses from the vascular compartment due to capillary leak that is generally related to infection.

Resuscitation Fluids

Resuscitation fluids are meant to replace large volumes of fluid in all compartments. The adequacy of the resuscitation depends on estimating the volume and specific composition of lost fluids, and the effects the resuscitation fluids will have on blood chemistry, pH, coagulation, and platelet and cellular responses as well as the result of changes in microvascular flow and end-organ Do_2/Vo_2.

On arrival at the trauma bay, trauma patients may have lost a combination of blood, sweat, interstitial fluid from open wounds, and/or gastric contents. Surgical patients become hypovolemic from blood loss, gastrointestinal (GI) losses from emesis/diarrhea or bowel preparations, decreased intake, as well as insensible losses from respiration, evaporation, or open body cavities. The amount of volume loss is frequently estimated by reports of or directly observed blood or fluid loss, or by noting any abnormalities in a patient's physiology at initial evaluation and then in response to ongoing resuscitation.

The goal of fluid resuscitation is plasma volume expansion (PVE) to maintain or regain adequate perfusion, so as to enable optimal organ function via oxygen delivery. Hypovolemia and decreased tissue oxygenation lead to anaerobic metabolism and increased production of lactic acid. With persistent tissue hypoxia, buffering ability is overwhelmed, leading to lactic acidosis. Acidosis directly reduces the activity of the extrinsic and intrinsic coagulation pathways as measured by prothrombin time and activated partial thromboplastin time, and also diminishes platelet function as measured by platelet aggregation and platelet factor III release assays. Acidosis speeds the progression to coagulopathy and organ failure, in particular after injury.

Goal-directed resuscitation therapy aims to correct physiologically and clinically relevant parameters to specific end points, the merits of which continue to be debated. Traditional end points include a systolic blood pressure greater than 120 mm Hg or mean arterial pressure greater than 70 mm Hg, urine output greater than 0.5 mL/kg/h, base deficit less than 2, or lactic acid level less than 2.5. Each of these traditional end points has been variably supported or discounted as a result of later investigations, many of which are reviewed herein. When military and trauma systems became overwhelmed with casualties in the setting of limited resources, the merits of permissive hypotension prior to definitive hemorrhage control were discovered. Whereas the initial theory cited preserving developed clots as a means of limiting hemorrhage, further investigation has revealed that avoiding overresuscitation and the subsequent cardiopulmonary and compartment strains improves survival.[1–4]

At present, a range of parameters from the most basic subjective temperature of a patient's extremities to invasive monitoring of cardiac performance are used, depending on the setting and cause of the patient's shock. Early goal-directed therapy (EGDT) for sepsis as described by Rivers and colleagues[5] involves infusion of crystalloid to a central venous pressure of 14 mm Hg, and transfusing packed red blood cells (PRBCs) to a hemoglobin of 8 g/dL to augment tissue oxygen delivery as measured by central (not mixed) venous oxygen saturation in either the superior vena cava or the subclavian vein. Similarly, in hypotensive injured patients, Advanced Trauma Life Support recommends the infusion of 2 L of crystalloid as an initial resuscitation bolus. Ongoing hypotension should prompt PRBCs for the management of hemorrhagic shock. Noninvasive (ie, near-infrared spectroscopy) or invasive tissue oxygenation probes are the subject of ongoing evaluation as a real-time monitor of these interventions.[6,7]

Many advances in shock resuscitation have occurred during military conflicts. During World War I, little preoperative resuscitation was administered and many soldiers died of overwhelming sepsis.[8] In World War II, misconceptions regarding resuscitation, including the need to address deficits in all fluid compartments as well as the failure to address hemoconcentration, led to large-volume colloid administration. With ongoing investigation, banked blood resuscitation became standard care in addition to colloid resuscitation. Early survival improved, but complications related to acute renal failure led to increased mortality.[8] Resuscitation with large-volume isotonic crystalloid solutions followed during the Vietnam War, introducing respiratory distress syndrome and acute lung injury as a major source of morbidity and mortality.[8] As intensive care units (ICUs) developed, survival in patients with organ failure improved, although controversies over the choice of initial resuscitation fluid continue to this day. Because patients generally require both resuscitation and maintenance, a discussion of maintenance fluids is in order.

Maintenance Fluids

The goal of administration of maintenance fluid is to provide water, electrolytes and, to a lesser extent, calories to the patient who is unable to ingest adequate quantities of these components on his or her own. Calories are provided as dextrose, decreasing the need for gluconeogenesis and in part retarding muscle catabolism. Dextrose is not used in resuscitation fluid, as it can lead to osmotic diuresis when administered in large quantity. A healthy adult ingests approximately 1 mL of free water per kilocalorie of energy (35–50 mL/kg of ideal body weight per day), and wide variations in fluid intake can be well tolerated without significant physiologic disturbance. Hospitalized patients may require less total fluid depending on their specific pathology. Patients with cardiopulmonary disease, liver disease, and renal failure, as well as trauma patients with closed head injuries are often managed with restricted fluid intake. By contrast, patients with ongoing GI losses or burns typically require more than body weight–based daily fluid administration.

SPECIFIC FLUID TYPES
Crystalloids

The purported advantages of crystalloid solutions are numerous. Such solutions are inexpensive, easy to store with a long shelf life, and readily available; they have a very low incidence of adverse reactions, are effective for use as replacement fluids or maintenance fluids, require no special compatibility testing, and there are no religious objections to their use. The most commonly used resuscitation crystalloids are 0.9% normal saline and lactated Ringer (LR), solutions that are isotonic to blood. Normal saline solution (NSS) is 0.9% sodium chloride solution, containing 154 mEq/L of both sodium and chloride. Normal saline is considered an isotonic solution because it has an osmotic pressure of 308 mOsm/L, similar to that of intravascular and interstitial fluid. This similarity in osmotic pressure reduces the likelihood of a rapid transcompartment shift of fluid following a large infusion.

In health, crystalloid fluids distribute though the body in a fashion parallel to body fluids, two-thirds intracellular and one-third extracellular, 20% of which is intravascular and 80% of which is interstitial. Because only a portion of the infused volume remains in the vascular space, large volumes may be required to raise and maintain adequate circulating volume and blood pressure following illness or injury due to capillary leak and reduced capillary oncotic pressure. In such a circumstance, normal saline's higher amount of sodium and significantly higher amount of chloride in comparison with plasma will predictably result in hyperchloremic acidosis when large volumes of fluid are administered for resuscitation.

LR consists of 130 mmol/L sodium, 4 mmol/L potassium, 3 mmol/L calcium, and 109 mmol/L chloride. Sidney Ringer, while studying the properties of various physiologic fluids in the 1800s, believed that potassium was necessary for any fluid that would be used to treat significant fluid losses, and subsequently developed Ringer solution from a normal saline base.[9,10] In 1910, after numerous studies on patients with severe diarrhea, it was determined that not only was there a significant electrolyte loss but there was also a loss of bicarbonate. Based on this research Alexis Hartmann added sodium lactate, a precursor to bicarbonate, to Ringer's formula, creating LR solution.[10] As the lactate in the solution is metabolized in the liver, a hydrogen atom is removed from the lactate molecule, leaving a hydroxide molecule free to combine with circulating CO_2 to form bicarbonate, HCO_3. As with normal saline, only 25% of infused volume will remain in the intravascular space, necessitating large volumes to maintain adequate blood pressure and perfusion in those with hypovolemia. Another buffered solution used in resuscitation is 0.45% normal saline with 75 mEq sodium bicarbonate. This solution is also isotonic with an elevated sodium concentration but contains far less chloride, mitigating against hyperchloremic acidosis. The physiologic underpinning for such acid-base changes is discussed in detail later.

As a result of identifying the physiology of capillary leak, there has been significant interest in using hypertonic crystalloid solutions in resuscitation to retain the fluid bolus in the vascular space and to draw fluid from the interstitial space into the vascular space. From the late 1980s through the early 1990s, several trials found survival outcome to be inconsistently improved but documented that a single bolus of hypertonic saline was safe in diverse patient types.[11–15] More specific analysis supports the use of safe hypertonic saline in patients with traumatic brain injuries, but identifies no outcome advantage compared with standard-of-care isotonic crystalloid fluids.[16–19]

Colloids

A colloid is a substance that is microscopically dispersed throughout a suspensory fluid. As a result of the fluid's oncotic pressure, it largely remains in the intravascular compartment longer in comparison with crystalloid solutions. Colloid solutions may be synthetic or biological. Synthetic colloids include dextrans, gelatins, and hetastarch. Dextrans are highly branched polysaccharide molecules that are produced using the bacterial enzyme dextran sucrase from the bacterium *Leuconostoc mesenteroides* (B512 strain). Although they are effective plasma volume expanders, the rheologic effects of dextrans limit their utility in the resuscitation of trauma patients and surgical patients. Dextrans can also cause severe anaphylactic reactions, due to dextran-reactive antibodies that trigger the release of vasoactive mediators including histamine. In addition, dextrans coat the surface of red blood cells, interfering with the ability to cross-match blood, and may accumulate in the renal tubules, causing tubular occlusions and acute kidney injury or renal failure.

Gelatin is a large molecular weight protein formed from the hydrolysis of collagen. Advantages of gelatin colloids include their low cost and decreased renal side effects in comparison with other colloids.[20,21] These smaller molecules are less effective than larger molecular weight colloids at PVE, but are easily excreted via glomerular filtration. Like dextrans, gelatin may induce severe anaphylactic responses.

Hydroxyethyl starches (HES) are derivatives of amylopectin, a highly branched compound of starch, and are derived from potato or maize. Different types of HES are typically described by their average molecular weight and their degree of molar substitution (the proportion of the glucose units on the starch molecule that have been replaced by hydroxyethyl units). A solution of hydroxyethyl starch may further be described by its concentration by percentage (ie, grams per 100 mL). Advantages include effective PVE, low cost, and immediate availability. Disadvantages include anaphylactoid reactions, decreases in hematocrit, and anticoagulant effects. There are 3 HES products currently approved in the United States: Hespan (6% hetastarch 600/0.75 in 0.9% sodium chloride), Hextend (6% hetastarch 670/0.75 in lactated electrolyte), and Voluven (6% hydroxyethyl starch 130/0.4 in 0.9% sodium chloride).

Biological colloids include whole blood, fresh frozen plasma (FFP), and albumin. Whole blood is the ultimate resuscitation fluid, and is used as part of the buddy-system transfusions in military emergencies when banked blood products are not readily available. The lack of availability of whole blood transfusion precludes its use except in civilian trauma. Moreover, given the shortages of blood product availability, blood component therapy is most efficacious in terms of providing the greatest amount of product to the greatest amount of needful patients. PRBCs, the first blood product requested in most hemorrhagic shock patients, is a red cell mass expander but not a plasma volume expander. FFP has been described as a volume-expanding resuscitation fluid, particularly in burn patients, and is increasingly used as part of a massive transfusion protocol in military and civilian trauma centers, in particular as target PRBC/FFP/platelet ratios are increasingly supported as 1:1:1.[22,23] The main advantage of blood product resuscitation is that the transfused components remain intravascular in the absence of ongoing hemorrhage. Disadvantages include the limited blood supply, alloimmunization, immune suppression related infection and risk of organ failure, and transfusion-related reactions.

Albumin

Albumin, with a molecular weight of 60 kDa, is a biologically active protein found in plasma. Used for PVE, 5% or 25% formulations are available in the United States. Its small size makes it suboptimal for use with septic shock physiology, as it is not able to remain intravascular when capillary leak is present. Albumin has been demonstrated to be an effective PVE with large-volume paracentesis (>5 L), acute hepatic failure in the pretransplant setting, and in combination with antimicrobials for the management of spontaneous bacterial peritonitis.[24–26] Multiple meta-analyses regarding the use of albumin versus crystalloid (normal saline) in critically ill adult patients concluded that albumin is equally as safe as saline in ICU patients with hypovolemia, burns, or hypoalbuminemia.[27,28] This drawback, in addition to the increased cost, potential for pulmonary edema, anticoagulant properties, and minor risk of infection makes albumin a less attractive resuscitation fluid than other colloids. Nonetheless, the widespread use of albumin persists, in particular in liver transplant and cardiac surgery patients.

Prescribing Resuscitation and Maintenance Fluids

It also important that patients with ongoing large volume losses may require the simultaneous infusions of both maintenance fluid and resuscitation fluid, each titrated to its own goal. Maintenance fluids are calculated based on weight and caloric needs, and are not meant to provide PVE. Resuscitative fluid response continues until appropriate tissue perfusion and oxygenation is restored.

SPECIFIC ELECTROLYTE ABNORMALITIES

Daily electrolyte requirements for an average healthy adult are listed in **Table 1**.

DISORDERS OF SODIUM BALANCE
Hyponatremia

Dilutional hyponatremia is the most common inpatient disorder of sodium (Na^+) balance. Because most patients have received maintenance fluid and many have also received resuscitation fluid in the ED, OR, or ICU, it is the rare patient who has not received water far in excess of their daily minimum requirements. This excess is complicated by a typically elevated antidiuretic hormone level that supports water retention, and may be especially marked in those with heart failure. Thus, a decreasing Na^+ generally indicates free water excess, rather than a true total body sodium deficit. In general, those with dilutional hyponatremia have a normal or nearly normal plasma chloride (Cl^-) and a high urinary Na^+ as well. The therapy for this disorder is fluid restriction to decrease free water, not the delivery of a higher Na^+ content fluid. Judicious diuretic use may also help correct dilutional hyponatremia, and particular efficacy may be realized with the use of the new class of diuretics, the aquaporins, based on their pure aquaretic effect. Data are currently lacking on the application of the aquaporins to this disorder.

Special note is made regarding the correction of hyponatremia with respect to timing. The Na^+ concentration may be corrected at the same rate as that with which

Table 1		
Typical adult baseline electrolyte requirements		
Electrolyte	**Normal Serum Value**	**Daily Requirements**
Sodium (chloride, acetate, or phosphate)	135–145 mmol/L	1–2 mEq/kg
Potassium (chloride, acetate, or phosphate)	3.5–5.0 mmol/L	0.7–0.9 mEq/kg
Calcium (chloride or gluconate)	7.6–10.8 mg/dL	1000 mg Pregnant females: 1300 mg Females >50 y: 1500 mg
Magnesium (sulfate)	1.5–2.5 mEq/L	Females: 310–320 mg Pregnant females: 350–400 mg Males: 400–420 mg
Phosphate (sodium or potassium)	2.4–4.5 mEq/L	700 mg In states of severe catabolism or prolonged absence of nutritional intake: 15–25 mM per 1000 kcal of glucose
Chloride (sodium or potassium)	98–108 mmol/L	1–2 mEq/kg

it was acquired. One should, however, avoid raising the Na^+ more rapidly than 0.5 to 1 mEq per hour to avoid the induction of central pontine myelinolysis (CPM), especially in those with a Na^+ less than 120 mEq/L for longer than 48 hours. Once this entity is established, it may have permanent neurologically devastating effects, including the locked-in syndrome. Extrapontine demyelination may also occur. These time rules also apply to true total body salt depletion. In general, the rapidity of correction is also driven by the presence or absence of neurologic symptoms. Three percent NSS is a fluid commonly used to raise the Na^+ concentration above 120 mEq/L in symptomatic patients, as it provides concentrated salt without a significant volume of concomitant free water.

Salt-Depletion Hyponatremia

True total body salt depletion leading to hyponatremia is less common than dilutional hyponatremia in the inpatient setting. However, this disorder is more common in those on chronic diuretic therapy coupled with a salt-restricted diet (<9 g NaCl per day). It may also accompany cerebral salt wasting as well as a variety of medical therapies that result in urinary salt loss; more rare causes include biliary drains and high-output proximal GI fistula with loss of bile salts. In these unique patient settings, both Na^+ and Cl^- are low, and are coupled with a low urine Na^+ concentration. Therapy is the provision of additional salt by the intravenous or oral route, or both. The following formula may be used to estimate the anticipated change in serum Na when correcting hyponatremia using intravenous fluids.

$$Na = [(\text{infusate Na} + \text{infusate K}) - \text{serum Na}]/[\text{Total body water} + 1]$$

Confounders of Sodium Concentration Measurement

The most common confounder is hyperglycemia, as occurs in diabetic ketoacidosis and in hyperglycemic, hyperosmolar nonketotic states. In both conditions, glucose is significantly elevated and the increased glucose concentration confounds determination of Na^+ concentration. Thus, the plasma Na^+ must be corrected for the glucose using the following formula:

$$Na_{corrected} = Na_{measured} + 0.016 \times (\text{Glucose} - 100) \text{ if the glucose is} < 400 \text{ mg\%}$$

For glucoses greater than 400 mg/dL the relationship is nonlinear and the following formula should instead be used:

$$Na_{corrected} = Na_{measured} + 0.024 \times (\text{Glucose} - 100)$$

Hypernatremia

Hypernatremia is a disorder of water metabolism, not sodium homeostasis. As such, the high Na^+ (>145 mEq/L) is secondary to a free water deficit. Like hyponatremia, hypernatremia is divided into acute and chronic states, with 48 hours as the dividing time. Some general rules apply to the safe correction of symptomatic hypernatremia:

1. Correct no more rapidly than 1 to 2 mEq/L per hour
2. Provide 50% of the water deficit in the first 12 to 24 hours and the rest over the next 24 hours
3. Measure electrolytes every 2 hours during correction to adjust the rate of correction to avoid cerebral edema

4. Asymptomatic chronic hypernatremia should be corrected at a rate not exceeding 0.5 mEq/L per hour, and not greater than 10 mEq/L over 24 hours.

Intravenous free water commonly provided as D5W (dextrose 5% in water) is most commonly used, but may be supplemented by GI luminal free water using either pure water or diluted tube feeds. The following formula may be used to calculate free water deficit:

$$\Delta \text{ Na} = [(\text{infusate Na} + \text{infusate K}) - \text{serum Na}]/[\text{Total body water} + 1]$$

where Total body water = weight (kg) × correction factor.

Correction factors:
   Children: 0.6
   Nonelderly men: 0.6
   Nonelderly women: 0.5
   Elderly men: 0.5
   Elderly women: 0.45.

DISORDERS OF POTASSIUM BALANCE
Hypokalemia

Hypokalemia is much more common than hyperkalemia in hospitalized patients. In those with normal renal function, hypokalemia is often related to diminished intake, the infusion of K^+ free fluids, or the use of kaliuretic diuretics (ie, loop diuretics such as furosemide). It is important to recall that serum K^+ deficit does not demonstrate linearity with the amount needed to restore a normal concentration when the measured K^+ is less than 3.0 mEq/L. Because K^+ is principally an intracellular cation, extracellular deficits draw on intracellular stores to maintain homeostasis. Thus, a total body deficit exists when serum K^+ is less than 3.0 mEq/L, and patients generally require 200 mEq K^+ (and often more) to replace intracellular and extracellular K^+ to normal, especially in the setting of ongoing renal or GI losses. As acute and potentially life-threatening dysrhythmias are common with K^+ less than 3.0 mEq/L, and the concentration of the replacement solutions is typically higher than may be administered on the general ward, continuous electrocardiographic monitoring is warranted, as is central access to avoid venosclerosis and tissue injury. In addition, restoration of normokalemia relies on the establishment of normomagnesemia, as both potassium and magnesium cotransport in the kidney.

Hyperkalemia

Therapy for hyperkalemia depends on achieving 3 goals: (1) reduction of plasma concentration, (2) preservation of myocardial conduction, and (3) reduction of total body potassium. The specific therapy undertaken depends in part on renal function, the ability to tolerate PVE, and the degree of hyperkalemia. Though often cited as a cause of hyperkalemia in those with renal dysfunction, infusion of LR with approximately 4 mEq K/L should not cause hyperkalemia. Even if the entirety of such a patient's plasma space was replaced with LR, the K^+ concentration would not exceed the concentration of potassium (K^+) in LR (4 mEq/L). Hyperkalemia in such a patient must instead derive from other sources, including K^+-rich enteral nutritional formulas, antibiotics, or other medication provided as a K^+-based salt, or from significant tissue destruction as in rhabdomyolysis. However, should hyperkalemia occur, the following therapies are generally useful after ceasing all potassium infusion or delivery.

Reduction of plasma concentration
Reduction of plasma concentration is most often accomplished by the infusion of 2000 mL 0.9% NSS, coupled with a bioappropriate dose of a kaliuretic diuretic (ie, furosemide). This medium dilutes the plasma concentration and has the added benefit of total body K^+ reduction. From an acid-base standpoint, the NSS will be acidifying and the loop diuretic alkalinizing, serving to create a balanced effect on pH. These therapies work for those who may tolerate PVE and who have a renal system capable of appropriately responding to a loop diuretic.

Preservation of myocardial conduction
This therapy relies on the membrane-stabilization properties of supplemental magnesium (Mg^{2+}), the cardiac conduction support of calcium (Ca^{2+}), and relocation of K^+ from the plasma space to the intracellular compartment. Empiric 4 g $MgSO_4$ plus 1 g $CaCl_2$ is common, relying on the fact that both Ca^{2+} and Cl^- are strong ions, rendering the Ca^{2+} immediately available for bioactivity; this is in sharp contradistinction to calcium gluconate, which requires hepatic processing by degluconases before freeing the Ca^{2+} for action. Relocation of K^+ takes advantage of the growth-hormone properties of insulin. In invertebrates, there is an insulin-like growth hormone whose major function is to incorporate K^+ into growing cells without any impact on glucose metabolism. In humans, insulin will also drive glucose out of plasma and into cells, and must therefore be accompanied by supplemental dextrose to avoid neuroglycopenia. Thus, 50 g dextrose (ie, 1 ampoule of D50W) is administered in conjunction with 10 IU of regular human insulin (intravenously).

Reduction of total body potassium
There are 3 methods for the reduction of total body K^+: kaliuresis, cation-exchange resin, and some form of hemodialysis (peritoneal dialysis is too slow and inefficient for acute therapy). Because kaliuresis is covered above, the focus here is on the latter 2 therapies. Kayexalate is a Na^+-K^+ cation-exchange resin that will bind a K^+ in exchange for the already bound Na^+. It is administered by mouth or per rectum in 15-g aliquots, and a common starting dose is 45 g. Of importance is that kayexalate, constructed in sorbitol, is an osmotic cathartic that will draw K^+-rich fluids into the GI lumen to allow for the cation exchange. Thus, one titrates the administered kayexalate to the generation of diarrhea, especially when administered by mouth.

For those unable to tolerate GI delivery of kayexalate (ileus, intestinal obstruction, recent GI anastomosis, *Clostridium difficile* colitis), and for those with life-threatening hyperkalemia and impending cardiac arrest, acute hemodialysis (HD) is the most efficient means of rapidly reducing total body K^+. The drawbacks to HD are the need for HD access, a dialysis nurse, the device, and the time required to put all of those elements into place. Thus, even for patients who require HD for life-threatening hyperkalemia, as many of the other therapies as are tolerable (including intubation to allow PVE to dilute the K^+ concentration) should be undertaken to initiate therapy before undertaking to begin HD.

DISORDERS OF CALCIUM BALANCE
Hypocalcemia

Hypocalcemia is commonly related to large-volume PVE, chelation, or the failure to correct the measured calcium for hypoalbuminemia in hospitalized patients. Although there is a myriad of other causes of hypocalcemia, including total thyroidectomy or subtotal (ie, 3-and-a-half gland) parathyroidectomy, hypocalcemia is most often related to fluid therapy or therapeutic undertakings. In a manner analogous to the therapy for hyperkalemia, plasma expansion with calcium free fluid is associated with the need for calcium supplementation on the basis of simple dilution.[29] Massive transfusion of banked blood preserved with a citrate-based anticoagulant may also establish hypocalcemia, and may lead to acute symptomatology just as may parathyroid or thyroid surgery, albeit by different mechanisms (chelation vs reduction of parathyroid hormone [PTH] concentration). In either case, one must assess by physical examination for evidence of hypocalcemia, including carpopedal spasm or Chvostek sign. Biochemical evidence may be derived from measuring the ionized Ca^{2+} or by assessing the serum Ca^{2+} in conjunction with the serum albumin. Because the ionized fraction is that with biological activity, one need only measure ionized calcium. However, not all devices routinely do so, and measuring the ionized portion requires a different tube from the basic tube for comprehensive metabolic profile so commonly obtained. The serum Ca^{2+} is obtained at the same time as the rest of the electrolytes using the same tube, and is more often measured for that reason. However, because Ca^{2+} is protein bound, the measurement must be adjusted for alterations in albumin from normal (4.0 g%) using the following formula to obtain the corrected calcium:

$$Ca_{corrected} = Ca_{measured} + 0.8 \times (4.0 - Albumin_{measured})$$

Therapy consists of calcium supplementation. For symptomatic patients, $CaCl_2$ should be used for the reasons already outlined. Asymptomatic patients may be managed using calcium gluconate by intermittent infusion (dilution or chelation) or continuous infusion (after endocrine surgery).

Hypercalcemia

Although it is most common in patients with cancer, hypercalcemia may also complicate the care of those with critical illness stemming from immobility. To establish hypercalcemia, calcium homeostasis must be perturbed by an excess of PTH (increased GI absorption and reduced renal calcium excretion at the distal tubule), calcitriol, a tumor-produced hormone-like product with similar activity to PTH, or a bio-inappropriately large Ca load. Therapy is similar to that for hyperkalemia and is targeted toward plasma space dilution, urinary loss using loop diuretic therapy, or acute HD for those with acute symptomatology. However, unlike hyperkalemia, hypercalcemia also has a long-term component, bisphosphonates, designed to reduce the driving force for release of calcium from bone hydroxyapatite stores. These compounds are analogues of pyrophosphate that act by binding to hydroxyapatite, thereby inhibiting crystal matrix dissolution. As such, bisphosphonates prevent osteoclast attachment to hydroxyapatite and interfere with both osteoclast recruitment and viability. Calcimimetics such as cinacalcet (Sensipar) enhance the responsivity of the parathyroid calcium receptor residing on the chief cells, in essence falsely increasing its activity and triggering a reduction in PTH output. Glucocorticoids have been used as adjunctive agents for managing the hypercalcemia of vitamin D intoxication, that associated with nonsolid tumor malignancies, and that associated with granulomatous disease.

Special mention should be made of hypercalcemic crisis (serum Ca^{2+} >15 mEq/L) combined with central nervous system (CNS) abnormalities as well as hemodynamic alterations including tachycardia and hypertension, as such patients also benefit from admission to the ICU, and the use of calcitonin to acutely reduce serum Ca^{2+} and inhibit osteoclast RNA synthesis. Phosphate salts have previously been used for hypercalcemia, but carry a significant risk for $CaPO_4$ precipitation and deposition, and should generally be avoided.

DISORDERS OF MAGNESIUM BALANCE
Hypomagnesemia

Hypomagnesemia is seemingly ubiquitous in the critically ill, and may occur less commonly in patients managed on the general ward. This disorder generally stems from the provision of Mg^{2+} free fluid in large quantity, establishing the target patient population as those with hemorrhagic or septic shock, as well as those with significant plasma deficits from environmental dehydration or iatrogenic overdiuresis. Magnesium is similar to calcium in that the biologically active portion is in the ionized fraction; however, unlike Ca^{2+}, ionized Mg^{2+} is difficult to measure and not widely available. Therefore, treatment is based on serum levels alone. Hypomagnesemia occurs most commonly in conjunction with hypokalemia, and concomitant therapy is the rule rather than the exception. Similar to hypokalemia, more magnesium is usually required to restore normal serum Mg^{2+} levels than would be anticipated, and providing 10 g $MgSO_4$ for a patient with a serum Mg^{2+} of 1.5 mEq/L in the ICU is not uncommon. Despite the large amounts infused, creating hypermagnesemia is difficult outside of the labor and delivery suite, where hypermagnesemia is useful for tocolysis as well as for the management of hypertension with preeclampsia.

Hypermagnesemia

Hypermagnesemia is rare outside of the labor and delivery suite, with the exception of those with renal failure who have received a bioinappropriate dose of magnesium. The mainstay of therapy is cessation of administration and PVE, to dilute the magnesium concentration and initiate urinary magnesium loss (similar to induced kaliuresis). It is important to recognize that hypermagnesemia is associated with CNS depression, hyporeflexia, and hypoventilation, and may require airway control and mechanical ventilation while the magnesium is cleared; such therapy is altogether rare. Of note, magnesium is dialyzable in the event of such a circumstance if PVE and forced diuresis fails to resolve the hypermagnesemia.

DISORDERS OF PHOSPHATE BALANCE
Hypophosphatemia

Hypophosphatemia occurs so commonly that texts addressing fluids and electrolytes previously recommended including 10 to 15 mmol PO_4^{2-} in each liter of maintenance fluid to help avoid this disorder. At present, with the widespread availability of PO_4^{2-} measurement, PO_4^{2-} is no longer regularly included in maintenance fluids with the sole exception of total parenteral nutrition (TPN). Administered as the Na^+ or K^+ salt, phosphate repletion may address more than one electrolyte problem. Of importance is that severe acute hypophosphatemia with serum PO_4^{2-} less than 1 mEq/L is associated with a 10% incidence of spontaneous and irreversible respiratory arrest. Such low levels are associated with 1 of 4 conditions: massive PVE, refeeding syndrome, inappropriate PO_4^{2-} removal during HD, and inappropriate PO_4^{2-} binding; the first 2 causes comprise the overwhelming majority of instances. Massive PVE causes both PO_4^{2-} dilution and excretion (urinary loss). Refeeding syndrome, as occurs with the provision of substrate after starvation, results in acute hypophosphatemia as PO_4^{2-} is primarily incorporated into phospholipids such as phosphatidylcholine to create new cell membranes, and to a lesser extent as part of high-energy phosphates and structural proteins.

Hyperphosphatemia

This entity primarily manifests in patients with acute or chronic renal failure, or as the result of inappropriate PO_4^{2-} administration (intravenous) in those without renal failure. For those with abnormal renal function who do not require HD, the use of oral phosphate binders usually suffices to control hyperphosphatemia. For those with HD-requiring renal failure, PO_4^{2-} binders supplement clearance via HD. In all circumstances of renal dysfunction, dietary modification to reduce PO_4^{2-} intake is also appropriate. One consequence of untreated hyperphosphatemia is the development and progression of secondary hyperparathyroidism. When the product of serum calcium and phosphorus (Ca × PO_4) is elevated, metastatic calcification of nonosseous tissues may also result. Both of these conditions may contribute to the increased morbidity and mortality seen in patients with end-stage renal disease.[30]

DISORDERS OF CHLORIDE BALANCE
Hypochloremia

Hypochloremia may result from extrarenal or renal abnormalities in chloride intake or losses, or from changes in volume of total body water. Extrarenal causes included decreased sodium chloride intake, GI losses such as emesis, nasogastric drainage, or diarrhea, or skin losses as in severe burns. In these instances of depletion of total body chloride, extracellular fluid compartment contraction occurs, with subsequent hypotension, tachycardia, and orthostasis. Urine studies will reveal decreased sodium and chloride.

Increased renal clearance of chloride may be the result of overdiuresis with loop diuretics or osmotic diuresis as with mannitol, or in states of diabetic ketoacidosis or hyperosmolar nonketotic coma. Salt-losing nephropathies, including interstitial nephritis, chronic renal insufficiency, or postobstructive diuresis, decrease serum chloride levels. Adrenal insufficiency is another cause of chloride loss that is extrarenal in origin. With absolute or relative adrenal insufficiency, extracellular fluid volume contraction occurs, but unlike hypochloremia from other extrarenal causes, urine chloride levels are increased because of enhanced urinary loss. Administration of hypertonic sodium chloride solutions (NSS, 3%), potassium chloride supplements or, in severe cases, hydrochloric acid, is corrective in conditions of severe hypochloremia because is it associated with severe metabolic alkalosis, which is generally chloride responsive.

Hyperchloremia

Hyperchloremia occurs with loss of pure water, loss of hypotonic fluids whereby the water deficit exceeds the sodium and chloride deficits, and inappropriate administration of chloride-containing fluids. Pure water deficits occur via skin losses as in fever or other hypermetabolic states, as a result of inadequate water intake, or renal losses such as with central or nephrogenic diabetes insipidus.

In cases of severe diarrhea, burns, diuretic use, and osmotic diuresis, more water than sodium is lost, leading to increases in both sodium and chloride. In both pure water and hypotonic fluid losses or deficits, symptoms include dry mucus membranes, hypotension, tachycardia and, when severe, orthostasis.

Disproportionate increases in serum chloride predictably occur with prolonged administration of sodium chloride in all hyperchloremic solutions, including NSS. Hypertonic tube feeds also result in increased sodium and chloride when adequate free water is not provided. If untreated, patients may experience hypertension, edema, congestive heart failure, or pulmonary edema.

Hyperchloremic metabolic acidosis occurs with absolute or relative hyperchloremia in comparison with sodium. Causes include interstitial nephritis and renal tubular acidosis, severe diarrhea, and ureteral diversion procedures in which interposed bowel absorbs additional chloride. More commonly, hyperchloremic metabolic acidosis is created by administration of hyperchloremic solutions including hypertonic saline, NSS, or other acidic chloride salts as in TPN. Prevention and correction of this abnormality is achieved by removing the underlying source, such as treatment of infectious diarrhea or cessation of inciting medications, as well as by infusing intravenous solutions containing low or no chloride. Solutions that have equal amounts of Na^+ and Cl^- will lead to hyperchloremic metabolic acidosis and may be ameliorated, corrected, or prevented by substituting one-half NSS + 75 mEq/L $NaHCO_3$ for resuscitation and D5W + 75 mEq/L $NaHCO_3$ for maintenance fluid.[31] The key element in these solutions is the lack of chloride, a strong anion that exerts a negative plasma charge. As a result, the net plasma charge is relatively positive, leading to proton consumption (reassociation to form water) and an induced alkalosis. A more detailed explanation of strong ions and their impact on acid-base balance is given later.

SPECIAL CONSIDERATIONS
Antibiotics

It is important to consider the fluid and electrolyte content of medications, especially antibiotics. The volume of these medications ranges from minimal to 1000 mL with each dose. When antibiotics are administered more than once daily, this intake may become significant. Antibiotics or other infusions delivered in normal saline contribute to the specific abnormalities associated with hyperchloremic fluid. Other medications are administered in hypotonic dextrose solutions, adding free water to a patient's daily intake. Medication concentrations and delivery fluids can be altered, and discussions with the hospital pharmacy are often helpful in the management of fluid and electrolyte imbalances in the critically ill patient.

Enteral Nutritional Supplementation

Enteral feeding is preferred over parenteral nutrition for a host of reasons beyond the scope of this article. However, tube-feed formulas can create or exacerbate preexisting fluid and electrolyte imbalances. The osmolality of tube feed formulas varies from isotonic formulas that are generally well tolerated to hypertonic concentrations that may slow gastric emptying, resulting in nausea, emesis, and distention. Hypertonic tube feeds that are given directly into small bowel should be advanced slowly, as the osmotic gradient draws water into the intestine. The small bowel must adapt and absorb the additional fluid, or cramping and diarrhea occur.

Tube-fed patients often have fluid and electrolyte disturbances associated with their underlying illness. The initiation of nutritional support in a previously starving patient may result in a refeeding syndrome that has a host of specific and preemptively manageable electrolyte abnormalities. An acute intracellular shift of potassium, phosphate, and magnesium, as well as an increased demand for phosphate for tissue anabolism, leads to a variety of life-threatening symptoms including cardiac dysrhythmias, respiratory failure, congestive heart failure, and rhabdomyolysis. Fluid retention, hyperglycemia, thiamine deficiency, and neurologic and hematologic complications also result. In the most severe states, refeeding syndromes can be fatal. Risk factors include limited enteral intake for more than 10 days and current weight less than 80% of ideal body weight.[32] Alcoholism, anorexia nervosa, malignancy, pancreatitis, diabetes, and recent major surgery also predispose a patient to refeeding syndrome.[33]

Pregnancy

Traditionally 5% dextrose (D5) LR solution has been used for maintenance fluid for gravid patients in labor. Although this practice is based more on dogma than on recent trials, it continues to be the initial fluid of choice in these patients based on the well-described fetal need for both dextrose and placental perfusion for viability. Because labor may decrease placental flow, the normotonic component of D5 LR helps support perfusion, at least in theory. Outside of the labor and delivery suite, D5 LR is a poor resuscitation fluid because it may induce osmotic diuresis when administered in large quantity, and is a poor maintenance fluid because it contains a gross excess of salt relative to dextrose and water for this indication.

A UNIFYING APPROACH

Although many methods are used to assess acid-base balance, only one directly links electrolyte charge with pH. This method, articulated by Peter Stewart in 1983, is termed the strong-ion approach, and is rooted in physical chemistry and 2 laws of thermodynamics (conservation of mass, electrical neutrality).[34] As such, 3 independent control mechanisms for pH are identified: CO_2, the strong-ion difference, and the sum of weak acids. The end result of the interaction of these 3 independent control mechanisms is to drive water dissociation to generate protons, or water association to consume protons. In this method, ions that are dissociated in an aqueous milieu at physiologic pH range are termed strong ions. Strong ions may be cationic (Na, K, Ca, Mg) or anionic (Cl, lactate); the net charge difference between these two groups is termed the strong-ion difference (SID) or the strong-ion difference apparent (SIDapparent, SIDa). While these charge differences yield a net positive charge, a counterbalancing negative charge to preserve electrical neutrality is exerted by the sum of the weak acids, known as ATOT; ATOT may also be known as the strong-ion difference effective (SIDeffective; SIDe). ATOT is the charge principally related to the negative charges of the total inorganic phosphates, serum proteins, and exposed histidine residues on albumin. In patients with renal failure, an additional negative charge from ATOT stems from sulfates as well (generally <2%). The foregoing discussion may be summarized by the following 3 equations:

1. $CO_2 + H_2O \leftrightarrow H_2CO_3 \leftrightarrow HCO_3^- + H^+$

2. $[A_{TOT}] = [A^-] + [AH]$

3. $[SID] = [Na^+] + [K^+] + [Ca^{2+}] + [Mg^{2+}] - [Cl^-] - [Lactate]$

This conceptual framework is useful, as it allows one to understand how changes in the strong ion component or the weak acid component of plasma interact with pCO_2 to regulate pH. Therefore, at a pCO_2 of 40 torr, with equal SIDa and SIDe, and a normal temperature, patients have a pH of exactly 7.4. As such, the delivery of fluids for resuscitation or maintenance that contain electrolytes will readily and predictably interact with the patient's plasma charge and influence pH.

Regardless of whether one resuscitates with NSS or LR, both fluids are hyperchloremic with regard to plasma. Because the plasma chloride concentration is less than the plasma sodium concentration, both NSS and LR will raise the chloride concentration, although NSS will do so to a greater extent than will LR. LR may decrease the plasma Na whereas NSS will raise plasma Na when delivered in large quantity. In a 70-kg patient, the infusion of 10 L of NSS will only raise the Na by 3 mEq/L but will raise the Cl by 11 mEq/L. The end result will decrease the SIDa and reduce the plasma positive charge. Reduced SID will drive water dissociation to generate plasma positive charge to restore electrical neutrality. The end result is a decrease in pH that is identified as metabolic acidosis. However, concomitant decreases in exchangeable or excretable negative charge also occur, leading to decreases in albumin as well as phosphate. Thus, hypoproteinemia is not simply a dilutional effect, but is understandable as an adaptive event designed to help restore electrical neutrality. In light of these well-described effects, colloid resuscitation makes greater sense when providing large volumes of resuscitation fluid, as colloids are generally 3 times as efficient as crystalloids with regard to PVE. Therefore, one may administer only one-third of the total fluid volume and one-third of the total chloride. Indeed, intraoperative studies of elderly patients undergoing major surgery using such a low (vs high) chloride regimen documents fewer acid-base abnormalities, less total volume, better indices of perfusion, and improved urine flow.[35]

Similarly, the well-described metabolic alkalosis from vomiting is readily understood as the converse of the situation described heretofore. However, one must also recall the law of conservation of mass. Because one loses both protons and chloride, and we maintain a proton concentration of 55 M, protons are readily regenerated but chloride is not. Therefore, the loss of chloride leads to a net increase in plasma positive charge; this should lead to water association decreasing the readily available pool of plasma positive charge, resulting in metabolic alkalosis. Accordingly, the repair strategy is to provide that which cannot be regenerated, chloride. This mechanism is the genesis of chloride-responsive alkalemia. Related to this, urinary losses of equal amounts of Na^+ and Cl^- will have the same effect on plasma positive charge, as the chloride concentration falls more rapidly than the sodium concentration. This circumstance is most often found in those on potent diuretics such as loop diuretics in combination with a salt-restricted diet, leading to true total body sodium depletion. These patients exhibit an induced metabolic alkalosis arising from the decrease in plasma positive charge and are repaired in a similar fashion, through administration of hyperchloremic saline. Of course, the plasma volume deficit that accompanies diuretic therapy is also managed by the free water that accompanies the Na^+ and Cl^-.

The aforementioned mechanisms may not be sufficient in isolation to restore plasma electrical neutrality. In such cases, SIDa and SIDe are not equal. In such circumstances there is a strong-ion gap (SIG) to restore electrical neutrality: SIG = SIDa − SIDe. In normal healthy volunteers, SIG ranges from −2 to +2. An increased SIG has been closely correlated with early mortality after major vascular injury as well as major trauma.[36,37] An increased SIG has been identified in various conditions of organ failure, including renal and hepatic failure. The origin of the charged entities that comprise the unmeasured anions or cations remains unclear. However, it is known that different resuscitation fluids can induce different unmeasured species after a similar episode of hemorrhagic shock.[38] Therefore, unmeasured species may be useful predictors of outcome, and should also be considered in selecting fluids for large-volume resuscitation (>5 L of crystalloid).

SUMMARY

Fluid and electrolyte goals and deficiencies must be defined for individual patients to provide the appropriate combination of resuscitation and maintenance fluids. Specific electrolyte abnormalities should be anticipated, identified, and corrected to optimize organ functions. Using the strong-ion approach to acid-base assessment, delivered fluids that contain calculated amounts of electrolytes will interact with the patient's plasma charge and influence the patient's pH, allowing the clinician to achieve a more precise end point.

REFERENCES

1. Morrison CA, Carrick MM, Norman MA, et al. Hypotensive resuscitation strategy reduces transfusion requirements and severe postoperative coagulopathy in trauma patients with hemorrhagic shock: preliminary results of a randomized controlled trial. J Trauma 2011;70(3):652–63.
2. Duchesne JC, Barbeau JM, Islam TM, et al. Damage control resuscitation: from emergency department to the operating room. Am Surg 2011;77(2):201–6.
3. Beekley AC. Damage control resuscitation: a sensible approach to the exsanguinating surgical patient. Crit Care Med 2008;36(Suppl 7):S267–74.
4. Hai SA. Permissive hypotensive resuscitation—an evolving concept in trauma. J Pak Med Assoc 2004;54(8):434–6.
5. Rivers E, Nguyen B, Havstad S, et al. Early goal-directed therapy in the treatment of severe sepsis and septic shock. N Engl J Med 2001;345(19):1368–77.
6. Crookes BA, Cohn SM, Bloch S, et al. Can near-infrared spectroscopy identify the severity of shock in trauma patients? J Trauma 2005;58(4):806–13.
7. Cohn SM, Nathens AB, Moore FA, et al. Tissue oxygen saturation predicts the development of organ dysfunction during traumatic shock resuscitation. J Trauma 2007;62:44–55.
8. Moore FA, McKinley BA, Moore EE. The next generation in shock resuscitation. Lancet 2004;363(9425):1988–96.
9. Moore B. In memory of Sidney Ringer [1835-1910]: Some account of the fundamental discoveries of the great pioneer of the bio-chemistry of crystallo-colloids in living cells. Biochem J 1911;5(6–7):i.b3–xix.
10. Lee JA. Sidney Ringer (1834-1910) and Alexis Hartmann (1898-1964). Anaesthesia 1981;36(12):1115–21.
11. Velasco IT, Pontieri V, Rocha e Silva M. Hypertonic NaCl and severe hemorrhagic shock. Am J Physiol 1980;239:H664–73.
12. Nakayama S, Sibley L, Gunther RA, et al. Small volume resuscitation with hypertonic saline resuscitation (2400 mOsm/l) during hemorrhagic shock. Circ Shock 1984;13:149–59.
13. Rocha e Silva M, Velasco IT, Nogueira da Silva RI, et al. Hyperosmotic sodium salts reverse severe hemorrhagic shock: other solutes do not. Am J Physiol 1987;253:H751–62.
14. Fallon WF. Trauma systems, shock, and resuscitation. Curr Opin Gen Surg 1993;40–5.
15. Krausz MM. Controversies in shock research: hypertonic resuscitation—pros and cons. Shock 1995;3(1):69–72.
16. Dubick MA, Atkins JL. Small-volume fluid resuscitation for the far-forward combat environment: current concepts. J Trauma 2003;54(Suppl 5):S43–5.
17. Wade CE, Grady JJ, Kramer GC, et al. Individual patient cohort analysis of the efficacy of hypertonic saline/dextran in patients with traumatic brain injury and hypotension. J Trauma 1997;42(Suppl 5):S61–5.
18. Bavir H, Clark RS, Kochanek PM. Promising strategies to minimize secondary brain injury after head trauma. Crit Care Med 2003;31(Suppl 1):S112–7.
19. White H, Cook D, Venkatesh B. The use of hypertonic saline for treating intracranial hypertension after traumatic brain injury. Anesth Analg 2006;102(6):1836–46.
20. Davidson IJ. Renal impact of fluid management with colloids: a comparative review. Eur J Anaesthesiol 2006;23(9):721–38.
21. Ragaller MJR, Theilen H, Koch T. Volume replacement in critically ill patient with acute renal failure. J Am Soc Nephrol 2001;12:533–9.

22. Holcomb JB, Wade CE, Michalek JE, et al. Increased plasma and platelet to red blood cell ratios improves outcome in 466 massively transfused civilian trauma patients. Ann Surg 2008;248:447–58.
23. Borgman MA, Spinella PC, Perkins JG, et al. The ratio of blood products transfused affects mortality in patients receiving massive transfusions at a combat support hospital. J Trauma 2007;63:805–13.
24. Umgelter A, Reindl W, Wagner KS, et al. Effects of plasma expansion with albumin and paracentesis on haemodynamics and kidney function in critically ill cirrhotic patients with tense ascites and hepatorenal syndrome: a prospective uncontrolled trial. Crit Care 2008;12(1):R4.
25. Choi CH, Ahn SH, Kim DY, et al. Long-term clinical outcome of large volume paracentesis with intravenous albumin in patients with spontaneous bacterial peritonitis: a randomized prospective study. J Gastroenterol Hepatol 2005;20(8): 1215–22.
26. Narula N, Tsoi K, Marshall JK. Should albumin be used in all patients with spontaneous bacterial peritonitis? Can J Gastroenterol 2011;25(7):373–6.
27. Alderson P, Bunn F, Li Wan Po A, et al. Human albumin solution for resuscitation and volume expansion in critically ill patients. Cochrane Database Syst Rev 2011; 10:CD001208.
28. Finfer S, Bellomo R, Boyce N, et al. A comparison of albumin and saline for fluid resuscitation in the intensive care unit. N Engl J Med 2004;350(22):2247–56.
29. Roche AM, James MF, Bennett-Guerrero E, et al. A head-to-head comparison of the in vitro coagulation effects of saline-based and balanced electrolyte crystalloid and colloid intravenous fluids. Anesth Analg 2006;102(4):1274–9.
30. Block GA, Hulbert-Shearon TE, Levin NW, et al. Association of serum phosphorus and calcium × phosphate product with mortality risk in chronic hemodialysis patients: a national study. Am J Kidney Dis 1998;31(4):607–17.
31. Kaplan LJ, Cheung NH, Maerz L, et al. A physiochemical approach to acid-base balance in critically ill trauma patients minimizes errors and reduces inappropriate plasma volume expansion. J Trauma 2009;66(4):1045–51.
32. Fuentebella J, Kerner JA. Refeeding syndrome. Pediatr Clin North Am 2009; 56(5):1201–10.
33. Byrnes MC, Stangenes J, et al. Refeeding in the ICU: an adult and pediatric problem [review]. Current Opinion in Clinical Nutrition & Metabolic Care 2011; 14(2):186–92.
34. Stewart PA. Modern quantitative acid-base chemistry. Can J Physiol Pharmacol 1983;61:1444–61.
35. Kaplan LJ, Kellum JA. Fluids, pH, ions, and electrolytes. Curr Opin Crit Care 2010;16(4):323–31.
36. Kaplan LJ, Kellum JA. Initial pH, base deficit, lactate, anion gap, strong ion difference, and strong ion gap predict outcome from major vascular injury. Crit Care Med 2004;32(5):1120–4.
37. Kaplan LJ, Kellum JA. Comparison of acid-base models for prediction of hospital mortality after trauma. Shock 2008;29(6):662–6.
38. Kaplan LJ, Philbin N, Arnaud F, et al. Resuscitation from hemorrhagic shock: fluid selection and infusion strategy drives unmeasured ion genesis. J Trauma 2006; 61(1):90–7.

Hypoperfusion, Shock States, and Abdominal Compartment Syndrome (ACS)

Koen Ameloot, MD[a,1], Carl Gillebert, MD[a,1], Nele Desie, MD[a],
Manu L.N.G. Malbrain, MD, PhD[a,b],*

KEYWORDS

• Shock • Abdominal compartment syndrome • Hypoperfusion

DEFINITIONS

Intra-abdominal pressure (IAP) varies from individual to individual and is influenced by body mass index, body position (head of bed elevation), and the severity of a patient's critical illness.[1,2] In general, normal adult IAP is considered 5 mm Hg to 7 mm Hg. Intra-abdominal hypertension (IAH) has been defined by the World Society of the Abdominal Compartment Syndrome (WSACS) (www.wsacs.org) as sustained increased IAP greater than or equal to 12 mm Hg and abdominal compartment syndrome (ACS) as IAP greater than or equal to 20 mm Hg with new organ dysfunction or failure.[1,2] Given the marked variation in IAP values that may be measured in critically ill patients and given that in some patients even a slight elevation of IAP can cause end-organ hypoperfusion, it is unlikely that a single threshold value of IAP is universally applicable to all critically ill patients. IAP in excess of 25 mm Hg, a level of IAH commonly associated with significant organ dysfunction, is generally accepted to suggest the need for abdominal decompression.[1,3]

EPIDEMIOLOGY OF IAH/ACS

A multicenter epidemiologic study reported IAH (defined as mean IAP ≥12 mm Hg) present in 32% of critically ill medical and surgical ICU patients and ACS present in

M.L.N.G.M. is member of the medical advisory board of Pulsion Medical Systems, a monitoring company. The other authors have nothing to disclose. No funding support.

[a] Intensive Care Unit, Ziekenhuis Netwerk Antwerpen, Campus Stuivenberg/Erasmus, Lange Beeldekensstraat 267, B-2060 Antwerpen 6, Belgium

[b] High Care Burn Unit, Ziekenhuis Netwerk Antwerpen, Campus Stuivenberg/Erasmus, Lange Beeldekensstraat 267, B-2060 Antwerpen 6, Belgium

[1] Drs Ameloot and Gillebert equally contributed to this work.

* Corresponding author. Intensive Care Unit, Ziekenhuis Netwerk Antwerpen, Campus Stuivenberg/Erasmus, Lange Beeldekensstraat 267, B-2060 Antwerpen 6, Belgium.

E-mail address: Manu.Malbrain@zna.be

4%.[4] The prevalence of elevated IAP in patients developing organ failure suggests that IAH may be a key factor in the development of multiple system organ failure, a major cause of ICU mortality.[5]

MEASUREMENT OF IAP

IAH is difficult to detect by clinical examination alone. Assessment of IAP, most commonly using the surrogate measurement of intravesicular or bladder pressure, has been identified as essential to accurate diagnosis and treatment of patients with IAH or ACS.[6–8] According to the WSACS consensus guidelines, IAP should be measured at end expiration in the complete supine position after ensuring that abdominal muscle contractions are absent and with the transducer zeroed at the level of the midaxillary line at the iliac crest after an instillation volume of maximal 20 mL to 25 mL.[1] Alternatively, IAP can be measured continuously via a balloon-tipped nasogastric tube (CiMON, Pulsion Medical Systems, Munich, Germany).[9] Given the high prevalence of IAH in critically Ill patients, the importance of routine measurement of IAP cannot be overemphasized.

PHYSIOLOGY

The organ dysfunctions that characterize IAH and ACS may be related to either direct compressive effects, such as occur with IAP-induced pulmonary or renal failure, or more commonly may be related to inadequate end-organ perfusion as a result of decreased abdominal perfusion pressure (APP) due to decreased cardiac output (CO) and increased IAP (**Fig. 1**).

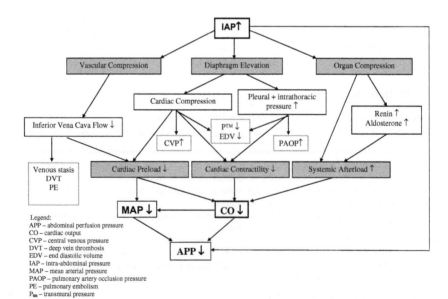

Fig. 1. Cardiovascular effects of IAH. DVT, deep vein thrombosis; EDV, end-diastolic volume; PE, pulmonary embolism; P_{tm}, transmural pressure.

Cardiovascular Implications of IAH

Decreased cardiac output in IAH/ACS

Cardiac function may be distilled into 3 essential components: preload, afterload, and contractility. Elevated IAP has a negative impact on all 3 of these interrelated components.

Decreased preload

It has been demonstrated that IAP of only 10 mm Hg can significantly reduce inferior vena cava (IVC) blood flow and cardiac preload.[10–16] Reduced venous return has the immediate effect of decreasing CO through decreased stroke volume by the Frank-Starling relation. In patients with IAH, multiple mechanisms are responsible for the reduced cardiac preload. First, as originally described by Coombs,[17] intrathoracic pressure (ITP) is increased as a result from a cephalad movement of the diaphragm due to increased IAP. This decreases blood flow through the IVC and limits blood return from below the diaphragm in a pressure-dependent manner.[10,12,17] Reducing ITP by limiting peak and mean airway pressures through pressure-limiting ventilatory strategies or institution of neuromuscular blockade to increase chest wall compliance improves venous return and cardiac function in this patient population.[1,18,19] Second, when IAP rises, this cephalad deviation of the diaphragm narrows the inferior vena cava as it passes through the diaphragm.[20] Finally, the concept of abdominal vascular zones analogous to the pulmonary vascular zone conditions described by West should be emphasized. According to this concept, increased IAP increases venous return when the transmural IVC pressure (defined as IVC pressure minus IAP) at the thoracic inlet significantly exceeds the critical closing transmural pressure (zone 3 abdomen). This is most often the case in hypervolemic patients with high IVC pressure. In zone 3 conditions, the abdominal venous compartment functions as a capacitor. By contrast, when the transmural IVC pressure at the thoracic inlet is below the critical closure transmural pressure (zone 2 abdomen), venous return is significantly decreased. This is most often the case in hypovolemic patients and by extension most noncardiogenic shock patients. In zone 2 conditions, the abdominal venous compartment functions as a collapsible starling transistor.[21] This model illustrates why hypovolemia (especially in combination with positive pressure ventilation and positive end-expiratory pressure [PEEP]) predisposes patients to lower CO in response to elevated IAP than does normovolemia.[21]

Decreased contractility

Diaphragmatic elevation and increased ITP can also have marked effects on cardiac contractility. Traditionally, the right ventricle has been considered solely a conduit for delivering blood to the lungs and left ventricle. Compression of the pulmonary parenchyma increases pulmonary artery pressure and pulmonary vascular resistance while simultaneously reducing left ventricular preload. As right ventricular afterload increases, the right side of the heart must play a more active role in maintaining CO.[22] In response to worsening right ventricular afterload, the thin-walled right ventricle dilates with decrease in RVEF and increase in ventricular wall tension and myocardial oxygen demand. This increased oxygen requirement, coinciding with an increase in right ventricular work requirement, places the myocardium at risk for subendocardial ischemia and further reductions in right ventricular contractility. Also, the interventricular septum may bulge into the left ventricular chamber impeding left ventricular function with further decreases in CO. Right ventricular dysfunction can become severe in the presence of marked IAH leading to significant reductions in left ventricular contractility as a result of this ventricular interdependence.[22,23] Reduced left ventricular output may contribute to the development of systemic hypotension, worsening right coronary artery blood flow, ischemia, and right ventricular contractility. This decrease in contractility results in a rightward and downward shift on the Frank-Starling curve (**Fig. 2**). Although initially responsive to fluid loading and inotropic support at lower levels of IAH, the reduced biventricular contractility of advanced IAH/ACS can effectively be treated only by abdominal decompression.

Increased afterload

Elevated IAP can cause increased systemic vascular resistance in 2 ways: first, through direct compressive effects on the aorta and systemic vasculature, and second, more commonly, as compensation for the reduced venous return and falling stroke volume (as stated above supra). As a result of this physiologic compensation, mean arterial pressure (MAP) typically remains stable in the early stages of IAH/ACS despite reductions in venous return and CO. These increases in afterload may be poorly tolerated by patients with marginal cardiac contractility or inadequate intravascular volume.[24–27] Preload augmentation through volume administration seems to ameliorate, at least partially, the injurious effects of IAH-induced increases in afterload. It has also been proposed that the use of a moderate PEEP might efficiently reduce the increase in ventricular afterload.[10–12,18]

Effects of IAH on Pulmonary Function

The interactions between the abdominal and the thoracic compartments pose a specific challenge for clinicians. The abdominal and thoracic compartments are linked through the diaphragm and, on average, 50% of the increase in IAP is transmitted to the thoracic compartment, increasing ITP.[28–30] IAH causes an increase in alveolar pressures, dead space, and shunt fraction and a decrease in tranpulmonary pressures, functional residual capacity and static compliance of the chest wall, resulting in hypoxemia and hypercapnia.[31] These effects already take place at IAP of 15 mm Hg and are accentuated by the presence of hypovolemia.[32]

In postoperative patients, the presence of capillary leak, positive fluid balance, and raised IAP put patients at exponential risk for lung edema. In a porcine model, for example,

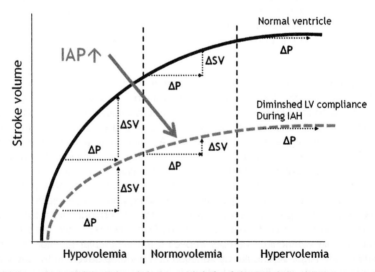

Fig. 2. IAH creates a rightward and downward shift of the Frank-Starling curve, so that for the same change in preload (ΔP) only a small change in stroke volume (ΔSV) can be observed.

the application of IAP of 15 mm Hg after oleic acid–induced lung injury resulted in a greater than 2-fold increase in pulmonary edema, as measured by extravascular lung water (EVLW).[33]

Effects of IAH on End-Organ Perfusion

Neurologic
A close relationship between IAP and intracranial pressure (ICP) has been observed in several animal and human studies.[34] As a result of IAH, cerebral perfusion pressure, defined as MAP minus ICP, decreases. The increased ITP in IAH (described previously) causes a functional obstruction of cerebral venous outflow. This, in combination with reduced systemic blood pressure as a result of the effect of IAH on cardiac function, causes a decrease in cerebral perfusion pressure. As a result, laparoscopic procedures should be performed with caution in patients with recent head injury.[35–37]

Kidney
After emergency abdominal surgery, IAH occurs in 33% to 41% of patients and is associated with acute kidney injury and mortality.[38,39] Elevated IAP significantly decreases renal venous and arterial blood flow, leading to renal dysfunction and failure. Oliguria develops at IAP of 15 mm Hg and anuria at 30 mm Hg in the presence of normovolemia and at lower levels of IAP in patients with hypovolemia.[40–42] Kidney perfusion pressure can be defined as MAP minus IAP.[43] Therefore, in theory, decreased kidney function can be prevented either by decreasing IAP or increasing MAP. Ulyatt[44] suggested that filtration gradient (FG) is a more appropriate parameter to explain acute kidney injury associated with IAH. The FG can be calculated as glomerular filtration pressure minus proximal tubular pressure, which in conditions of IAH can be simplified as $FG = MAP - (2 \times IAP)$. Thus, changes in IAP have a greater impact on renal function and urine production than do changes in MAP. It is not surprising, therefore, that decreased renal function, as evidenced by development of oliguria, is one of the first visible signs of IAH. Also, in patients admitted with advanced systolic heart failure, IAH on admission (in this study defined as IAP >8 mm Hg) was associated with increased creatinine and after treatment with diuretics or renal replacement therapy both IAP and creatinine decreased.[45,46] This finding was confirmed in a small case series were patients with refractory ascites due to heart failure were successfully treated by large fluid paracentesis with significant improvement in renal function.[47]

Gastrointestinal
Virtually all intra-abdominal and retroperitoneal organs demonstrate a decrease in blood flow in the presence of IAH.[12] It seems that through worsening the mesenteric perfusion, IAH and ACS may serve as the second hit in the 2-hit model for the causation of multiple organ dysfunction syndrome, by triggering a vicious cycle from gut hypoperfusion leading to intestinal edema, ischemia, and bacterial translocation.[2] In the presence of hypovolemia or hemorrhage, these negative effects of increased IAP are augmented.

Hepatic
Experimental data have demonstrated a decrease in hepatic arterial blood flow, caused by extrinsic compression, with IAP of only 10 mm Hg.[48,49] Changes in portal venous blood flow were only seen with IAP of 20 mm Hg. In another study, a strict association between IAH and liver dysfunction was not found although a correlation between the degree of IAH and the degree of hyperbilirubinemia existed.[50] Recent studies also show an inverse relation between IAP and the plasma disappearance rate of indocyanine green.[51,52]

CLINICAL PRACTICE
Cardiopulmonary Monitoring in Patients with IAH

Do not use intracardiac filling pressures to assess fluid responsiveness
According to the Frank-Starling principle, ventricular preload is defined as myocardial muscle fiber length at end diastole. Ideally, the appropriate clinical correlate is left ventricular end-diastolic volume (LVEDV). Because LVEDV cannot be easily measured, pressure-based parameters (baroindicators), such as left ventricular end-diastolic pressure, left atrial pressure (LAP), and pulmonary artery occlusion pressure (PAOP), have long been used clinically as surrogate estimates of intravascular volume. Although likely valid in normal healthy individuals, the multiple assumptions necessary to use PAOP and central venous pressure (CVP) as estimates of left ventricular preload status and right ventricular preload status, respectively, are not necessarily true in critically ill patients with IAH/ACS.[16] These patients commonly demonstrate multiple significant aberrations in cardiac function that can interfere with the accuracy of PAOP and CVP measurements as estimates of intravascular volume **(Fig. 3)**.

First, both PAOP and CVP are measured relative to atmospheric pressure and are the sum of intravascular pressure and ITP. As a result, in patients with IAH/ACS, cephalad elevation of the diaphragm and secondary elevated ITP, PAOP, and CVP also tend to be erroneously elevated despite decreased LVEDV due to decreased venous return.[11,13,15,23,24,53] Transmural PAOP ($PAOP_{tm}$) (ie, measured PAOP minus pleural pressure) has been identified as decreasing with rising ITP, correctly reflecting the inherent decreased venous return and cardiac preload. Other studies found that 20% to 80% of IAP, or, on average, 50%, is transmitted to the thorax.[28] As a rule of thumb, a quick estimate of transmural filling pressures can be obtained by subtracting half the IAP from the measured filling pressure (eg, $PAOP_{tm} = PAOP - IAP/2$).[54] Alternatively, the index of transmission can be calculated, although this might be a bit complicated for bedside use. This can be done by looking at changes in IAP (ΔIAP) (eg, by means of a Velcro belt) versus changes in CVP (ΔCVP). The index of transmission can then be calculated as ΔCVP divided by ΔIAP. It has not been shown that real measurement of pleural pressure by an esophageal catheter improves the ability of PAOP alone to predict volume recruitable increases in CO.[16,54]

Second, ventricular compliance is dynamically changing from beat to beat in critically ill patients, resulting in a variable relationship between pressure and volume.[55]

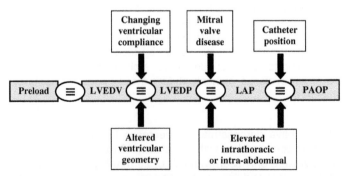

Fig. 3. The PAOP assumption: why intracardiac filling pressures do not accurately estimate preload status. LVEDP, left ventricular end-diastolic pressure; LAP, left atrial pressure. (*Adapted from* Cheatham ML. Right ventricular end-diastolic volume measurements in the resuscitation of trauma victims. Int J Intens Care 2000;7:165–76; with permission.)

As a result, changes in intravascular pressure no longer reflect changes in intravascular volume, further reducing the accuracy of intracardiac filling pressures, such as PAOP and CVP, as estimates of preload status. In general, the presence of IAH causes a flattening and rightward shift of the ventricular compliance curve.[20]

Third, patients with IAH-induced pulmonary hypertension or acute lung injury demonstrate increased pulmonary vascular resistance and are at significant risk for tricuspid valve regurgitation.

Finally, in patients with IAH/ACS, proper placement of the pulmonary artery catheter (PAC) tip in West lung zone 3 may be difficult. Compression of the pulmonary parenchyma as a result of elevated IAP can markedly alter the normal progression of alveolar distention. The use of PEEP to restore alveolar volume, oxygenation, and ventilation increases the relative size of West zone 1 at the expense of zones 2 and 3.[16]

Hemodynamic monitoring can only improve patient care and outcome when clinicians thoroughly understand both the appropriate use as well as the potential measurement errors associated with the use of parameters, such as PAOP and CVP. Resuscitation to absolute PAOP and CVP in patients with IAH/ACS should be avoided because such a practice can lead to under-resuscitation, inappropriate administration of diuretics, and inappropriate end-organ perfusion.

Use volumetric monitoring to assess fluid status

Continuous right ventricular end-diastolic volume obtained with PAC The new generation of PACs allows continuous determination of CO, right ventricular ejection fraction (RVEF), and right ventricular end-diastolic volume index (RVEDVI) (Vigilance monitor, Edwards Lifesciences, Irvine, CA, USA).[22,24,56–59] Continuous CO monitoring provides a beat-to-beat assessment of patient response to therapeutic interventions. RVEF is used to calculate the RVEDVI using the equation, RVEDVI = SVI/RVEF, where *SVI* indicates stroke volume index. Independent of the effects of changing ventricular compliance and increased ITP or IAP, RVEDVI has been reported in several studies as an accurate indicator of preload recruitable increases in cardiac index (CI) in a variety of patient populations, including hemorrhagic, cardiogenic, and septic shock. Moreover, it has been shown that RVEDVI goal-directed fluid resuscitation leads to a reduction of hard clinical endpoints, such as multiple organ failure and death.[24] Many studies report that at high levels of PEEP, RVEDVI consistently maintained a highly significant correlation with CI, whereas PAOP and CVP frequently exhibited inverse correlations with CI.[22,58] Although some investigators have raised concern that mathematical coupling, the interdependence of 2 variables when one is used to calculate the other, may explain the significant correlation between RVEDVI and CI, 3 separate studies have confirmed the validity of RVEDVI as a predictor of preload recruitable increases in CI.[60,61]

Intermittent global end-diastolic volume obtained with PiCCO Pulse contour analysis uses a dedicated PiCCO thermistor-tipped arterial catheter (Pulsion Medical Systems, Munich, Germany) to continuously analyze patient heart rate and arterial pressure waveform. By calculating the change in pressure over time from end diastole to end systole and making several assumptions regarding the elastic and mechanical properties of the arterial tree, continuous beat-to-beat SVI can be estimated and CI calculated. This technology can also be used to measure stroke volume variation (SVV), the variation in beat-to-beat stroke volume during a single respiratory cycle, and pulse pressure variation (PPV), which have been suggested as valuable predictors of fluid responsiveness.[62] Due to the unique mechanical characteristics of each patient's arterial tree, initial calibration of the monitoring system using the transpulmonary thermodilution technique and the Stewart-Hamilton equation greatly improves the accuracy of the stroke volumes subsequently calculated.

Pulse contour analysis has several advantages over traditional intermittent thermo-dilution PAC monitoring. First, it is less invasive, only requiring an arterial catheter and a central venous catheter. Second, it provides an estimate of global end-diastolic volume (GEDV) and global ejection fraction as opposed to RVEDV and RVEF. Third, PiCCO allows calculation of EVLW index (EVLWI) as surrogate predictor of capillary leak.

Fluid Resuscitation in Patients with IAH/ACS

Use volumetric measurements

As discussed previously, volumetric measurements should be used because only GEDVI index (GEDVI) and RVEDVI correctly reflect ventricular filling in IAH/ACS because traditional intracardiac filling pressures (PAOP and CVP) tend to be errone-ously elevated despite intravascular fluid depletion in patients with IAH/ACS.[63]

Use continuous hemodynamic monitoring

Cardiac contractility in critically ill patients changes dynamically from beat to beat and can be described as a series of ventricular function curves.[55] Each curve has an associated ejection fraction and associated optimal LVEDV. Resuscitation to this plateau LVEDV is widely believed to optimize patient intravascular volume, cardiac function, and end-organ perfusion. As a result of this constantly changing ventricular compliance there cannot be a single value of RVEDVI or GEDVI that can be considered the goal of fluid resuscitation in every patient with IAH/ACS. Each patient must, therefore, be resus-citated to the LVEDV that optimizes the circulation at that specific moment of time. Because this optimal volume varies in response to a patient's improving or deteriorating cardiac status, the true value of continuous hemodynamic monitoring becomes clear.

Use abdominal perfusion pressure as resuscitation target

APP is defined as MAP minus IAP.[64] Because patients with IAH/ACS have end-organ hypoperfusion due to the combination of reduced MAP and increased IAP with secondary increased end-organ pressure, it seems reasonable to use APP in stead of MAP in combination with arterial lactate and urinary output as primary resuscitation targets. APP has been demonstrated to exceed the clinical prediction of IAP alone in 2 clinical trials. In a retrospective trial of surgical/trauma patients, Cheatham and colleagues[64] reported that APP greater than 50 mm Hg optimized survival. Moreover APP was superior to MAP, arterial pH, lactate, and base deficit and hourly urinary output as predictor of patient outcome. Cheatham[16] reported, in a mixed surgical/medical population, that failure to maintain APP greater than 60 mm Hg by day 3 discriminated between survivors and nonsurvivors. As a resuscitation endpoint, APP has yet to be subjected to a prospective, randomized clinical trial.

Use pulse pressure variation as predictor of fluid responsiveness

Target APP values should be achieved through a balance of judicious fluid resuscita-tion to reach optimal LVEDV and through application of appropriate vasopressive and/or inotropic medications. Indiscriminate fluid administration should be avoided because it places patients at risk for secondary ACS and because it increases EVLWI in patients with capillary leak. Because in patients with IAH/ACS the increased IAP prevents venous return from the legs and the mesenteric veins, the classical passive leg-raising test may be false negative.[65,66] The Trendelenburg position has a beneficial effect on IAP and results in a more pronounced venous return from the legs and mesenteric veins but has the disadvantage of increased risk of ventilator-associated pneumonia and increased ICP. SVV and definitely PPV are better predictors of fluid responsiveness in patients with IAH/ACS than classical passive leg raising. Increased IAP results in concomitant increased ITP, however, and thus increased SVV and PPV also. This means that the classical 10% to 12% SVV/PPV cutoff cannot be used. A 20% to 25% SVV/PVV cutoff has been proposed to determine fluid responsiveness in patients with ACS. Moreover, PPV has been demonstrated superior to SVV for predicting fluid responsiveness in the patients.[67–69]

Mechanical Ventilation in Patients with IAH/ACS

Recruitment and PEEP setting

Compression of the pulmonary parenchyma as a result of elevated IAP and cephalad deviation of the diaphragm reduces functional residual capacity of the lungs.[31] Therefore, higher opening pressures are needed to recruit the lungs (40 + IAP/2). PEEP should be set equal to IAP to counteract IAP to counteract the deleterious effects on respiratory function caused by IAP while at the same time avoiding overinflation of already well-aerated lung regions.[31] Moreover, the increased left ventricle afterload induced by increased IAP may be counteracted by moderate PEEP, as reported in a recent French echocardiographic study.[70]

Use transmural plateau pressures

IAH decreases total respiratory system compliance by a decrease in chest wall compliance whereas lung compliance remains unchanged.[31] Because tidal volume equals compliance $\times$ (plateau pressure [Pplat] − PEEP), this reduced compliance together with increased PEEP reduces tidal volumes during pressure-controlled ventilation. During lung-protective ventilation, inspiratory pressure can be safely elevated if transmural Pplat ($Pplat_{tm}$ = Pplat − IAP/2) is not higher then 35 cm H_2O.[2]

Monitor extravascular lung water

EVLWI should be monitored because patients with IAH/ACS are at increased risk for pulmonary edema and patients with primary ACS often develop a secondary acute respiratory distress syndrome.[31,33] The PAOP criterion in acute respiratory distress syndrome consensus definition is futile in patients with IAH/ACS because PAOP is erroneously elevated.

Use of neuromuscular blockers

Consideration of neuromuscular blockers should balance the potentially beneficial effects on abdominal muscle tone, resulting in decreased IAP and improved APP against the potentially detrimental effect on respiratory muscles and lung mechanics, resulting in atelectasis and superinfection.[54]

Treatment of ACS

Immediate abdominal decompression should be considered in any patient who demonstrates evidence of ACS. In surgical patients, this is best achieved by either performing a decompressive laparotomy or revising a patient's temporary abdominal closure if the abdomen is already open.[71] The decompressive laparotomy can be performed either in the operating room or at a patient's bedside in the ICU based on current hemodynamic stability. Such a procedure should not be feared or delayed because rapid decompression after the diagnosis of ACS dramatically improves cardiac function and results in improved organ perfusion and survival. Once a patient's abdomen in open, both IAP and APP should continue to be monitored. In patients with an open abdomen, inability to maintain adequate APP is an indication to decompress the patient's abdomen further through either a larger laparatomy or placement of a looser, more compliant temporary abdominal closure. In medical patients whose IAH is secondary to accumulation of ascites or resuscitation fluid, paracentesis should be considered a viable alternative to open abdominal decompression. Leaving the paracentesis catheter in place until a patient's condition stabilizes allows ongoing drainage of peritoneal fluid, continued reduction in IAP, and a reduced incidence of recurrent ACS. In medical patients with IAH without ACS, ileus should be corrected and diuretics or renal replacement therapy in combination with albumin considered. Patients whose IAH is secondary to retroperitoneal hemorrhage, visceral edema, or ileus are best served by open abdominal decompression because paracentesis is not effective in reducing the severity of IAH or restoring end-organ perfusion. The timing of closing a patient's abdomen after decompression should be guided by measurements of IAP and APP.

SUMMARY

IAH and ACS have been increasingly recognized as causes of significant morbidity and mortality in critically ill patients. Cardiovascular dysfunction, as a result of elevations in ITP and IAP, plays a major role in the systemic organ dysfunction and failure that characterizes IAH/ACS. Aggressive hemodynamic monitoring and optimization of both systemic and regional perfusion are essential to improve patient outcome. Traditional measures of intravascular volume, such as PAOP and CVP, are erroneous in patients with IAH and reliance on such measurements may lead to inappropriate fluid resuscitation and administration of diuretics, leading to end-organ hypoperfusion. Volumetric estimates of preload recruitable increases in CO, such as RVEDVI and GEDVI, should be used in such patients with changing ventricular compliance and elevated ITP and IAP. Clinicians must be aware of the interactions between IAP, ITP, PEEP, and intracardiac filling pressures to correctly resuscitate these patients. Patients should be resuscitated to maintain APP of 50 mm Hg to 60 mm Hg through judicious fluid resuscitation and application of vasopressive/inotropic agents. When adequate APP cannot be maintained or a patient demonstrates evidence of ACS, strong consideration should be given to performing abdominal decompression to relieve severe IAH and restore adequate cardiovascular function.

REFERENCES

1. Malbrain M, Cheatham M, Kirkpatrick A, et al. Results from the international conference of experts on intra-abdominal hypertension and abdominal compartment syndrome. I. Definitions. Intensive Care Med 2006;32(11):1722–32.
2. Malbrain M, De laet I. Intra-abdominal hypertension: evolving concepts. Clin Chest Med 2009;30(1):45–70, viii.
3. Cheatham M, Malbrain M. Cardiovascular implications of elevated intra-abdominal pressure. In: Ivatury R, Cheatham M, Malbrain M, et al, editors. Abdominal compartment syndrome. Georgetown (TX): Landes Bioscience; 2006. p. 89–104.
4. Malbrain M, Chiumello D, Pelosi P, et al. Incidence and prognosis of intraabdominal hypertension in a mixed population of critically ill patients: a multiple-center epidemiological study. Crit Care Med 2005;33(2):315–22.
5. Malbrain M, Chiumello D, Pelosi P, et al. Prevalence of intra-abdominal hypertension in critically ill patients: a multicentre epidemiological study. Intensive Care Med 2004;30(5):822–9.
6. Malbrain M. You don't have any excuse, just start measuring abdominal pressure and act upon it! Minerva Anestesiol 2008;74(1–2):1–2.

7. Kirkpatrick A, Brenneman F, McLean R, et al. Is clinical examination an accurate indicator of raised intra-abdominal pressure in critically injured patients? Can J Surg 2000;43(3):207–11.

8. Sugrue M, Bauman A, Jones F, et al. Clinical examination is an inaccurate predictor of intraabdominal pressure. World J Surg 2002;26(12):1428–31.

9. Malbrain M, De laet I, Viaene D, et al. In vitro validation of a novel method for continuous intra-abdominal pressure monitoring. Intensive Care Med 2008;34(4):740–5.

10. Richardson JD, Trinkle JK. Hemodynamic and respiratory alterations with increased intra-abdominal pressure. J Surg Res 1976;20(5):401–4.

11. Kashtan J, Green JF, Parsons EQ, et al. Hemodynamic effect of increased abdominal pressure. J Surg Res 1981;30(3):249–55.

12. Caldwell CB, Ricotta JJ. Changes in visceral blood flow with elevated intraabdominal pressure. J Surg Res 1987;43(1):14–20.

13. Ridings PC, Bloomfield GL, Blocher CR, et al. Cardiopulmonary effects of raised intra-abdominal pressure before and after intravascular volume expansion. J Trauma 1995;39(6):1071–5.

14. Barnes G, Laine G, Giam P, et al. Cardiovascular responses to elevation of intra-abdominal hydrostatic pressure. Am J Physiol 1985;248(2 Pt 2):R208–13.

15. Schachtrupp A, Graf J, Tons C, et al. Intravascular volume depletion in a 24-hour porcine model of intra-abdominal hypertension. J Trauma 2003;55(4): 734–40.

16. Cheatham M, Malbrain M. Cardiovascular implications of abdominal compartment syndrome. Acta Clin Belg Suppl 2007;62(1):98–112.

17. Coombs HC. The mechanism of the regulation of intra-abdominal pressure. Am J Physiol 1922;61:159–70.

18. Bloomfield G, Dalton J, Sugerman H, et al. Treatment of increasing intracranial pressure secondary to the acute abdominal compartment syndrome in a patient with combined abdominal and head trauma. J Trauma 1995;39(6):1168–70.

19. Bloomfield G, Blocher C, Fakhry I, et al. Elevated intra-abdominal pressure increases plasma renin activity and aldosterone levels. J Trauma 1997;42(6): 997–1004 [discussion: 1004–5].

20. Diamant M, Benumof JL, Saidman LJ. Hemodynamics of increased intra-abdominal pressure: interaction with hypovolemia and halothane anesthesia. Anesthesiology 1978;48(1):23–7.

21. Takata M, Wise RA, Robotham JL. Effects of abdominal pressure on venous return: abdominal vascular zone conditions. J Appl Physiol 1990;69(6):1961–72.

22. Cheatham ML, Nelson LD, Chang MC, et al. Right ventricular end-diastolic volume index as a predictor of preload status in patients on positive end-expiratory pressure. Crit Care Med 1998;26(11):1801–6.

23. Cullen DJ, Coyle JP, Teplick R, et al. Cardiovascular, pulmonary, and renal effects of massively increased intra-abdominal pressure in critically ill patients. Crit Care Med 1989;17(2):118–21.

24. Cheatham M, Safcsak K, Block E, et al. Preload assessment in patients with an open abdomen. J Trauma 1999;46(1):16–22.

25. Malbrain ML. Intra-abdominal pressure in the intensive care unit: clinical tool or toy? In: Vincent JL, editor. Yearbook of intensive care and emergency medicine. Berlin: Springer-Verlag; 2001. p. 547–85.

26. Cheatham M. Intra-abdominal hypertension and abdominal compartment syndrome. New Horiz 1999;7:96–115.

27. Malbrain ML. Abdominal pressure in the critically ill. Curr Opin Crit Care 2000;6: 17–29.

28. Wauters J, Wilmer A, Valenza F. Abdomino-thoracic transmission during ACS: facts and figures. Acta Clin Belg Suppl 2007;62(1):200–5.
29. Malbrain ML, De laet I. A new concept: the polycompartment syndrome—part 1. Int J Intensive Care 2008;Autumn:19–24.
30. Malbrain ML, De laet I. A new concept: the polycompartment syndrome—part 2. Int J Intensive Care 2009;Spring:19–25.
31. Pelosi P, Quintel M, Malbrain ML. Effect of intra-abdominal pressure on respiratory mechanics. Acta Clin Belg Suppl 2007;62(1):78–88.
32. Simon RJ, Friedlander MH, Ivatury RR, et al. Hemorrhage lowers the threshold for intra-abdominal hypertension-induced pulmonary dysfunction. J Trauma 1997; 42(3):398–403 [discussion: 404–5].
33. Quintel M, Pelosi P, Caironi P, et al. An increase of abdominal pressure increases pulmonary edema in oleic acid-induced lung injury. Am J Respir Crit Care Med 2004;169(4):534–41.
34. De laet I, Citerio G, Malbrain ML. The influence of intraabdominal hypertension on the central nervous system: current insights and clinical recommendations, is it all in the head? Acta Clin Belg Suppl 2007;62(1):89–97.
35. Irgau I, Koyfman Y, Tikellis JI. Elective intraoperative intracranial pressure monitoring during laparoscopic cholecystectomy. Arch Surg 1995;130(9):1011–3.
36. Joseph DK, Dutton RP, Aarabi B, et al. Decompressive laparotomy to treat intractable intracranial hypertension after traumatic brain injury. J Trauma 2004;57(4): 687–93 [discussion: 693–5].
37. Josephs L, Este-McDonald J, Birkett D, et al. Diagnostic laparoscopy increases intracranial pressure. J Trauma 1994;36(6):815–8 [discussion: 818–9].
38. Sugrue M, Buist M, Hourihan F, et al. Prospective study of intra-abdominal hypertension and renal function after laparotomy. Br J Surg 1995;82(2):235–8.
39. Sugrue M, Jones F, Deane S, et al. Intra-abdominal hypertension is an independent cause of postoperative renal impairment. Arch Surg 1999;134(10): 1082–5.
40. Bradley S, Mudge G, Blake W, et al. The effect of increased intra-abdominal pressure on the renal excretion of water and electrolytes in normal human subjects and in patients with diabetes insipidus. Acta Clin Belg 1955;10(3):209–23.
41. Kirkpatrick A, Colistro R, Laupland K, et al. Renal arterial resistive index response to intraabdominal hypertension in a porcine model. Crit Care Med 2007;35(1):207–13.
42. Harman P, Kron I, McLachlan H, et al. Elevated intra-abdominal pressure and renal function. Ann Surg 1982;196(5):594–7.
43. De Waele J, De Laet I, Kirkpatrick A, et al. Intra-abdominal hypertension and abdominal compartment syndrome. Am J Kidney Dis 2011;57(1):159–69.
44. Ulyatt DB. Elevated intra-abdominal pressure. Australian Anaes 1992;108–14.
45. Mullens W, Abrahams Z, Skouri H, et al. Elevated intra-abdominal pressure in acute decompensated heart failure: a potential contributor to worsening renal function? J Am Coll Cardiol 2008;51(3):300–6.
46. Caldwell CB, Ricotta JJ. Evaluation of intra-abdominal pressure and renal hemodynamics. Curr Surg 1986;43(6):495–8.
47. Vivier E, Metton O, Piriou V, et al. Effects of increased intra-abdominal pressure on central circulation. Br J Anaesth 2006;96(6):701–7.
48. Diebel L, Saxe J, Dulchavsky S. Effect of intra-abdominal pressure on abdominal wall blood flow. Am Surg 1992;58(9):573–5.
49. Wendon J, Biancofiore G, Auzinger G. Intra-abdominal hypertension and the liver. In: Ivatury R, Cheatham M, Malbrain M, et al, editors. Abdominal compartment syndrome. Georgetown (TX): Landes Bioscience; 2006. p. 138–43.

50. Dalfino L, Malcangi V, Cinnella G, et al. Abdominal hypertension and liver dysfunction in intensive care unit patients: an "on-off" phenomenon? Transplant Proc 2006;38(3):838–40.

51. Inal M, Memis D, Sezer Y, et al. Effects of intra-abdominal pressure on liver function assessed with the LiMON in critically ill patients. Can J Surg 2011;54(2):42709.

52. Michelet P, Roch A, Gainnier M, et al. Influence of support on intra-abdominal pressure, hepatic kinetics of indocyanine green and extravascular lung water during prone positioning in patients with ARDS: a randomized crossover study. Crit Care 2005;9(3):R251–7.

53. Luca A, Cirera I, Garcia-Pagan JC, et al. Hemodynamic effects of acute changes in intra-abdominal pressure in patients with cirrhosis. Gastroenterology 1993; 104(1):222–7.

54. De laet I, Malbrain ML. ICU management of the patient with intra-abdominal hypertension: what to do, when and to whom? Acta Clin Belg Suppl 2007; 62(1):190–9.

55. Calvin JE, Driedger AA, Sibbald WJ. Does the pulmonary capillary wedge pressure predict left ventricular preload in critically ill patients? Crit Care Med 1981; 9(6):437–43.

56. Chang MC, Meredith JW. Cardiac preload, splanchnic perfusion, and their relationship during resuscitation in trauma patients. J Trauma 1997;42(4):577–82 [discussion: 582–74].

57. Diebel LN, Wilson RF, Tagett MG, et al. End-diastolic volume. A better indicator of preload in the critically ill. Arch Surg 1992;127(7):817–21 [discussion: 821–2].

58. Diebel LN, Myers T, Dulchavsky S. Effects of increasing airway pressure and PEEP on the assessment of cardiac preload. J Trauma 1997;42(4):585–90 [discussion: 590–1].

59. Durham R, Neunaber K, Vogler G, et al. Right ventricular end-diastolic volume as a measure of preload. J Trauma 1995;39(2):218–23 [discussion: 223–4].

60. McNamee JE, Abel FL. Mathematical coupling and Starling's law of the heart. Shock 1996;6(5):330.

61. Nelson LD, Safcsak K, Cheatham ML, et al. Mathematical coupling does not explain the relationship between right ventricular end-diastolic volume and cardiac output. Crit Care Med 2001;29(5):940–3.

62. Malbrain ML, De Potter P, Deeren D. Cost-effectiveness of minimally invasive hemodynamic monitoring. In: Vincent J-L, editor. Yearbook of Intensive Care and Emergency Medicine. Berlin: Springer-Verlag; 2005. p. 603–31.

63. Malbrain ML, Van Mieghem N, Verbrugghe W, et al. PiCCO derived parameters versus filling pressures in intra-abdominal hypertension. 2003;29(Suppl 1):S130.

64. Cheatham M, White M, Sagraves S, et al. Abdominal perfusion pressure: a superior parameter in the assessment of intra-abdominal hypertension. J Trauma 2000;49(4):621–6 [discussion: 626–7].

65. Mahjoub Y, Touzeau J, Airapetian N, et al. The passive leg-raising maneuver cannot accurately predict fluid responsiveness in patients with intra-abdominal hypertension. Crit Care Med 2010;38(9):1824–9.

66. Malbrain M, Reuter D. Assessing fluid responsiveness with the passive leg raising maneuver in patients with increased intra-abdominal pressure: be aware that not all blood returns! Crit Care Med 2010;38(9):1912–5.

67. Duperret S, Lhuillier F, Piriou V, et al. Increased intra-abdominal pressure affects respiratory variations in arterial pressure in normovolaemic and hypovolaemic mechanically ventilated healthy pigs. Intensive Care Med 2007; 33(1):163–71.

68. Jacques D, Bendjelid K, Duperret S, et al. Pulse pressure variation and stroke volume variation during increased intra-abdominal pressure: an experimental study. Crit Care 2011;15(1):R33.
69. Malbrain M, de Laet I. Functional hemodynamics and increased intra-abdominal pressure: same thresholds for different conditions. Crit Care Med 2009;37(2):781–3.
70. Fellahi JL, Caille V, Charron C, et al. Hemodynamic effects of positive end-expiratory pressure during abdominal hyperpression: a preliminary study in healthy volunteers. J Crit Care 2011. [Epub ahead of print].
71. De Laet I, Ravyts M, Vidts W, et al. Current insights in intra-abdominal hypertension and abdominal compartment syndrome: open the abdomen and keep it open! Langenbecks Arch Surg 2008;393(6):833–47.

Massive Transfusion of Blood in the Surgical Patient

Jordan M. Raymer, MD[a], Lisa M. Flynn, MD, RVT[b],
Ronald F. Martin, MD[a,c],*

KEYWORDS

- Blood transfusion • Trauma • Blood products
- Transfusion-related injury

It could reasonably be argued that the history of surgery and the history of war are completely intertwined. Although not all advances in surgical thought come from war, the pace of advance in surgical understanding and practice is markedly increased during times of prolonged armed conflict. The United States, with its coalition partners, is now engaged in 2 of the most protracted armed conflicts in the relatively short history of the republic. The current armed conflicts, as those that came before, have provided an opportunity to vastly increase our understanding of treating victims of traumatic injury.

While all armed conflicts have produced significant gains in medical knowledge, albeit at tragic cost, these most recent and ongoing hostile operations have presented some unique opportunities. Perhaps most important is our ability to gather and analyze data, both medical and nonmedical, from the battlesphere, in real time or near real time. Advances in technology allow unparalleled access to communication from the most forward (if that really exists in asymmetric conflict) locations to the most developed definitive care facilities in the continental United States. Real-time teleconferencing and reliable access for data transfer have allowed those of us who have worked in these forward-operating conditions to have access to information and clinical follow-up on patients who, in previous eras, would have been lost to follow-up for those who provide initial and in-transit care. The 2 senior investigators of this article (L.M.F. and R.F.M.) have benefited tremendously from these advances.

Hemorrhage remains a leading cause of morbidity and death in both civilian and military trauma patients. It is responsible for almost 50% of deaths occurring within

---

[a] Department of Surgery, Marshfield Clinic and Saint Joseph's Hospital, 1000 North Oak Avenue, Marshfield, WI 54449, USA
[b] Department of Surgery, Wayne State University, 4201 Saint Antoine, Detroit, MI 48201, USA
[c] University of Wisconsin School of Medicine and Public Health, 750 Highland Avenue, Madison, WI 53705, USA
* Corresponding author. Department of Surgery, Marshfield Clinic and Saint Joseph's Hospital, 1000 North Oak Avenue, Marshfield, WI 54449.
E-mail address: martin.ronald@marshfieldclinic.org

Surg Clin N Am 92 (2012) 221–234
doi:10.1016/j.suc.2012.01.008
0039-6109/12/$ – see front matter © 2012 Elsevier Inc. All rights reserved.

24 hours of injury, and up to 80% of intraoperative trauma mortalities.[1] The end point of resuscitation in these patients is the restoration of effective end-organ perfusion by stopping hemorrhage and restoring intravascular volume, done in such a way that minimizes acidosis, hypothermia, and coagulopathy. This end point almost always requires the use of blood and/or blood component therapy. The best way to manage life-threatening hemorrhage is either to avoid the circumstance that prompted it or to mitigate blood loss early in the injury cycle, in the absence of which blood replacement must suffice. In this article, the authors review the current understanding of massive transfusion, and its attendant unintended consequences, in the management of patients with profound hemorrhage. The authors do so with the greatest respect and gratitude to those who have suffered, and by doing so have provided clinicians with some increased capability to perhaps reduce the suffering of others.

DEFINITION

It is estimated that 10% of military trauma patients and 3% to 5% of civilian trauma patients receive massive transfusions.[1] Massive transfusion is generally defined as administration of 10 or more units of packed red blood cells (PRBCs) to an individual patient within 24 hours.[2,3] For massive transfusion guidelines to be useful, a recognition and anticipation of ongoing blood loss over a specific period is required. Much of the data on the blood component ratio are gathered from populations who conform to the traditional definition. Some investigators object that this definition may exclude groups of patients who die early, specifically underrepresenting the acute resuscitation phase.[2] This criticism has generated other dynamic definitions that use lower volumes and shorter time frames, such as transfusion of greater than 4 units of PRBCs in 1 hour with anticipation of continued need, or the replacement of 50% total blood volume in 3 hours.[3]

HISTORICAL PERSPECTIVE

As alluded to in the introduction, much of what we know about large-volume transfusion has been learned from wartime experience. The first warm blood transfusion in a human was administered in 1667 by Dr Jean-Baptiste Denis in France, when he directly transfused blood from the femoral artery of a lamb into the vein of a demented man, theorizing that the lamb's blood would cure his illness. The man died shortly thereafter secondary to tuberculosis; however, at the time his demise was attributed to the blood transfusions.[4] Following this, the concept of bloodletting dominated for some time and the practice of transfusing blood in humans did not occur again until the nineteenth century.[4,5]

The discovery of ABO compatibility and the development of citrate storage solutions made the process of collecting blood and transfusing it easier and more frequent. By the time of World War I, the capacity to collect and store viable blood made it possible to deliver blood to the battlefield for the first time.[5,6] The etiology and understanding of shock, however, was still a matter of controversy. Some considered death to be attributable to wound shock, an entity thought to be distinct from hemorrhagic shock. Blood transfusions for resuscitation therapy were accepted by the British Forces in 1918, and by the time they entered World War II, the British had a functioning blood-banking system. The Americans, however, were slower to adopt these practices.

Dr Edward D. Churchill, a thoracic surgeon from Harvard, played an integral role in the US Military blood program. He was appointed chief surgical consultant in the North Africa campaign during the United States' early involvement in World War II. On assumption of his duties, which were largely not described, he found that not only was there no plan for the collection of blood, there was also a push to use plasma for resuscitation.[7] The consensus of US Military medical opinion had not yet dismissed the idea of wound shock, and therefore was not fully engaged with red cell transfusion as a primary form of resuscitation. More than 5 million collected units of blood were converted into either plasma or albumin during this period.[7]

Churchill remained skeptical and came to the conclusion that wound shock was hypovolemic shock resulting from hemorrhage. He believed that the British were basically correct and that whole blood collection and transfusion was the ideal solution for this problem. He petitioned for a laboratory, established a blood-banking center, and eventually headed a research team to evaluate the physiologic consequences of injury and shock.[5,6] The actual story of how Churchill managed this is too long to recall in this article, but it is a worthwhile read for those who like stories of perseverance and discovery despite minimal support from the higher-ups.

STORAGE AND COMPATIBILITY CONSIDERATIONS

In 1914, Adolph Hustin discovered that adding citrate to blood prevented it from clotting and that the citrated blood could be safely transfused into dogs. In 1915, Richard Lewisohn determined the maximum amount of citrate that could be transfused into dogs without toxicity. Richard Weil then showed that citrated blood could be stored for 2 days and still be effective when transfused into dogs and guinea pigs. In 1916, work on rabbits by Rous and Turner showed that blood could be stored for 14 days and successfully transfused.[8–11] Shortly thereafter, during World War I, separated red blood cells (RBCs) were stored in a similar solution for up to a month and then used to resuscitate wounded soldiers in the British Forces. Blood transfusion became the accepted resuscitation therapy for the British; however, US Army officials became concerned about bacterial contamination secondary to the glucose storage medium, and eventually decided to reduce the storage time of RBCs to only 5 days, which greatly limited their widespread use.[5,12]

The initial standards for RBC storage were that the cells did not hemolyze in the bottle, and that they appeared to recirculate when transfused. The same storage principles essentially hold true today. The current consensus is that 75% of cells must remain in circulation at 24 hours posttransfusion, with less than 1% hemolysis.[13] However, the controversy surrounding lengthening of storage time to build inventory versus optimizing safety and efficacy of blood products continues.

The current standards and procedures for storage of blood products include rigorous quality measures. There are, however, inherent problems with storing living RBCs in a closed plastic bag. The authors permit a unit of PRBCs to be stored for up to 42 days, during which time several biochemical changes occur. Decreases in pH lead to lower levels of adenosine triphosphate and 2,3-diphosphoglycerate. Acidosis contributes to changes in the shape of red cells. As storage time increases, membranes become rigid secondary to phospholipid asymmetry, leading to accumulation and release of biologically active lipids, as well as oxidative damage. Hypothermic storage and cryopreservation also contribute to increased membrane permeability, loss of cation pumping, and hemolysis.[14,15] The reported effects of RBC age on clinical outcomes are mixed. Lelubre and colleagues[16] reviewed the literature and identified 24 studies that evaluated the effects of RBC age on outcomes. Their analysis of the published data did not support a clinically relevant relationship between the age of transfused RBCs and morbidity or mortality, except perhaps on trauma patients who have undergone massive transfusions. It is difficult to discern the impact of older blood from the effects of severe injuries requiring massive volumes of transfused blood. Total volume of transfused blood seems to serve as the primary risk factor for transfusion-related mortality.[17]

Duration of blood component storage may also be a contributing factor in multiorgan failure. Zallen and colleagues,[18] in a prospective analysis, identified trauma patients who received significantly more units of RBCs that were stored for longer than 14 to 21 days. The investigators observed that patients who developed multiorgan failure received significantly older red cell units, and concluded that age of PRBC units is an independent predictor of developing multiorgan failure. There is also support in the literature to suggest a relationship between the age of RBCs transfused and the development of complicated sepsis. An association between the number of units of older blood transfused, not simply the total amount of blood, and the development of sepsis suggests that the immunomodulatory effect of allogenic blood is influenced by the duration of storage.[17] Other studies demonstrate that the use of units older than 14 to 21 days remains an independent risk factor for major infections.[13,16,19] Potential mechanisms for this effect come from in vitro studies showing that incubating normal neutrophils with plasma from blood stored for 21 to 42 days increases production of interleukin (IL)-8, IL-1β, tumor necrosis factor α, and secretory phospholipase.[20] Further randomized prospective trials are needed to evaluate these relationships in patients receiving massive transfusions and to more fully understand the process.

Another potential problem related to the prolonged storage of blood is the potential for bacterial contamination. This problem was among the earliest recognized transfusion risks, as blood components were originally collected in reusable glass bottles. With the advent of sterile containment devices and refrigeration systems, this risk dropped dramatically.[21] Today, approximately 1 in 30,000 stored RBC units can be demonstrated at some point to be bacterially contaminated, accounting for about 1 in 5 transfusion-related deaths per year.[13] Platelets are more susceptible to this risk because of a storage temperature that can facilitate microbial growth (20°–24°C). The implementation of bacterial testing has significantly decreased this risk.[21]

Given the large volume of blood products received by patients who are massively transfused, it is not always feasible to use fully cross-matched, type-specific blood products. One of the earliest civilian experiences with uncross-matched PRBCs, by Blumberg and Bove[22] in the 1970s, reported the use of more than 200 units of PRBCs without any "untoward effects." Similarly, in several prospective studies of patients requiring massive transfusion using uncross-matched PRBCs, no acute transfusion reactions were reported.[23,24] The largest use of uncross-matched PRBCs comes again from the military experience. In Vietnam, the US Army used more than 100,000 units of uncross-matched blood without any reportable deaths as a result of transfusion reactions.[23]

In another large study of more than 25,000 trauma patients,[25] increased mortality was noted in the group receiving uncross-matched PRBC transfusions. The mortality impact persisted even after correcting for differences in demographics, injury severity, and the amount of blood products received. The investigators concluded that the requirement for uncross-matched blood during the acute resuscitation of trauma patients is an independent predictor of mortality and the need for massive transfusion. In their analysis they attributed the increase in mortality to the transfusion of uncross-matched PRBCs as a marker for acute active hemorrhage, but not to the uncross-matched blood itself.[25] Collectively these results suggest that the use of uncross-matched PRBCs may be a predictor of the need for massive transfusion.

Overall, the literature supports that uncross-matched red cells are safe for patients with acute hemorrhage, and certainly safer than the risk associated with uncompensated anemia or persistent hypovolemia. The risk of an acute hemolytic transfusion reaction is low, and the risk of creating alloantibodies that interfere with future cross-matching is also low. The indications and thresholds for transfusion with uncross-matched blood products are continuing to evolve; however, their safety seem to be acceptable at present.

TEMPERATURE, BASE DEFICIT, AND pH

Massive transfusion is associated with several metabolic and hemostatic consequences. Uncontrolled hemorrhage and the subsequent massive resuscitation can result in the development of coagulopathy, hypothermia, and acidemia in the postinjury period. The etiology of coagulopathy is multifactorial, and involves a combination of both dilutional and consumptive factors. The total volume of blood loss, as well as the blood component products used for resuscitation, contributes to this lethal triad. Shock and tissue injury seem to be the main driving forces early in the development of coagulopathy, and once resuscitation is initiated, hemodilution further exacerbates these derangements.[12] Also, the physical process of separating whole blood into component products results in dilution of RBCs, clotting factors, and platelets, which further contributes to these physiologic changes.[26]

Hypothermia may be induced by several mechanisms in the postinjury period, including prehospital environmental conditions, evaporative losses in the operating room, or iatrogenic prevention of endogenous heat production by use of paralytics. In patients, hypothermia from all causes, to the degree that core temperature decreases to less than 32°C, is associated with 21% mortality.[27] In trauma patients who develop similar hypothermia, the mortality rate increases. One study demonstrated a 100% mortality rate at core temperatures lower than 32°C. In the hypothermic and traumatized patient, this was noted to be independent of the presence of shock, volume of fluid resuscitation, and injury severity.[28] The systemic response to hypothermia, specifically at temperatures lower than 35°C, induces coagulopathy by affecting hemostasis, mainly by its effect on platelets, coagulation factors, and the fibrinolytic system.[29] Decreased enzymatic activity as an integral mechanism in hypothermia-induced coagulation stems from studies in which clotting assays were performed at temperatures lower than 37°C. Prothrombin time (PT) and activated partial thromboplastin time (aPTT) are significantly increased at temperatures lower than 33° to 35°C. The activity of tissue factor, or factor VIIa complex, decreases with dropping temperatures. In animal studies, hypothermia increases fibrinolysis by its inhibitory effects on plasminogen activator inhibitor.[27] Furthermore, platelet function is affected mainly secondary to the reduced effect of von Willebrand factor, which mediates platelet adhesion and activation.[12]

Rapid transfusion of large quantities of blood products or infusion of other fluids that are cooler than ideal core temperature will either create or exacerbate hypothermia. Blood products are usually stored at temperatures between 1° and 6°C. For every 1°C drop in core temperature of the patient there is a 10% reduction in coagulation factor activity. Warming blood products to 37°C before administration and close monitoring of the patient's temperature are recommended to mitigate this effect.[29,30]

Acidemia in the massively transfused patient is usually an indicator of end-organ hypoperfusion with subsequent metabolic acidosis, caused by either low-flow states or excessive use of chloride-containing resuscitative products. Acidemia impairs the generation of thrombin, increases the degradation of fibrinogen, impairs the function of plasma proteases, and reduces the activity of coagulation factor complexes.[12,30,31] Specifically, a drop in pH from 7.4 to 7.0 reduces the activity of factor VIIa by 90%, factor VIIa/tissue factor complex by 55%, and factor Xa/Va complex by 70%.[31]

Correlating these deficiencies with clinical outcomes is difficult. A patient's calculated plasma base deficit on hospital admission and transfusion requirements in the first 24 hours has been associated with postinjury organ failure and death.[32,33] The overall effects of acidemia and base deficit on outcomes, however, have not been well defined.

WHOLE BLOOD

The practice of transfusing fresh whole blood has been used in almost every military conflict since World War I, as well in situations in which certain fractionated blood product components are not available.[34] Since the development of citrate storage solutions, the process of collecting blood and subsequently transfusing it at a later date has become easier and more frequent. As the fractionation process developed and improved between the 1940s and 1980s, transfusion of blood components increased while the use of stored whole blood diminished.[34]

One advantage of transfusing fresh whole blood is that it provides replacement of each blood component in the same ratio that it was lost, and is not affected by the storage process. Current practice in forward military environments is to use warm fresh blood transfusions for patients who require any blood component that is not immediately available, most notably platelets or cryoprecipitate. A recent analysis of combat-related trauma patients receiving 1 or more units of blood reported that fresh whole blood was associated with improved survival when compared with component therapy.[35]

Between March 2003 and July 2007, more than 6000 units of whole blood were transfused in Afghanistan and Iraq. The donor pool consists generally of hospital and military personnel, as well as government contractors, who have been pre-screened. The units are transfused warm without leukoreduction or irradiation within 20 to 30 minutes.[35] One review that evaluated more than 2000 units of warm fresh whole blood transfused between 2003 and 2005 found that no patient contracted human immunodeficiency virus (HIV). The risk is low, as all military donors are screened for HIV within 2 years before deployment and are immunized against hepatitis B. In the same study, the incidence of hepatitis C measured in military donors was 0.11%, and the risk of transfusing a unit contaminated with hepatitis C was 1 in 69,930 units. Rapid screening for hepatitis C in this scenario prevented the transfusion of 2 contaminated units. Based on these data, there is currently discussion regarding the utility of screening for hepatitis C as well.[36]

Transfusion of whole blood has largely been abandoned, probably for good reason, by the civilian medical community. Blood component therapy has proved to be safe and readily available. The logistic considerations in delivering blood products in the civilian sector or even well-supplied and connected aspects of the military medical system are quite different to those in forward austere operating environments. When blood product availability is not an issue, it is difficult to make a case for the use of whole blood. Also, austere forward environments have a fairly captive population of donors, which markedly improves one's ability to draw from a relatively safe donor population. The military experience clearly suggests that there is still a place for the use of fresh whole blood in patient resuscitation.

Perhaps the largest whole blood drive in the United States followed the September 11, 2001 terrorist attacks. Roughly 5000 units of whole blood were collected by United States civilian blood systems, and almost 40,000 units of PRBCs were collected. Specifically, whole blood was collected in preference to apheresis units for ease and speed of collection immediately after the attack.[37] While this demonstrates that the civilian capability to collect fresh whole blood exists, it does not provide insight into the utility of it or need for it under less than highly unusual circumstances.

BLOOD PRODUCTS BY COMPONENT AND RATIOS DATA

Although fresh whole blood has been used historically in the military setting, and more recently during the conflicts in Iraq and Afghanistan, component therapy is the standard for transfusion of blood products. Blood component therapy optimizes the use of resources by allowing components to be used in different patients.

There are generally 2 different approaches to blood component replacement in managing coagulopathy: prophylactic transfusion of fresh frozen plasma (FFP) and platelets in patients expected to have or develop coagulopathy versus transfusion only when there is clinical and laboratory evidence of coagulopathy.[38] If using laboratory data, guidelines generally recommend transfusion of the appropriate blood components based on the following values: PT greater than 1.5 times normal, aPTT greater than 1.5 times normal, fibrinogen less than 1.0 g/L, and platelet count less than 50×10^9. Motivation to standardize resuscitation has generated the development of massive transfusion protocols, which facilitates administration of blood components in standardized ratios.

Much of the early data on blood component ratio have been generated by military studies. Mixing of components in a 1:1 ratio of plasma to RBCs creates a unit of whole blood with a hematocrit of 29%, a platelet count of 88,000, and 62% clotting activity.[6] The available data suggest an FFP/RBC ratio approaching 1:1 is associated with improved survival and decreased early hemorrhagic death. In patients predicted to require or who do require massive transfusion, current US Military practice is administration of FFP, platelets, and PRBCs in a 1:1:1 ratio, which approximates that of whole blood.[39–41]

Numerous multicenter prospective studies have supported these recommendations, documenting a survival benefit and reduction in mortality for patients who receive more FFP and platelets as part of the resuscitation.[30,42–44] There is, however, a limit, as this survival benefit is not seen at very high ratios of FFP/PRBC.

When examining the effect of blood component ratio on the coagulation response, beneficial effects are observed at FFP/RBC ratios between 1:2 and 3:4. These benefits were confined to patients with coagulopathy and were seen to diminish at ratios of greater than 1:3. The survival benefit can also be extended to platelet/RBC ratios, with optimal levels of 1:1, similar to that of plasma and red cells.[45–47]

In blunt trauma patients with hemorrhagic shock undergoing massive transfusion, FFP/RBC ratios approaching 1:1.5 are associated with a significantly lower risk of mortality. The mortality reduction is most relevant within the first 48 hours from the time of injury. These results suggest that the risk occurs early, and likely secondary to ongoing coagulopathy and hemorrhage.[47]

TRANSFUSION-RELATED ACUTE LUNG INJURY

Transfusion-related acute lung injury, or TRALI, is a clinical syndrome manifesting as hypoxia and bilateral noncardiogenic pulmonary edema after transfusion of blood products. Although the term TRALI was initially coined by Popovsky and colleagues in 1983, the literature on this subject dates back much earlier. In the early 1950s, the *New York State Medical Journal* describes lung "hypersensitivity" to transfusion, and *JAMA* also reported on this new disease in 1957. The first case series later followed in 1966, but not until 2003 were clinical criteria proposed and agreed on for the diagnosis of TRALI.[48,49]

TRALI is currently defined as a new episode of acute lung injury (ALI) occurring during or within 6 hours of a completed transfusion, which is not related to a competing cause of ALI. This diagnosis is based on clinical and radiographic evidence alone, including hypoxemia with a Pao_2/Fio_2 ratio of 300 or less, bilateral pulmonary infiltrates, and no evidence of left atrial hypertension.[50] TRALI is now the second leading reported cause of mortality from transfusion, and the leading cause of transfusion-related death reported to the US Food and Drug Administration. Mortality rates of up to 6% to 9% have been reported.[48,49] The incidence of TRALI varies, and the reported risk varies by type of blood product transfused. Reports range from 1 in 5000 units of PRBCs, 1 in 2000 plasma-containing components, 1 in 7900 units of FFP, and 1 in 432 units of whole blood–derived platelets.[48] In one large study of 90 cases of TRALI, the prevalence was 1 in 1120 for all cellular components, which is a significant increase from the accepted statistics.[51] Despite the consensus on a common definition for TRALI, these numbers may be much higher after considering the occurrence of underrecognition, variable expression of the reaction, and underreporting.

The pathophysiology of TRALI is not well understood, and there are currently 2 potential mechanisms for TRALI: antibody-mediated and non–antibody-mediated. In the antibody-mediated model, donor antibodies interact with recipient leukocytes via anti-HLA class I, anti-HLA class II, and antigranulocyte antibodies. These antibody interactions activate complement, leading to pulmonary sequestration and activation of neutrophils, endothelial damage, and capillary leak in the lungs. Usually the alloantibodies are present in the transfused product, are of donor origin, and react with the recipient's granulocytes.[49] Multiparous women are at highest risk as carriers, due to their greater alloantigen exposure, which causes higher titers of anti-HLA antigen and antigranulocyte antibodies.[48,52] The other hypothesis is a 2-hit model.

The first hit is related to the patient's preexisting condition or underlying illness that primes and sequesters neutrophils to the lungs. It is thought that critical care is a general risk, and specific situations such as cardiac surgery and sepsis are the first hits that make the patient more vulnerable to developing TRALI.[53] The second hit is the transfusion of biologically active substances that activate neutrophils, and subsequently lead to an inflammatory cascade ultimately causing increased pulmonary microvascular permeability.[49,50] These 2 hypotheses are not mutually exclusive in that the second hit could be the antibody in the antibody-mediated TRALI.[48,49] Numerous in vitro animal studies on rabbits and rat lungs are attempting to further elucidate these mechanisms, but there is as yet no in vivo model.

Although TRALI can be caused by any blood component, data suggest that plasma is the most common culprit. Age of the blood component also plays a role. Older platelet concentrates are associated with increased incidence and severity of reactions, which may be as result of the accumulation of cytokines during storage. Specifically, IL-6 and IL-8 levels are shown to increase as a function of storage time, and higher IL-6 posttransfusion levels have been demonstrated in TRALI patients when compared with pretransfusion levels and controls.[51]

Efforts to prevent TRALI have focused on characterizing high-risk patients, donor screening and evaluation, and blood product modification. At present, donors associated with TRALI events are implicated after being tested for an antibody that corresponds to the recipient antigen. The current recommendation is screening of blood from implicated donors for detection of antibodies for major histocompatibility antigen class I and class II, and testing for neutrophil antibodies.[49] These current strategies are only helpful in confirming TRALI after it has already occurred. There is no screening test available for blood banks; however, the American Red Cross is deferring all donors previously implicated with episodes of TRALI.

The mainstay of treatment for TRALI remains supportive. The suspected blood product should be discontinued and the appropriate reporting systems notified. In patients requiring ventilatory support, smaller tidal volumes and optimization of positive end-expiratory pressure are advised. Because TRALI is caused by microvascular injury and not fluid overload, diuretics are not recommended. The use of corticosteroids in those with TRALI but not relative or absolute adrenal insufficiency is not well defined.[54]

FACTOR VIIa

As discussed earlier, the lethal triad of coagulopathy, acidemia, and hypothermia accounts for a mortality rate among trauma patients of approximately 50% to 60%.[55] Efforts to reduce mortality rates are aimed at stopping hemorrhage, correcting acidosis, preventing hypothermia, and transfusing appropriate blood products. Recombinant activated factor VII (rFVIIa, NovoSeven) has been proposed as one adjunctive form of therapy to accomplish these goals. Although it was first developed for treatment of patients with hemophilia, its use in the trauma population requiring massive transfusion is less well established. At present, rFVIIa is a damage-control tool in coagulopathic patients refractory to standard treatment, and is often coupled with massive transfusion protocols. The mechanism of action of factor VIIa is through activation of the extrinsic pathway of the coagulation cascade. It binds to exposed tissue factor at the site of endothelial injury and facilitates the conversion of factor IX to factor IXa, and factor X to Xa, to promote thrombin formation and coagulation (**Fig. 1**).[56]

The CONTROL trial was the first multicenter randomized trial using rFVIIa in the setting of bleeding trauma patients. Severely bleeding patients (those aged 16–65 years requiring 6 units of PRBCs within 4 hours of admission) were randomized to rFVIIa or placebo. The first dose was given after the eighth unit of packed cells, the second dose 1 hour later, and the third dose 3 hours after the first. The primary end point of the study was the number of units of PRBCs transfused within 48 hours of the first dose of factor rFVIIa. In the patients with blunt trauma who received rFVIIa, the number of units of PRBCs transfused was significantly fewer, with an estimated reduction of 2.6 units. Similar trends were observed in the penetrating trauma group; however, these were not statistically significant.[57,58] The investigators did not demonstrate a survival benefit in either group, particularly when bleeding was associated with acidemia and hypothermia.

A post hoc analysis by Rizoli and colleagues[59] analyzed the effects of rFVIIa on coagulopathic patients. The investigators noted that the rFVIIa-treated coagulopathic group received fewer blood products including packed cells, FFP, and platelets, and also observed a decreased incidence of multiorgan failure and acute respiratory distress syndrome in these patients. Other reports suggest that the efficacy of rFVIIa may be reduced in acidemic patients. One in vitro study examined the activity of rFVIIa on platelets, and showed that a pH drop from 7.4 to 7.0 reduced rFVIIa activity by 90%.[60]

If much of the data support that rFVIIa can reduce the number of PRBCs used in the massively transfused patient, then being able to predict when to optimally give rFVIIa may be of benefit. Methods that have emerged to help predict the optimal use of FVIIa include severe hemorrhage scores to determine the probability of a patient needing massive transfusion. One such scoring system is the Trauma Associated Severe Hemorrhage (TASH) score.[61] Variables include blood pressure, gender, hemoglobin, focused abdominal sonography for trauma (FAST), heart rate, base excess, and extremity or pelvic fractures, with a score range from 0 to 28 points. Yucel and colleagues[61] concluded that increasing TASH scores were associated with increasing

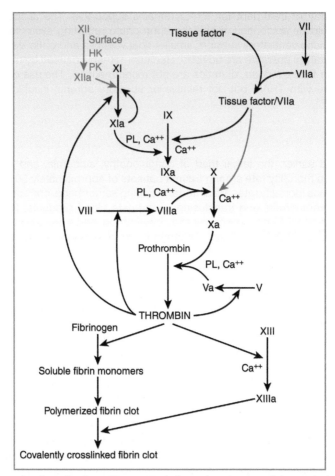

Fig. 1. The mechanism of action of factor VIIa is through activation of the extrinsic pathway of the coagulation cascade. It binds to exposed tissue factor at the site of endothelial injury and facilitates the conversion of factor IX to factor IXa, and factor X to Xa, to promote thrombin formation and coagulation. (*From* Miller JL. Coagulation and fibrinolysis. In: McPherson R, Pincus MR, eds. Henry's clinical diagnosis and management by laboratory methods. 22nd edition. Philadelphia: Saunders, 2011; with permission.)

probability for massive transfusion. The ABC (assessment of blood consumption) score proposed by Nunez and colleagues,[62] a 4-component scoring system that accounts for penetrating mechanism, emergency department systolic blood pressure of 90 mm Hg or less, heart rate of 120 or greater, and a positive FAST, showed higher accuracy than the TASH score.

The military has also contributed to the pool of knowledge regarding the use of rFVIIa as treatment for massive hemorrhage. Spinella and colleagues[63] performed a retrospective review of combat casualties (defined as Injury Severity Score >15 and received ≥10 units PRBC/24 hours) from Baghdad Hospital from December 2003 to October 2005. These investigators identified 124 patients, of whom 49 received rFVIIa and 75 did not. The main end point of mortality was statistically significant in the rFVIIa group at 24 hours and 30 days. Death from hemorrhage was lower in the rFVIIa group but did not reach statistical significance. Mechanism and location of injury were not different between the groups, and most of the laboratory results and vital signs were similar. Adverse thrombotic events were also equal between the 2 groups.[63] Recombinant activated factor VII appears to have a beneficial effect as a damage-control therapy in patients requiring massive transfusion. The cost will remain somewhat prohibitive for more routine use until level 1 evidence shows efficacy.

SUMMARY

Much of what is known about the physiology and management of significant hemorrhage has been learned during wartime. Large-volume hemorrhage with significant hypovolemia is not just the result of an injury but creates an injury cycle of its own. Conversely, restoration of intravascular volume with blood products, especially when used in large quantities, is not just a therapy but also induces significant physiologic alterations.

One thing is abundantly clear from our wartime experience: early control of hemorrhage is far more effective than trying to replace blood that has been spilled. Despite our best efforts and intentions, people will continue to engage in activities that may result in significant blood loss during times of hostility or peace. The rational, prompt, and judicious use of the correct components of blood under the correct circumstances can and does meaningfully prolong lives.

The authors respectfully acknowledge the suffering of those who allowed this information to be gathered, and applaud those who studied these matters under exceptional conditions.

REFERENCES

1. Kauvar D, Lefering R, Wade C. Impact of hemorrhage on trauma outcome: an overview of epidemiology, clinical presentation, and therapeutic considerations. J Trauma 2006;60:S3–11.
2. Mitra B, Cameron P, Gruen RL, et al. The definition of massive transfusion in trauma: a critical variable in examining evidence for resuscitation. Eur J Emerg Med 2011;18:137–42.
3. Sihler KC, Napolitano LM. Massive transfusion. Chest 2009;136:1654–67.
4. Spinella P. Warm fresh whole blood transfusion for severe hemorrhage: U.S. military and potential civilian applications. Crit Care Med 2008;36:S340–5.
5. Hoyt D. Blood and war—lest we forget. J Am Coll Surg 2009;209:681–6.
6. Hess JR, Zimrin AB. Massive blood transfusion for trauma. Curr Opin Hematol 2005;12:488–92.
7. Cannon J, Fischer JE, Edward D. Churchill as a combat consultant. Ann Surg 2010;251:566–72.
8. Hustin A. Principe d'une nouvelle method de transfusion. Journal Medical de Bruxelles 1914;2:436.
9. Lewisohn R. Blood transfusion by citrate method. Surg Gynecol Obstet 1915;21:37–47.
10. Weil R. Sodium citrate in the transfusion of blood. JAMA 1915;64(5):425–6.
11. Rous P, Turner J. The transfusion of kept cells. J Exp Med 1916;23:239–47.
12. Hess JR, Brohi K, Dutton RP, et al. The coagulopathy of trauma: a review of mechanisms. J Trauma 2008;65:748–54.
13. Zimrin AB, Hess JR. Current issues relating to the transfusion of stored red blood cells. Vox Sang 2009;96:93–103.

14. Gilliss B, Looney M. Reducing noninfectious risk of blood transfusion. Anesthesiology 2011;115:635–49.
15. Stoll C, Wolkers W. Membrane stability during biopreservation of blood. Transfus Med Hemother 2011;38:89–97.
16. Lelubre C, Piagnerelli M, Vincent JL. Association between duration of storage of transfused red blood cells and morbidity and mortality in adult patients: myth or reality? Transfusion 2009;49:1384–9.
17. Hassan M, Pham T, Cuschieri J, et al. The association between the transfusion of older blood and outcomes after trauma. Shock 2011;35:3–8.
18. Zallen G, Offner P, Moore E, et al. Age of transfused blood is an independent risk factor for postinjury multiple organ failure. Am J Surg 1999;178:570–2.
19. Offner P, Moore E, Biffl W, et al. Increased rate of infection associated with transfusion of old blood after severe injury. Arch Surg 2002;137:711–7.
20. Malone D, Dunne J, Tracy K, et al. Blood transfusion, independent of shock severity, is associated with worse outcome in trauma. J Trauma 2003;54:898–907.
21. Alter H, Klein H. The hazards of blood transfusion in a historical perspective. Blood 2008;112:2617–26.
22. Blumberg N, Bove J. Uncrossmatched blood for emergency transfusion. JAMA 1978;240:2057–9.
23. Dutton R, Shih D, Edelman B, et al. Safety of uncrossmatched type-O red cells for resuscitation from hemorrhagic shock. J Trauma 2005;59:1445–9.
24. Schwab C. Immediate trauma resuscitation with type O uncrossmatched blood: a two-year prospective experience. J Trauma 1986;26:897–902.
25. Inaba K, Pedro GR, Shulman I, et al. The impact of uncross-matched blood transfusion on the need for massive transfusion and mortality: analysis of 5166 uncross-matched units. J Trauma 2008;65:1222–6.
26. Sebesta MA. Special lessons learned from Iraq. Surg Clin North Am 2006;86:711–26.
27. Tsuei B, Kearney P. Hypothermia in the trauma patient. Injury 2004;35:7–15.
28. Jurkovich G, Greiser W. Hypothermia in trauma victims: an ominous predictor of survival. J Trauma 1987;27:1019–24.
29. Sihler KC, Napolitano LM. Complications of massive transfusion. Chest 2010;137:209–20.
30. Johansson P, Ostrowsk R, Secher N. Management of major blood loss: an update. Acta Anaesthesiol Scand 2010;54:1039–49.
31. Meng Z, Wolberg A, Monroe D. The effect of temperature and pH on the activity of factor VIIa: implications for the efficacy of high dose factor VIIa in hypothermic and acidotic patients. J Trauma 2003;55:886–91.
32. Davis J, Parks S, Kaups K, et al. Admission base deficits predicts transfusion requirement and risks of complications. J Trauma 1996;41:769–74.
33. Thorsen K, Ringdal KG, Soreide E, et al. Clinical and cellular effects of hypothermia, acidosis and coagulopathy in major injury. Br J Surg 2011;98:894–907.
34. Repine TB, Perkins JG, Kauvar DS, et al. The use of fresh whole blood in massive transfusion. J Trauma 2006;60:S59–69.
35. Spinella P, Perkins J, Grathwohl K, et al. Warm fresh blood is independently associated with improved survival for patients with combat-related traumatic injuries. J Trauma 2009;66:S69–76.
36. Spinella P, Perkins J, Grathwohl K, et al. Risks associated with fresh whole blood transfusions in a combat support hospital. Crit Care Med 2007;35:2576–81.
37. Linden J, Davey R, Burch J, et al. The September 11th, 2001 disaster and the New York blood supply. Transfusion 2002;42:1385–7.

38. Spahn DR, Rossaint R. Coagulopathy and blood component transfusion in trauma. Br J Anaesth 2005;95:130–9.
39. Jansen J, Thomas R, Louson M, et al. Damage control resuscitation for patients with major trauma. BMJ 2009;338:1436–40.
40. Mitra B, Mori A, Cameron PA, et al. Fresh frozen plasma use during massive blood transfusion in trauma resuscitation. Injury 2010;41:35–9, Int J Care Injured.
41. Zink KA, Sambasivan CN, Holcomb JB, et al. A high ratio of plasma and platelets to packed red blood cells in the first 6 hours of massive transfusion improves outcomes in a large multicenter study. Am J Surg 2009;197:565–70.
42. Borgman MA, Spinella PC, Perkins JG, et al. The ratio of blood products transfused affects mortality in patients receiving massive transfusions at a combat support hospital. J Trauma 2007;63:805–13.
43. Johansson P, Stensalle J. Hemostatic resuscitation for massive bleeding: the paradigm of plasma and platelets—a review of the current literature. Transfusion 2010;50:701–10.
44. Duschesne JC, Hunt JP, Wahl G, et al. Review of the current blood transfusions strategies in a mature level I trauma center: were we wrong for the last 60 years? J Trauma 2008;65:272–6.
45. Davenport R, Curry N, Manson J, et al. Hemostatic effects of fresh frozen plasma may be maximal at red cell ratios of 1:2. J Trauma 2011;70:90–6.
46. Holcomb JB, Wade CE, Michalek CE, et al. Increased plasma and platelet to red blood cell ratios improves outcome in 466 massively transfused civilian trauma patients. Ann Surg 2008;248:447–58.
47. Sperry JL, Ochoa JB, Gunn SR, et al. An FFP:PRBC transfusion ratio >1:1.5 is associated with a lower risk of mortality after massive transfusion. J Trauma 2008;65:986–93.
48. Toy P, Popovsky M, Abraham E, et al. Transfusion related acute lung injury: definition and review. Crit Care Med 2005;33:721–6.
49. Sheppard C, Lodgberg L, Zimring J, et al. Transfusion related acute lung injury. Hematol Oncol Clin North Am 2007;21:163–76.
50. Kleinman S, Caulfield T, Chan P, et al. Toward an understanding of transfusion related acute lung injury: statement of a consensus panel. Transfusion 2004;44:1774–89.
51. Silliman C, Boshkov L, Mehdizadehkashi Z, et al. Transfusion related acute lung injury: epidemiology and prospective analysis of etiologic factors. Blood 2003; 101:454–62.
52. Looney M, Gillis B, Matthay M. Pathophysiology of transfusion-related acute lung injury. Curr Opin Hematol 2010;17:418–23.
53. Hess JR. Translating research in the intensive care unit into effective educational strategies. Crit Care Med 2010;38:981–2.
54. Cherry T, Steciuk M, Reddy V, et al. Transfusion related acute lung injury: past and present. Am J Clin Pathol 2008;129:287–97.
55. Mitra B, Cameron P, Phillips L. Recombinant factor VIIa in trauma patients with the triad of death. Injury 2011;1:1–6.
56. Gonzalez E, Jastrow K, Holcomb J, et al. Schwartz's principles of surgery. 9th edition. Available at: http://www.accesssurgery.com. Accessed January 9, 2012.
57. Boffard K, Riou B, Warren B, et al. Recombinant factor VIIa as adjunctive therapy for bleeding in severely injured trauma patients: two parallel randomized, placebo-controlled, double-blind clinical trials. J Trauma 2005;59:8–18.
58. Dutton R, Hauser C, Boffard K, et al. Scientific and logistical challenges in designing the CONTROL trial: recombinant factor VIIa in severe trauma patients with refractory bleeding. Clin Trials 2009;6:467–79.

59. Rizoli S, Boffard K, Riou B, et al. Recombinant activated factor VII as an adjunctive therapy for bleeding control in severe trauma patients with coagulopathy: subgroup analysis from two randomized trials. Crit Care 2006;10:R178.

60. Meng Z, Wolberg A, Monroe D, et al. The effect of temperature and pH on factor VIIa: implications for the efficacy of high dose factor VIIa in hypothermic and acidotic patients. J Trauma 2003;55:855–61.

61. Yucel N, Lefering R, Maegele M, et al. Trauma associated severe hemorrhage (TASH)-score: probability of mass transfusion as surrogate for life threatening hemorrhage after multiple trauma. J Trauma 2006;60:1228–37.

62. Nunez T, Vosckrensensky I, Dossett L, et al. Early prediction of massive transfusion in trauma: simple as ABC (assessment of blood consumption)? J Trauma 2009;66:346–52.

63. Spinella P, Perkins J, McLaughlin D, et al. The effect of recombinant activated factor VII on mortality in combat-related casualties with severe trauma and massive transfusion. J Trauma 2008;64:286–94.

Postoperative Gastrointestinal Hemorrhage

Seon Jones, MD, Addison K. May, MD*

KEYWORDS

- Gastrointestinal bleeding • Hemorrhage
- Postoperative complications

Significant gastrointestinal (GI) bleeding in the postoperative period is an uncommon complication of both GI and non-GI surgery. Although uncommon, the management of GI bleeding within the postoperative period is more complex than that occurring outside the perioperative period because of a larger differential for the source of bleeding and a more complex risk/benefit analysis. There is minimal published literature specific to the management of postoperative GI bleeding, and the infrequency, complexity, and variability of the clinical setting of this complication confound simplistic consideration of its cause and therapy. Postoperative GI bleeding may be considered to occur secondary to 3 scenarios: (1) those in which the surgery or complications of the surgery are the predominate pathophysiologic cause of bleeding, (2) bleeding that occurs from causes unrelated to surgery and that predominately occur serendipitously in the postoperative period, and (3) surgical stress or complications of surgery contribute to the exacerbation of a preexisting GI bleeding source. GI bleeding in the immediate or early postoperative period is more frequently the result of the first scenario outlined, particularly when the patient has a critical illness or has other postoperative complications. Thus, this article focuses on situations in which the GI bleeding occurs secondary to surgery or surgical complications, and outlines a systematic evaluation of the patient, treatment options, and assessment of risk/benefit ratio for various treatment options.

Although most occurrences of postoperative GI bleeding are self-limiting, consideration of whether or not bleeding indicates another unrecognized postoperative complication is paramount to allow appropriate therapy. Minor postoperative bleeding likely occurs frequently and without recognition. Significant GI bleeding, generally defined as overt bleeding (nasogastric drainage with coffee-ground appearance or frank blood, hematemesis, hematochezia, or melena) complicated by hemodynamic

---

The authors have nothing to disclose.

Division of Trauma and Surgical Critical Care, Vanderbilt University Medical Center, 1211 21st Avenue South, 404 MAB, Nashville, TN 37212-3755, USA

* Corresponding author.

E-mail address: addison.may@vanderbilt.edu

Surg Clin N Am 92 (2012) 235–242

doi:10.1016/j.suc.2012.01.002

0039-6109/12/$ – see front matter surgical.theclinics.com

instability, a decrease in hemoglobin of 2 g/dL or more, a need for transfusion of blood products, or requiring invasive therapeutic intervention, occurs much less frequently but is associated with significant morbidity and mortality. For severe bleeding that requires therapeutic intervention, the risks and benefits of various therapeutic options must be considered in each postoperative setting.

INCIDENCE

The incidence of postoperative GI bleeding is low but increases with increasing magnitude of the surgical intervention, severity of illness, and underlying comorbid conditions of the patient population. For most elective cases of GI surgery, postoperative GI bleeding is not reported in case series of operative complications. Although minor suture-line bleeding occurs with some frequency after GI anastomoses, significant bleeding is uncommon. Suture-line bleeding from hand-sewn anastomoses seems to be rare (<1%) and is difficult to identify in any large series. In one large series of resections for gastric cancer, 0.4% of patients experienced significant bleeding requiring intervention.[1] Significant bleeding has been reported to occur in 0.3% to 0.9% of patients after elective bariatric surgery,[2] and significant GI bleeding has been reported in up to 3% of patients undergoing percutaneous endoscopic gastrostomy procedures. For colon resection with stapled colorectal anastomosis, the incidence is also low, with significant bleeding in 0.6% of 2166 colorectal procedures reported in recent series[3,4] and 1.8% in older series.[5] Significant suture-line hemorrhage may be more common in laparoscopic left-sided colorectal resections, reported to be 4% in one series.[6]

Significant GI bleeding also occurs after nonintestinal surgery. Pseudoaneurysm rupture with enteric communication or vascular erosion into the GI anastomosis occurs after pancreatic and hepatobiliary procedures in roughly 2% of cases.[7–9] Following cardiac surgery, roughly 0.3% of patients develop GI bleeding that requires transfusion of 2 or more units of blood.[10,11] The incidence of GI bleeding seems to be greater after aortic reconstruction procedures, with up to 4% of patients developing significant GI bleeding in the early postoperative period, all secondary to upper GI sources.[12] This high incidence is hypothesized to be related to the association of vascular disease and hypoperfusion of the enteric organs in these cases. Late bleeding complications after aortic and abdominal vascular surgical procedures also occur as a result of vascular-enteric fistulas (0.4%–2% incidence).[12–14] These fistulas typically occur months to years after surgery and have been reported after open and endovascular aortic procedures and repair of other abdominal vascular structures. Postoperative GI bleeding is more common in critically ill than in noncritically ill postoperative surgical patients. In critically ill patients undergoing either GI tract or non-GI tract surgery, significant GI bleeding occurs in 1.5% to 6% of patients, depending on the number of risk factors present, most cases being related to upper GI sources.[15,16]

CAUSES

GI bleeding in the postoperative period is predominately related to 3 causal categories including (1) stress-related mucosal damage in the upper GI tract; (2) suture-line bleeding; and (3) infectious, inflammatory, or ischemic complications. A small minority of patients have GI bleeding related to sources that coincidentally occur in the postoperative period. In all surgical procedures, both enteric and nonenteric, the upper GI tract (proximal to the ligament of Treitz) is the most common site of significant postoperative GI bleeding, accounting for more than 80% of all cases. Upper GI bleeding in this setting carries significant mortality, ranging from 20% to 30%.[17,18] Mortality for patients with upper GI bleeding in the postoperative period is up to 4 times that of matched patients without bleeding. Of these cases, bleeding related to stress-related mucosal damage (SRMD) of the stomach, duodenum, and esophagus is the most common source of significant GI bleeding. Other causes of upper GI tract post-operative bleeding include suture-line bleeding, which is typically noted less than 48 hours after surgery, disruption of suture lines because of infection or ischemia, vascular-enteric communications resulting from inflammatory or infectious processes eroding into vascular structures, and exacerbation of preexisting peptic ulcer disease, all of which typically present greater than 48 hours after surgery. Bleeding may also occur from hemobilia after hepatic injury or instrumentation, as well as Mallory-Weiss tears produced by postoperative vomiting or from the exacerbation of esophageal or gastric varices.

Lower GI tract sources also cause postoperative GI bleeding, but much less commonly. Suture-line bleeding of enteroenteric, enterocolonic, or colocolonic anastomoses may occur early after surgery and is usually self-limited. Bleeding from anastomoses that occurs after the initial postoperative period is usually secondary to an anastomotic disruption caused by infection or ischemia and mandates interventions to address the underlying cause in addition to the bleeding itself. Lower GI bleeding in the postoperative period may occur secondary to colonic ischemia, usually complicating cardiac or vascular procedures, or to vascular-enteric fistulas complicating aortic and other vascular procedures. Other causes of postoperative lower GI bleeding include diverticulosis, rectal ulcers, varices, and arteriovenous malformations.

SRMD

As noted earlier, the most common site of significant postoperative GI bleeding is the upper GI tract, and these cases are predominately secondary to SRMD. The incidence of stress-related upper GI bleeding varies greatly depending on the definition used to define the complication and the severity of illness of the patient population. Although rare, bleeding secondary to SRMD accounts for nearly all of the postoperative GI bleeding complications seen in cardiothoracic cases, vascular cases, and critically ill surgical patients.[10–12,15,16] Nearly all critically ill patients develop some degree of SRMD in the postoperative period.[15,19] However, the current incidence of clinically significant bleeding secondary to SRMD ranges from 1.5% to 6% depending on the population studied. Bleeding from SRMD may result from stress-induced gastritis, duodenitis, and esophagitis, stress-induced gastric and duodenal ulcers, or gastric, duodenal, and esophageal erosions.[15] The presence of clinically significant SRMD is associated with increased length of intensive care unit (ICU) stay and up to a 4-fold increase in mortality.[18] Several factors are thought to contribute to the pathophysiology of SRMD, including mucosal ischemia resulting from splanchnic hypoperfusion, gastric acid secretion, reflux of upper intestinal contents into the stomach or esophagus, and Helicobacter pylori. Of these, splanchnic hypoperfusion seems to be the major contributor.[19] With improved resuscitation techniques and intraoperative and postoperative management of patients, the incidence of significant SRMD and bleeding has decreased in the past several decades.

Major risk factors for GI bleeding from SRMD in critically ill patients were defined in a landmark study by Cook and colleagues,[16] published in 1994, in which 2252 patients from 4 medical-surgical ICUs were followed prospectively for evidence of overt and clinically significant GI bleeding. Of the 2252, 674 received prophylaxis and 1578 received no prophylaxis. Overt bleeding occurred in 4.4% of the patient population and clinically significant bleeding occurred in 1.5%. Two factors were significant in multiple regression analysis: mechanical ventilation for greater than 48 hours and coagulopathy. For patients with either or both of these 2 risk factors, clinically significant bleeding occurred in 3.7%, whereas bleeding occurred in only 0.1% of those without these risk factors. Other risk factors identified in univariate analysis included sepsis, shock, peritonitis, preexisting liver or renal failure, burns, and trauma. The incidence of bleeding increases with the number of risk factors present and is as high as 10% of patients with prophylaxis and 40% without prophylaxis if 3 to 6 risk factors are present.[20] In another study of 720 critically ill postoperative patients performed in the 1980s, 20% had overt GI bleeding and 9% had clinically significant bleeding.[21] A large portion of these patients had peritonitis as their admitting diagnosis, and sepsis seemed to be a significant contributing risk factor for bleeding. The cause of bleeding was erosive gastritis (75%), duodenal ulcer (14%), gastric ulcer (7%), and esophageal bleeding (4%).[21] Thus, all patients requiring mechanical ventilation, those with coagulopathy, and those with combinations of other risk factors should undergo stress ulcer prophylaxis.

GENERAL APPROACH TO POSTOPERATIVE GI BLEEDING

Patients with overt postoperative GI bleeding should be considered to have clinically significant and potentially life-threatening bleeding until adequate data exist to determine otherwise. Determining the significance and magnitude of bleeding may be made more complex by preexisting postoperative anemia and volume shifts, perioperative β-blockade that may blunt the heart rate response to acute blood loss, or preexisting tachycardia resulting from pain or the systemic inflammatory response. Hematocrit is not useful for determining the degree of hemorrhage in the acute setting because the red cell and plasma volume lost is constant. Gastric and intestinal ileus may delay the presentation of hematemesis, hematochezia, or melena. Thus, a high index of suspicion should be maintained and adequate monitoring should be instituted. The association of postoperative GI bleeding with significantly increased mortality supports management of these patients in the ICU setting. That new-onset postoperative GI bleeding may result from another unrecognized complication such as infection and sepsis should be considered.

The basic principles of management of significant postoperative GI bleeding include

- Initial assessment of airway, vascular access, and hemodynamics
- Fluid resuscitation for the restoration of intravascular volume
- Transfusion of blood products based on hemodynamic response to fluid resuscitation and laboratory evaluation
- Evaluation and correction of coagulation and clotting abnormalities
- Identification and control of the bleeding source
- Identification and treatment of disorders contributing to the bleeding source.

Initially, all patients should undergo evaluation of their ability to safely maintain their airways without aspiration hypoxia or hypercarbia, evaluation and establishment of adequate intravenous access, and establishment of appropriate monitoring. Patients who have unstable hemodynamics, alteration in mental status, are having significant hematemesis, or who are to undergo invasive diagnostic or therapeutic procedures should be considered for placement of an endotracheal tube to prevent acute airway compromise. These patients should all be considered as high risk during the intubation process because of the risk of aspiration, hypotension, and acute desaturation. All patients should have two 18-gauge or larger intravenous catheters placed and adequate monitoring with continuous or intermittent blood pressure assessment initiated including continuous electrocardiogram and heart rate monitoring, and a Foley catheter to assess urine output. Elderly patients and patients with preexisting or new-onset organ dysfunction or coexisting sepsis should be considered for placement of a central venous or pulmonary artery catheter and an arterial catheter for closer monitoring of end points of resuscitation. Serum lactate should be assessed; increased levels most frequently indicate inadequate organ perfusion and incomplete resuscitation even in the setting of normal hemodynamics.

Patients with evidence of significant volume depletion or a change in their hemodynamics should undergo volume resuscitation with isotonic crystalloid solutions. Initial volume resuscitation may be up to 2 L. If hemodynamic response to this volume of fluid is not complete or overt ongoing hemorrhage is present, then packed red blood cells should be transfused. The rate and volume of transfusion is based on the patient's hemodynamic response, evidence of ongoing active hemorrhage, hemoglobin levels, and the presence of active cardiovascular disease. Patients with significant hypotension have typically lost greater than 30% of their blood volume and transfusion of blood components should be strongly considered at the time that the diagnosis of hemorrhagic shock is established. Patients with active cardiovascular disease are commonly transfused with a goal to maintain hemoglobin at 10 g/dL, whereas those without can generally tolerate levels as low as 6 to 7 g/dL. However, estimation of the rate of bleeding is typically difficult and evidence of active hemorrhage generally mandates transfusion to higher levels. During volume resuscitation, normothermia should be maintained to prevent the exacerbation of coagulopathy. Patients undergoing significant volume resuscitation should have warm fluids instilled and blood-warming devices used. Forced-air warming devices should be placed on the patient and intubated patients should have a heated humidifier used in the ventilator circuit. Evaluation of coagulation and clotting profiles should be undertaken. Abnormalities may require correction with fresh frozen plasma, vitamin K, and platelet transfusion.

LOCALIZATION OF THE BLEEDING SOURCE

Once the patient has had adequate initial evaluation and stabilization, identification of the bleeding site should be undertaken. The diagnostic and therapeutic approach is similar, but not identical, to that of GI bleeding in the nonpostoperative period because the causes are different and more frequently related to suture-line bleeding in the early postoperative period and to SRMD or postoperative complications such as infection or pseudoaneurysm formation with bleeding as a presenting manifestation. Without considering other factors, upper GI bleeding is more common than lower GI bleeding. For non-GI surgery in the early postoperative period, stress-related bleeding from the upper GI tract is the most common source of blood. Endoscopic diagnosis of the bleeding site is the most appropriate initial localization technique in most cases and may allow therapeutic intervention with low risk. The choice of whether to perform upper versus lower endoscopy first is determined by the estimated likely source. The authors suggest the following algorithmic approach to locate the bleeding source:

1. An estimation of the likely bleeding site can be formulated by considering the character of the presenting symptoms (ie, hematemesis, nasogastric tube blood, melena vs hematochezia, or clots per rectum), the patient's severity of illness and risk factors for SRMD, the operation itself, the timing of bleeding since the index operative procedure, and accompanying clinical signs and symptoms of nonbleeding complications such as infection and pancreatitis.

2. Unless clearly from a lower GI source, nasogastric tube placement should be performed and may assist in determining an upper GI source, but a lack of bloody return does not rule out duodenal bleeding. The return of blood, coffee-ground material,. or a lack of bile should all prompt upper endoscopy. If clear bile is produced, bleeding from sources distal to the duodenum is more likely.
3. If upper GI sources are not suspected or identified, lower endoscopy should generally be performed.
4. If upper and lower endoscopy do not identify the active source, then subsequent studies should be chosen based on the clinical setting.
   a. In the early postoperative period, if bleeding is not visualized or appears proximal to the colon and an enteroenteric anastomosis is present, then bleeding from the suture line is most commonly the source. Angiographic localization may be undertaken if the rate of bleeding is thought to be significant (>0.5–1.0 mL/min)[22] and may be therapeutic but the risk of angiography should be weighed against relaparotomy.
   b. In the late postoperative period, inflammatory and infectious complications causing intermittent bleeding may be present. Computed tomography with intravenous contrast may identify inflammation, abscesses, and pseudoaneurysms, all of which may require therapy beyond hemorrhage control. For rapidly bleeding patients (>0.5–1 mL/min), angiography may identify the source and allow therapeutic intervention. However, the underlying pathophysiologic process of the bleeding may still require diagnostic evaluation and therapy.

CONTROL OF HEMORRHAGE

Three basic modalities are indicated for the control of GI hemorrhage in the postoperative period: endoscopy, arteriography, and surgery. These modalities may be used in conjunction with each other to facilitate definitive control of hemorrhage and to address other underlying disorders. Endoscopy is the most commonly used modality for both localization and control of hemorrhage. Endoscopic control of bleeding can be achieved through a variety of techniques including injection of epinephrine, electrocoagulation, laser coagulation, heater probe, clip application, and banding. Endoscopic therapy may successfully control hemorrhage related to SRMD if the bleeding points are discrete and amenable to therapy. Endoscopic control of suture-line bleeding in the early postoperative period is safe and effective in most patients.[1,3–6,23–27] In the late postoperative period, the underlying disorder leading to bleeding may limit the effectiveness and should be considered. Angiography may be used to control bleeding safely using several different techniques[28–31] but the risk of ischemia and contrast nephropathy must be considered. Techniques vary depending on the clinical setting, the need for permanent vessel occlusion, and the risk of ischemia; techniques include infusion of vasoconstrictive agents and embolization with Gelfoam, autologous clot, and coils. Surgical therapy is typically indicated for patients in whom bleeding cannot be controlled by other measures successfully or without significant risk and for treatment of delayed complications that present with GI bleeding. Morbidity and mortality increase as the volume of blood loss increases, and a prospectively determined plan for intervention should be set early in the course of bleeding to limit adverse outcomes. Specific surgical therapy is determined by location and clinical setting and is beyond the scope of this article.

IDENTIFICATION OF DISORDER CONTRIBUTING TO THE BLEEDING SOURCE

In patients with GI bleeding that occurs outside the immediate postoperative period, identification of the underlying disorder contributing to delayed bleeding should be undertaken. Patients in whom stress-related upper GI bleeding presents days to weeks after surgery frequently have other postoperative complications that contribute to the pathophysiology, such as pneumonia or a change in cardiac function. A search for the cause contributing to the acute clinical change should be undertaken to enable appropriate therapy. In addition, patients in whom GI bleeding occurs in a delayed fashion at or near the surgical site should be considered to have ischemic, inflammatory, or infectious changes that present as GI bleeding. Thus, a directed evaluation should be undertaken to establish other contributing disorders and considered in the decision-making process for the most appropriate therapeutic intervention.

REFERENCES

1. Tanizawa Y, Bando E, Kawamura T, et al. Early postoperative anastomotic hemorrhage after gastrectomy for gastric cancer. Gastric Cancer 2010;13:50–7.
2. Abell TL, Minocha A. Gastrointestinal complications of bariatric surgery: diagnosis and therapy. Am J Med Sci 2006;331:214–8.
3. Malik AH, East JE, Buchanan GN, et al. Endoscopic haemostasis of staple-line haemorrhage following colorectal resection. Colorectal Dis 2008;10:616–8.
4. Martinez-Serrano MA, Pares D, Pera M, et al. Management of lower gastrointestinal bleeding after colorectal resection and stapled anastomosis. Tech Coloproctol 2009;13:49–53.
5. Cirocco WC, Golub RW. Endoscopic treatment of postoperative hemorrhage from a stapled colorectal anastomosis. Am Surg 1995;61:460–3.
6. Linn TY, Moran BJ, Cecil TD. Staple line haemorrhage following laparoscopic left-sided colorectal resections may be more common when the inferior mesenteric artery is preserved. Tech Coloproctol 2008;12:289–93.
7. Beyer L, Bonmardion R, Marciano S, et al. Results of non-operative therapy for delayed hemorrhage after pancreaticoduodenectomy. J Gastrointest Surg 2009; 13:922–8.
8. Yekebas EF, Wolfram L, Cataldegirmen G, et al. Postpancreatectomy hemorrhage: diagnosis and treatment: an analysis in 1669 consecutive pancreatic resections. Ann Surg 2007;246:269–80.
9. Vernadakis S, Christodoulou E, Treckmann J, et al. Pseudoaneurysmal rupture of the common hepatic artery into the biliodigestive anastomosis. A rare cause of gastrointestinal bleeding. JOP 2009;10:441–4.
10. Andersson B, Nilsson J, Brandt J, et al. Gastrointestinal complications after cardiac surgery. Br J Surg 2005;92:326–33.
11. Sakorafas GH, Tsiotos GG. Intra-abdominal complications after cardiac surgery. Eur J Surg 1999;165:820–7.
12. Valentine RJ, Hagino RT, Jackson MR, et al. Gastrointestinal complications after aortic surgery. J Vasc Surg 1998;28:404–11.
13. Baril DT, Carroccio A, Ellozy SH, et al. Evolving strategies for the treatment of aortoenteric fistulas. J Vasc Surg 2006;44:250–7.
14. Peck JJ, Eidemiller LR. Aortoenteric fistulas. Arch Surg 1992;127:1191–3.
15. Hiramoto JS, Terdiman JP, Norton JA. Evidence-based analysis: postoperative gastric bleeding: etiology and prevention. Surg Oncol 2003;12:9–19.

16. Cook DJ, Fuller HD, Guyatt GH, et al. Risk factors for gastrointestinal bleeding in critically ill patients. Canadian Critical Care Trials Group. N Engl J Med 1994;330: 377–81.
17. Cohen M, Sapoznikov B, Niv Y. Primary and secondary nonvariceal upper gastrointestinal bleeding. J Clin Gastroenterol 2007;41:810–3.
18. Cook DJ, Griffith LE, Walter SD, et al. The attributable mortality and length of intensive care unit stay of clinically important gastrointestinal bleeding in critically ill patients. Crit Care 2001;5:368–75.
19. Stollman N, Metz DC. Pathophysiology and prophylaxis of stress ulcer in intensive care unit patients. J Crit Care 2005;20:35–45.
20. Hastings PR, Skillman JJ, Bushnell LS, et al. Antacid titration in the prevention of acute gastrointestinal bleeding: a controlled, randomized trial in 100 critically ill patients. N Engl J Med 1978;298:1041–5.
21. Bumaschny E, Doglio G, Pusajo J, et al. Postoperative acute gastrointestinal tract hemorrhage and multiple-organ failure. Arch Surg 1988;123:722–6.
22. Baum ST. Arteriographic diagnosis and treatment of gastrointestinal bleeding. In: Baum ST, Pentecost MJ, editors. Abram's angiography and interventional radiology. Philadelphia: Lippincott Williams & Wilkins; 2006. p. 488.
23. Lee YC, Wang HP, Yang CS, et al. Endoscopic hemostasis of a bleeding marginal ulcer: hemoclipping or dual therapy with epinephrine injection and heater probe thermocoagulation. J Gastroenterol Hepatol 2002;17:1220–5.
24. Perez RO, Sousa A Jr, Bresciani C, et al. Endoscopic management of postoperative stapled colorectal anastomosis hemorrhage. Tech Coloproctol 2007;11: 64–6.
25. Trottier DC, Friedlich M, Rostom A. The use of endoscopic hemoclips for postoperative anastomotic bleeding. Surg Laparosc Endosc Percutan Tech 2008;18: 299–300.
26. Umano Y, Horiuchi T, Inoue M, et al. Endoscopic microwave coagulation therapy of postoperative hemorrhage from a stapled anastomosis. Hepatogastroenterology 2005;52:1768–70.
27. Wisniewski B, Rautou PE, Drouhin F, et al. Endoscopic hemoclips in postoperative bleeding. Gastroenterol Clin Biol 2005;29:933–4.
28. Atabek U, Pello MJ, Spence RK, et al. Arterial vasopressin for control of bleeding from a stapled intestinal anastomosis. Report of two cases. Dis Colon Rectum 1992;35:1180–2.
29. Bulakbasi N, Kurtaran K, Ustunsoz B, et al. Massive lower gastrointestinal hemorrhage from the surgical anastomosis in patients with multiorgan trauma: treatment by subselective embolization with polyvinyl alcohol particles. Cardiovasc Intervent Radiol 1999;22:461–7.
30. Kim J, Kim JK, Yoon W, et al. Transarterial embolization for postoperative hemorrhage after abdominal surgery. J Gastrointest Surg 2005;9:393–9.
31. Kramer SC, Gorich J, Rilinger N, et al. Embolization for gastrointestinal hemorrhages. Eur Radiol 2000;10:802–5.

Damage Control for Intra-Abdominal Sepsis

Brett H. Waibel, MD*, Michael F. Rotondo, MD

KEYWORDS

- Damage control • Abdominal sepsis • Complications

HISTORY AND EVOLUTION OF DAMAGE CONTROL

Formalized only 20 years ago, damage control was developed in response to the poor outcomes associated with truncal injury with uncontrolled hemorrhage. The need for altering the treatment paradigm was a direct result of taking a traditional elective surgical mindset of attempting definitive repair at the initial operation in patients unable to tolerate such operations. Fundamental differences in physiology, as well as some anatomic issues, made the traumatically injured patient recalcitrant to such treatment approaches. Attempting definitive repair in these patients led to ongoing hemorrhage from an acquired coagulopathy, physiologic failure from nonresuscitatable shock, or multiple organ system failure.[1–3] Although some discussion of these problems can be found dating back to the civil war and the world wars, Stone and Burch laid the true foundations for the damage-control approach in the 1980s.[4,5] However, the descriptive term, along with definition and refinement of the process, came in the 1990s with Rotondo and Schwab.[6–9]

Damage control focuses on the abbreviation of the initial laparotomy after control of hemorrhage and contamination. Resuscitation is then performed in the intensive care unit (ICU) before attempting definitive repair of injuries and abdominal closure. This simple concept proved successful in treating those with uncontrolled hemorrhage arising from truncal trauma. Since this time, the use of these core concepts has expanded into other areas of surgery including vascular, orthopedic, and emergent general surgery.[10,11]

In emergent general surgery, the damage-control concepts are applied to patients with similar physiology, resulting in an intolerance of the shock state.[12–16] The aggressive resuscitation needed in the septic abdomen has led to an increased incidence in abdominal compartment syndrome in the open abdomen, along with the related issues of enterocutaneous fistula.[17,18] However, it is probably better recognition and

No funding source.
The authors have nothing to disclose.
Department of Surgery, The Brody School of Medicine, East Carolina University, 600 Moye Boulevard, Greenville, NC 27834, USA
* Corresponding author.
E-mail address: brett.waibel@pcmh.com

Surg Clin N Am 92 (2012) 243–257
doi:10.1016/j.suc.2012.01.006
0039-6109/12/$ – see front matter © 2012 Elsevier Inc. All rights reserved.
surgical.theclinics.com

treatment of abdominal compartment syndrome, a by-product of resuscitation research through the last 2 decades, which has improved outcomes in the septic abdominal patient.[15,17,19]

INDICATIONS FOR DAMAGE CONTROL

At the core of the damage-control philosophy is the limitation of the initial laparotomy to hemorrhage and contamination control before the progression to physiologic exhaustion noted by the development of acidosis, coagulopathy, and hypothermia.[20] Resuscitation in the ICU takes precedence over definitive repair of the injuries. In addition, closure of the abdominal wall often is further delayed to prevent the development of abdominal compartment syndrome by ongoing resuscitative needs or closure over distended viscera. Although in practice the aforementioned sequence is not completely applicable to the septic abdomen, the underlying concept of earlier termination of the initial laparotomy after control of contamination to allow for further resuscitation before definitive repair can be applied. Furthermore, the techniques of open-abdomen management so commonly found in damage control have many advantages in the septic abdomen.

The decision to limit the initial laparotomy should be made early in the procedure, before the development of hypothermia, acidosis, or coagulopathy.[21] No definitive values exist for consideration of performing a damage-control procedure, but commonly discussed values include temperatures lower than 35°C, pH less than 7.20, or base deficit exceeding 8, and laboratory or clinical evidence of coagulopathy.[22–24] Though initially discussed for injury, these values represent patients failing to compensate for the shock state, and are generally transferable to emergent general surgery cases in patients with similar physiologic instability. The open-abdomen techniques commonly used with damage control also allow for control of the peritoneal effluent associated with the septic process while allowing for easier reentry when source control is tenuous. Furthermore, use of the open abdomen allows for potential prevention of abdominal compartment syndrome associated with the large volume resuscitation of the septic abdomen.[15,17,19] It is the recognition and prevention of physiologic instability, temporary source control with open-abdomen techniques, and avoidance of abdominal compartment syndrome that are the cornerstones of damage control in the septic abdomen. As such, the physiology of the patient should dictate the need for using damage-control and open-abdomen techniques.

DAMAGE-CONTROL SEQUENCE FOR ABDOMINAL SEPSIS

The sequence of damage control for trauma follows a predetermined order of prehospital resuscitation/initial evaluation period (ground zero) followed by a truncated initial laparotomy focused on hemorrhage and contamination control (part 1). This stage is followed by ICU resuscitation (part 2), before definitive repair of injuries (part 3). Closure of the abdominal wall (part 4) can be further delayed when necessary. Patients with a septic abdomen have many of the same management focuses as the damage-control trauma patient, allowing for easy adoption of damage-control and open-abdomen techniques in this population.

However, the sequence for damage control in the septic abdomen needs to be slightly altered from the traditional trauma sequence. A longer initial resuscitation phase is used in the septic abdomen patient than in the trauma patient in preparation for induction of anesthesia. Usually this is achieved rapidly in a few hours. The operative goal at the initial laparotomy is control of the infectious source, including wide drainage. In general, a temporary abdominal closure is used at the end of the initial laparotomy. This dressing allows for easy, instantaneous access to the abdominal cavity while providing effluent control and measurement.[15] It is rapidly placed, allowing for reduced operative times in hemodynamically unstable patients. In addition, it reduces the chance that abdominal compartment syndrome might develop during the ongoing resuscitation. A second resuscitative phase is then performed in the ICU in preparation for further surgery. Overall, this alteration can be easily integrated into the Surviving Sepsis Campaign guidelines.[25]

In the current literature on comparison between open- and closed-abdomen techniques, only small studies have been published, often using mixed populations of trauma, medical, and abdominal sepsis patients, with widely variable mortalities.[12–14,16,26,27] It is thought that prevention of abdominal compartment syndrome is the primary influence on positive outcomes in the use of damage control for abdominal sepsis.

Part 0: Initial Resuscitation

Before the initial laparotomy, a focused resuscitative period is implemented to prevent hemodynamic collapse on induction of anesthesia. Furthermore, correction of hypothermia, acidosis, and coagulopathy should be started during this period.

The resuscitative goals are to reestablish preload and systemic blood pressure to allow for adequate organ perfusion, and this process can be begun in the emergency department.[28] However, no single end point of resuscitation measurement is ideal.[29,30] Moreover, even after normalization of vital signs is achieved, most patients will continue to have evidence of inadequate tissue perfusion and oxygenation.[31] However, the goal of the initial resuscitation is to reestablish adequate organ perfusion, not necessarily optimal organ perfusion. Once adequate preload and systemic pressure are established, the patient may proceed to operative intervention to obtain source control.

At present, no evidence exists to support one type of fluid over another for this resuscitation, but the fluid chosen can have significant effects on physiology. For example, large volumes of normal saline will lead to a hyperchloremic metabolic acidosis, whereas Ringer lactate may stimulate proinflammatory mediator production.[32–34] Colloids, while more expensive, are associated with reduced edema for the same resuscitative goal points but are not associated with improved survival rates in comparison with crystalloid resuscitation.[35–38] Hypertonic saline is another option under investigation, but at present has failed to show improved outcomes.[39]

In addition to volume resuscitation, vasoactive medications may be required. Dopamine and norepinephrine are the first-line agents for septic shock, with epinephrine being a second-line agent.[25] Vasopressin is a potential adjunct in sepsis, due to its decline as sepsis progresses (relative vasopressin deficiency), but should be used in conjunction with norepinephrine.[40] Vasoactive medications are not a replacement for adequate volume resuscitation, as their use in volume-depleted patients leads to tissue ischemia.

Hypothermia correction should begin during this period. Although the use of induced hypothermia has been noted in numerous elective cases, spontaneous hypothermia is associated with energy depletion and poorer outcomes.[41–44] In addition, hypothermia causes alterations in drug metabolism and clearance, altered renal function, and electrolyte shifts, and induces both coagulopathy and platelet dysfunction.[45] A variety of both invasive and noninvasive techniques for rewarming are available, including the use of heat-exchange catheters.[46] Fortunately, most patients can be rewarmed using environmental control, forced air-warming devices, and warmed intravenous fluids.

Acidosis correction generally will follow active and adequate resuscitation as organ perfusion improves. The Surviving Sepsis Campaign does not recommend the use of bicarbonate in the septic patient for the purpose of improving hemodynamics or reducing vasopressor requirements when treating hypoperfusion-induced lactic acidosis with pH greater than 7.15, based on 2 randomized trials.[47,48] Bicarbonate or an alternative alkalinizing agent, such as tromethamine, may be needed in patients with severe acidosis (pH <7.15) secondary to catecholamine receptor resistance–induced hypotension.

Part 1: Initial Surgical Intervention

The initial surgical management for abdominal sepsis will obviously depend on the etiology. Most abdominal sepsis patients will have a hepatobiliary issue, pancreatic necrosis/infection, or hollow viscus perforation/necrosis. Traditionally the surgical focus in damage control was to go to the compelling source of hemorrhage; in the septic abdomen, it should be on obtaining source control using a combination of resection and wide drainage. Without source control resuscitative efforts are for naught, as failure to achieve source control is associated with increased mortality.[49,50] Definitive repair is not necessary, especially if obtaining such would lead to a prolonged operation. Moreover, the patient can be initially left in intestinal discontinuity with a subsequent ostomy, especially given the high failure rates for anastomosis in this unstable population.

Once source control is obtained, the operation should be truncated. The closure technique preferably should be rapid, contain the viscera while preventing injury, avert further peritoneal contamination, control and quantify peritoneal effluent, provide adequate tension relief to avoid abdominal compartment syndrome, and preserve fascial integrity for later abdominal wall closure. The abdominal vacuum pack and commercial vacuum-assisted abdominal dressings both allow for rapid, easy reentry into the peritoneal cavity, control and quantification of effluent, and preservation of the fascia for latter definitive closure.[51–55] In addition, they are quicker than suture closure techniques (primary fascial closure or interpositional mesh) and lack the radiographic artifacts of towel-clip closures (as well as the fascial injury and peritoneal space limitation).[56] The dynamic properties of the vacuum-assisted closures are being evaluated, including ongoing studies comparing the Barker style of closure (abdominal vacuum pack) with commercial vacuum-assisted closure devices for superiority.[57–60] Given the ease of placement and dynamic properties of these dressings, they have come to dominate temporary closure dressings in use today.

The crux of the issue beyond source control is prevention of abdominal compartment syndrome, secondary to the aggressive volume resuscitation seen in various disease processes.[17,61–64] Although abdominal compartment syndrome is more common in tighter abdominal closures, the use of temporary abdominal closures does not assure prevention.[65–67] It is through delays in recognition and treatment that increased morbidity and mortality occur.[68] When identified and treated, improvements in organ perfusion and function ensue.[69,70] With an aggressive approach for monitoring and treatment, the mortality of patients with an open abdomen approached that of the closed-abdomen patients in one prospective study.[19] In those patients at high risk of developing abdominal compartment syndrome or already displaying evidence of visceral edema, the use of a temporary abdominal closure should be considered requisite.

Part 2: Subsequent Resuscitation

Resuscitation is continued after the initial laparotomy in the ICU. It is at this point that optimal dynamics should be achieved. A period of distributive shock is very common and should be anticipated after surgical manipulation of the septic source.

Fortunately, this is generally time limited to 24 to 72 hours with aggressive resuscitation. No single end point of resuscitation is ideal; therefore, multiple end points have been developed and should be used. Such methods include right ventricular end-diastolic volume index (RVEDVI) pulmonary catheters, arterial pulse contour analysis, shock index, and heart rate variability.[71–80] Both RVEDVI and global end-diastolic volume index can provide volumetric measurements independent of traditional barometric measurements, which are altered with intra-abdominal hypertension, a common entity with septic abdomen.[81]

In addition to electrolyte abnormalities and aforementioned acid-base disturbances, hyperglycemia is typically found. Since 2001, aggressive insulin therapy to achieve strict glycemic control has become commonplace.[82] However, studies since this landmark article have generally failed to obtain the same results, but may reflect increased issues of hypoglycemia during this aggressive therapy.[82–88] One recent meta-analysis did note a survival benefit with strict glycemic control in the surgical population.[89] At present, the Surviving Sepsis Campaign recommends maintenance of glucose levels below 150 mg/dL.[25]

Poor therapeutic decisions can induce iatrogenic injury. Inappropriate ventilator-management strategies can produce or extend a pulmonary injury.[90–93] As such, a lung-protective strategy along with plateau airway pressure limitation should be initiated. Although the use of analgesia and sedation are commonly needed to promote synchrony, routine neuromuscular blockade should be avoided because of the potential for polyneuropathy, especially in patients with asthma or renal or hepatic dysfunction.[94–99]

Nutritional support is of great importance because of the catabolic stress in these patients. Initiation of enteral feeds should be delayed in the unstable patient, due to the potential for visceral ischemia; however, once stable physiology is restored, enteral feeds are preferred because of the reduction in infectious complications.[100–102] In addition, feeding of the open abdomen is feasible and is associated with earlier primary fascial closure rates, lower fistula rates, and decreased cost compared with delayed (>4 days) enteral feeding.[103]

Monitoring for the development of abdominal compartment syndrome cannot be understated. The clinical entity is described with hypotension, increased ventilatory pressures, and oliguria in the presence of intra-abdominal hypertension, but has global effects beyond simple pressure-volume relationships.[104] Clinical examination and abdominal wall measurements do not correlate with intra-abdominal pressure; therefore some measurement of this pressure, generally bladder pressure, should be routinely made.[105–110] The World Society of Abdominal Compartment Syndrome have defined it as sustained intra-abdominal pressure greater than 20 mm Hg with an attributable organ failure.[106] Although decompressive celiotomy is often needed in this situation, various other techniques have been described to help reduce its necessity in abdominal compartment syndrome.[111,112]

Part 3: Subsequent Operations

Control of the septic source should be obtained, if not done at the initial operation. As already stated, failure to achieve control initially is associated with increased death rates. A great deal of debate concerning on-demand (relaparotomy for clinical deterioration or failure to advance) versus planned relaparotomy (reoperation regardless of clinical status) has occurred, and is complicated by various issues, including how one incorporates patients with open abdomens to avoid abdominal compartment syndrome but have source control at the initial operation. These open-abdomen patients are probably fundamentally different from patients who undergo an a priori planned relaparotomy or on-demand relaparotomy with source control and closure at the initial operation. Because of the high variability of patients and definitions used, it is difficult to identify a superiority of one technique (open abdomen vs relaparotomy) over another for the septic abdomen.[26,113] Use of open abdominal techniques should be reserved for patients at greatest risk for development of abdominal compartment syndrome or physiologic instability. Those patients not at such risk generally do not need damage-control techniques applied to their care.

Planned relaparotomy does not have a survival benefit compared with on-demand laparotomy based on several studies, including one meta-analysis.[114–116] However, on-demand laparotomy is associated with decreased costs and health care use.[117,118] Unfortunately, the studies demonstrate substantial variability, and further studies are needed. Nevertheless, frequent operative interventions are associated with increased complications, such as bleeding, fistula, and worsening of the cytokine response.[119–121]

Part 4: Definitive Abdominal Wall Closure

The time to definitive abdominal wall closure can be variable because of a multitude of concerns, including visceral edema, need to prevent abdominal compartment syndrome from ongoing resuscitation, and continued debridement or efforts at source control. Approximately 40% to 70% of abdomens in trauma patients are unable to be closed initially.[51,52,122] One would expect at least similar rates in the septic abdomen given the similar resuscitation but, compared with patients with injury, fascial closure rates may be lower in the septic abdomen.[123] When fascial closure is delayed because of visceral edema, approximately 1 week usually is needed for it to significantly reduce to allow closure, and generally correlates with resolution of the acute inflammatory phase. During this time the fascia is attempting to retract laterally, the visceral block is beginning to fuse, and adhesions are forming between these organs and the abdominal wall. Thus, a limited window of time exists before development of the fused visceral block to the abdominal wall at approximately 10 to 14 days prevents primary closure. However, preservation of the peritoneal space between the visceral organs and abdominal wall can be achieved using vacuum pack/vacuum-assisted closure devices, extending the time of primary fascial closure from a few days to up to 1 month.[124] In addition, vacuum-assisted devices can provide some medial traction on the fascial edges to help prevent its lateral retraction. A multitude of other suture devices and meshes can also be used to provide medial traction on the fascial edge with gradual tightening over time. More complex closures, such as component separation, extensive tissue flap mobilization, or nonabsorbable mesh closures, are generally not performed in the acute setting because of increased wound complication rates and impediment of reconstruction options at later dates.[55]

Ultimately, if primary closure is not attainable a planned ventral hernia, with subsequent abdominal wall reconstruction approximately 6 to 12 months after the visceral inflammatory process has resolved, is performed. This method involves the use of absorbable mesh to obtain visceral coverage until the defect can undergo skin grafting. After 6 to 12 months the underlying viscera will detach from the skin graft, allowing reconstruction. A subfascial or retrorectus underlay mesh (allograft or prosthetic) and/or component separation is often required to bridge the defect at this time.[125–131]

COMPLICATIONS

Beyond the expected issues of nosocomial infections and abdominal compartment syndrome, enterocutaneous fistula and intra-abdominal infections are commonplace complications for this patient population. The rates of fistula range considerably, but up to one-third of the patients with an open abdomen might suffer this complication.[27,53,122,123,132] In addition, these fistulas tend to occur within the granulating wound bed of an open abdomen, dramatically increasing the difficulty of treatment with a significant decrease in closure rate.[133] Beyond the usual therapies of bowel rest and parenteral nutrition, control of the caustic drainage has occupied the greater part of the discussion. Sundry techniques have been described to obtain control, but no single technique is perfect, and often several need to be tried before identifying the optimal treatment modality that best suits an individual patient.[134–139] With control of the effluent, ultimately a skin graft can be applied and the wound treated as an ostomy until definitive repair can be obtained. Fistula closure is generally performed at the time of abdominal wall reconstruction in these patients, and complicates this issue further.[140]

Tertiary peritonitis, a persistent or recurrent intra-abdominal infection despite adequate initial surgical source control, has historically occurred in approximately 20% of patients with secondary peritonitis.[141,142] However, as definitions used in past reports have varied greatly, a true rate is difficult to determine.[143] Despite this variability, tertiary peritonitis seems to reside on a clinical spectrum with secondary peritonitis, generally affecting sicker patients and being associated with multiple drug-resistant organisms and increased complications, especially infectious in nature (both local and remote).[132,144–146] The presenting signs and symptoms can be subtle, because a definitive event time point is often not present as the process develops over days. In one series, the use of open-abdomen techniques did reduce the need for percutaneous drainage.[132] The use of repeated abdominal washouts might reduce the rate of abscess formation, but does lead to increased bowel manipulation and fistula formation. Although standard surveillance methods should be used, liberal use of imaging modalities may be required to identify forming abscesses, especially in patients who fail to progress as anticipated, or with persistent fever or unexpected leukocytosis.

SUMMARY

Following the success of damage-control surgery for the treatment of exsanguinating truncal trauma, it has been adapted to other surgical diseases associated with shock states, such as severe secondary peritonitis. The structured approach of damage control is easily adapted to and can incorporate the fundamental elements of the Surviving Sepsis Campaign. It complements tried and true surgical principles, such as source control, and serves as a usable framework in managing the complicated circumstances seen with these patients. At its core is the concept of early termination of the initial laparotomy after adequate source control is achieved, so as to regain the patient's exhausted physiology before definitive repairs or abdominal closure. The use of open-abdomen techniques has some preferable features, including reduction in abdominal compartment syndrome, and may be the source of improved outcomes in these patients. However, the trade-off for improved survival is increases in other complications, especially enteroatmospheric fistula.

REFERENCES

1. Ciesla DJ, Moore EE, Johnson JL, et al. A 12-year prospective study of postinjury multiple organ failure: has anything changed? Arch Surg 2005;140:432–8 [discussion: 438–40].

2. Cinat ME, Wallace WC, Nastanski F, et al. Improved survival following massive transfusion in patients who have undergone trauma. Arch Surg 1999;134: 964–8 [discussion: 968–70].

3. Krishna G, Sleigh JW, Rahman H. Physiological predictors of death in exsanguinating trauma patients undergoing conventional trauma surgery. Aust N Z J Surg 1998;68:826–9.

4. Burch JM, Ortiz VB, Richardson RJ, et al. Abbreviated laparotomy and planned reoperation for critically injured patients. Ann Surg 1992;215:476–83 [discussion: 483–4].

5. Stone HH, Strom PR, Mullins RJ. Management of the major coagulopathy with onset during laparotomy. Ann Surg 1983;197:532–5.

6. Hoey BA, Schwab CW. Damage control surgery. Scand J Surg 2002;91:92–103.

7. Johnson JW, Gracias VH, Schwab CW, et al. Evolution in damage control for exsanguinating penetrating abdominal injury. J Trauma 2001;51:261–9 [discussion: 269–71].

8. Rotondo MF, Schwab CW, McGonigal MD, et al. 'Damage control': an approach for improved survival in exsanguinating penetrating abdominal injury. J Trauma 1993;35:375–82 [discussion: 382–3].

9. Rotondo MF, Zonies DH. The damage control sequence and underlying logic. Surg Clin North Am 1997;77:761–77.

10. Pape HC, Giannoudis P, Krettek C. The timing of fracture treatment in polytrauma patients: relevance of damage control orthopedic surgery. Am J Surg 2002;183:622–9.

11. Porter JM, Ivatury RR, Nassoura ZE. Extending the horizons of "damage control" in unstable trauma patients beyond the abdomen and gastrointestinal tract. J Trauma 1997;42:559–61.

12. Cipolla J, Stawicki SP, Hoff WS, et al. A proposed algorithm for managing the open abdomen. Am Surg 2005;71:202–7.

13. Finlay IG, Edwards TJ, Lambert AW. Damage control laparotomy. Br J Surg 2004;91:83–5.

14. Horwood J, Akbar F, Maw A. Initial experience of laparostomy with immediate vacuum therapy in patients with severe peritonitis. Ann R Coll Surg Engl 2009;91:681–7.

15. Schecter WP, Ivatury RR, Rotondo MF, et al. Open abdomen after trauma and abdominal sepsis: a strategy for management. J Am Coll Surg 2006;203:390–6.

16. Stawicki SP, Brooks A, Bilski T, et al. The concept of damage control: extending the paradigm to emergency general surgery. Injury 2008;39:93–101.

17. Balogh Z, McKinley BA, Cocanour CS, et al. Supranormal trauma resuscitation causes more cases of abdominal compartment syndrome. Arch Surg 2003;138: 637–42 [discussion: 642–3].

18. Maxwell RA, Fabian TC, Croce MA, et al. Secondary abdominal compartment syndrome: an underappreciated manifestation of severe hemorrhagic shock. J Trauma 1999;47:995–9.

19. Cheatham ML, Safcsak K. Is the evolving management of intra-abdominal hypertension and abdominal compartment syndrome improving survival? Crit Care Med 2010;38:402–7.

20. Moore EE. Thomas G. Orr Memorial Lecture. Staged laparotomy for the hypothermia, acidosis, and coagulopathy syndrome. Am J Surg 1996;172:405–10.

21. Aoki N, Wall MJ, Demsar J, et al. Predictive model for survival at the conclusion of a damage control laparotomy. Am J Surg 2000;180:540–4 [discussion: 544–5].

22. Asensio JA, McDuffie L, Petrone P, et al. Reliable variables in the exsanguinated patient which indicate damage control and predict outcome. Am J Surg 2001; 182:743–51.
23. Asensio JA, Petrone P, Roldan G, et al. Has evolution in awareness of guidelines for institution of damage control improved outcome in the management of the posttraumatic open abdomen? Arch Surg 2004;139:209–14 [discussion: 215].
24. Moore EE, Burch JM, Franciose RJ, et al. Staged physiologic restoration and damage control surgery. World J Surg 1998;22:1184–90 [discussion: 1190–1].
25. Dellinger RP, Levy MM, Carlet JM, et al. Surviving Sepsis Campaign: international guidelines for management of severe sepsis and septic shock: 2008. Crit Care Med 2008;36:296–327.
26. Adkins AL, Robbins J, Villalba M, et al. Open abdomen management of intra-abdominal sepsis. Am Surg 2004;70:137–40 [discussion: 140].
27. Christou NV, Barie PS, Dellinger EP, et al. Surgical Infection Society intra-abdominal infection study. Prospective evaluation of management techniques and outcome. Arch Surg 1993;128:193–8 [discussion: 198–9].
28. Rivers E, Nguyen B, Havstad S, et al. Early goal-directed therapy in the treatment of severe sepsis and septic shock. N Engl J Med 2001;345:1368–77.
29. Bendjelid K, Romand JA. Fluid responsiveness in mechanically ventilated patients: a review of indices used in intensive care. Intensive Care Med 2003; 29:352–60.
30. Cheatham ML, Safcsak K, Block EF, et al. Preload assessment in patients with an open abdomen. J Trauma 1999;46:16–22.
31. Tisherman SA, Barie P, Bokhari F, et al. Clinical practice guideline: endpoints of resuscitation. J Trauma 2004;57:898–912.
32. Rhee P, Burris D, Kaufmann C, et al. Lactated Ringer's solution resuscitation causes neutrophil activation after hemorrhagic shock. J Trauma 1998;44:313–9.
33. Walters JM, Tieu BH, Todd SR, et al. Fluid resuscitation increases inflammatory gene transcription after traumatic injury. J Trauma 2006;61:300–8 [discussion: 308–9].
34. Ho AM, Karmakar MK, Contardi LH, et al. Excessive use of normal saline in managing traumatized patients in shock: a preventable contributor to acidosis. J Trauma 2001;51:173–7.
35. Schierhout G, Roberts I. Fluid resuscitation with colloid or crystalloid solutions in critically ill patients: a systematic review of randomised trials. BMJ 1998;316:961–4.
36. Choi PT, Yip G, Quinonez LG, et al. Crystalloids vs. colloids in fluid resuscitation: a systematic review. Crit Care Med 1999;27:200–10.
37. Perel P, Roberts I. Colloids versus crystalloids for fluid resuscitation in critically ill patients. Cochrane Database Syst Rev 2007;4:CD000567.
38. Finfer S, Bellomo R, Boyce N, et al. A comparison of albumin and saline for fluid resuscitation in the intensive care unit. N Engl J Med 2004;350:2247–56.
39. Bunn F, Roberts I, Tasker R, et al. Hypertonic versus near isotonic crystalloid for fluid resuscitation in critically ill patients. Cochrane Database Syst Rev 2004;3: CD002045.
40. Sharshar T, Blanchard A, Paillard M, et al. Circulating vasopressin levels in septic shock. Crit Care Med 2003;31:1752–8.
41. Eidelman Y, Glat PM, Pachter HL, et al. The effects of topical hypothermia and steroids on ATP levels in an in vivo liver ischemia model. J Trauma 1994;37: 677–81.
42. Hildebrand F, Giannoudis PV, van Griensven M, et al. Pathophysiologic changes and effects of hypothermia on outcome in elective surgery and trauma patients. Am J Surg 2004;187:363–71.

43. Johannigman JA, Johnson DJ, Roettger R. The effect of hypothermia on liver adenosine triphosphate (ATP) recovery following combined shock and ischemia. J Trauma 1992;32:190–5.

44. Seekamp A, van Griensven M, Hildebrandt F, et al. Adenosine-triphosphate in trauma-related and elective hypothermia. J Trauma 1999;47:673–83.

45. Polderman KH. Mechanisms of action, physiological effects, and complications of hypothermia. Crit Care Med 2009;37:S186–202.

46. Giesbrecht GG. Emergency treatment of hypothermia. Emerg Med (Fremantle) 2001;13:9–16.

47. Cooper DJ, Walley KR, Wiggs BR, et al. Bicarbonate does not improve hemodynamics in critically ill patients who have lactic acidosis. A prospective, controlled clinical study. Ann Intern Med 1990;112:492–8.

48. Mathieu D, Neviere R, Billard V, et al. Effects of bicarbonate therapy on hemodynamics and tissue oxygenation in patients with lactic acidosis: a prospective, controlled clinical study. Crit Care Med 1991;19:1352–6.

49. Barie PS, Williams MD, McCollam JS, et al. Benefit/risk profile of drotrecogin alfa (activated) in surgical patients with severe sepsis. Am J Surg 2004;188:212–20.

50. Wacha H, Hau T, Dittmer R, et al. Risk factors associated with intraabdominal infections: a prospective multicenter study. Peritonitis Study Group. Langenbecks Arch Surg 1999;384:24–32.

51. Barker DE, Green JM, Maxwell RA, et al. Experience with vacuum-pack temporary abdominal wound closure in 258 trauma and general and vascular surgical patients. J Am Coll Surg 2007;204:784–92 [discussion: 792–3].

52. Barker DE, Kaufman HJ, Smith LA, et al. Vacuum pack technique of temporary abdominal closure: a 7-year experience with 112 patients. J Trauma 2000;48:201–6 [discussion: 206–7].

53. Brock WB, Barker DE, Burns RP. Temporary closure of open abdominal wounds: the vacuum pack. Am Surg 1995;61:30–5.

54. Schein M, Saadia R, Jamieson JR, et al. The 'sandwich technique' in the management of the open abdomen. Br J Surg 1986;73:369–70.

55. Campbell A, Chang M, Fabian T, et al. Management of the open abdomen: from initial operation to definitive closure. Am Surg 2009;75:S1–22.

56. Feliciano DV, Burch JM. Towel clips, silos, and heroic forms of wound closure. In: Maull KI, Cleveland HC, Feliciano DV, editors. Advances in trauma and critical care, vol. 6. St Louis (MO): Mosby-Year Book; 1991. p. 231–50.

57. Argenta LC, Morykwas MJ. Vacuum-assisted closure: a new method for wound control and treatment: clinical experience. Ann Plast Surg 1997;38:563–76 [discussion: 577].

58. Morykwas MJ, Argenta LC, Shelton-Brown EI, et al. Vacuum-assisted closure: a new method for wound control and treatment: animal studies and basic foundation. Ann Plast Surg 1997;38:553–62.

59. Mullner T, Mrkonjic L, Kwasny O, et al. The use of negative pressure to promote the healing of tissue defects: a clinical trial using the vacuum sealing technique. Br J Plast Surg 1997;50:194–9.

60. Garner GB, Ware DN, Cocanour CS, et al. Vacuum-assisted wound closure provides early fascial reapproximation in trauma patients with open abdomens. Am J Surg 2001;182:630–8.

61. Ertel W, Oberholzer A, Platz A, et al. Incidence and clinical pattern of the abdominal compartment syndrome after "damage-control" laparotomy in 311 patients with severe abdominal and/or pelvic trauma. Crit Care Med 2000;28:1747–53.

62. Malbrain ML, Chiumello D, Pelosi P, et al. Prevalence of intra-abdominal hypertension in critically ill patients: a multicentre epidemiological study. Intensive Care Med 2004;30:822–9.
63. Ivy ME, Atweh NA, Palmer J, et al. Intra-abdominal hypertension and abdominal compartment syndrome in burn patients. J Trauma 2000;49:387–91.
64. Wong K, Summerhays CF. Abdominal compartment syndrome: a new indication for operative intervention in severe acute pancreatitis. Int J Clin Pract 2005;59: 1479–81.
65. Ivatury RR, Porter JM, Simon RJ, et al. Intra-abdominal hypertension after life-threatening penetrating abdominal trauma: prophylaxis, incidence, and clinical relevance to gastric mucosal pH and abdominal compartment syndrome. J Trauma 1998;44:1016–21 [discussion: 1021–3].
66. Mayberry JC, Mullins RJ, Crass RA, et al. Prevention of abdominal compartment syndrome by absorbable mesh prosthesis closure. Arch Surg 1997;132:957–61 [discussion: 961–2].
67. Offner PJ, de Souza AL, Moore EE, et al. Avoidance of abdominal compartment syndrome in damage-control laparotomy after trauma. Arch Surg 2001;136:676–81.
68. Biffl WL, Moore EE, Burch JM, et al. Secondary abdominal compartment syndrome is a highly lethal event. Am J Surg 2001;182:645–8.
69. Meldrum DR, Moore FA, Moore EE, et al. Prospective characterization and selective management of the abdominal compartment syndrome. Am J Surg 1997;174:667–72 [discussion: 672–3].
70. De Laet IE, Ravyts M, Vidts W, et al. Current insights in intra-abdominal hypertension and abdominal compartment syndrome: open the abdomen and keep it open! Langenbecks Arch Surg 2008;393:833–47.
71. Chang MC, Miller PR, D'Agostino R Jr, et al. Effects of abdominal decompression on cardiopulmonary function and visceral perfusion in patients with intra-abdominal hypertension. J Trauma 1998;44:440–5.
72. Cheatham ML, Nelson LD, Chang MC, et al. Right ventricular end-diastolic volume index as a predictor of preload status in patients on positive end-expiratory pressure. Crit Care Med 1998;26:1801–6.
73. Wiedemann HP, Wheeler AP, Bernard GR, et al. Comparison of two fluid-management strategies in acute lung injury. N Engl J Med 2006;354:2564–75.
74. Birkhahn RH, Gaeta TJ, Terry D, et al. Shock index in diagnosing early acute hypovolemia. Am J Emerg Med 2005;23:323–6.
75. Morris JA Jr, Norris PR, Ozdas A, et al. Reduced heart rate variability: an indicator of cardiac uncoupling and diminished physiologic reserve in 1,425 trauma patients. J Trauma 2006;60:1165–73 [discussion: 1173–4].
76. Norris PR, Ozdas A, Cao H, et al. Cardiac uncoupling and heart rate variability stratify ICU patients by mortality: a study of 2088 trauma patients. Ann Surg 2006;243:804–12 [discussion: 812–4].
77. Rady MY, Nightingale P, Little RA, et al. Shock index: a re-evaluation in acute circulatory failure. Resuscitation 1992;23:227–34.
78. Rady MY, Smithline HA, Blake H, et al. A comparison of the shock index and conventional vital signs to identify acute, critical illness in the emergency department. Ann Emerg Med 1994;24:685–90.
79. Zarzaur BL, Croce MA, Fischer PE, et al. New vitals after injury: shock index for the young and age × shock index for the old. J Surg Res 2008;147:229–36.
80. Rady MY, Rivers EP, Nowak RM. Resuscitation of the critically ill in the ED: responses of blood pressure, heart rate, shock index, central venous oxygen saturation, and lactate. Am J Emerg Med 1996;14:218–25.

81. Malbrain ML, de Laet I. Functional hemodynamics and increased intra-abdominal pressure: same thresholds for different conditions...? Crit Care Med 2009;37:781–3.
82. Van den Berghe G, Wouters P, Weekers F, et al. Intensive insulin therapy in the critically ill patients. N Engl J Med 2001;345:1359–67.
83. Arabi YM, Dabbagh OC, Tamim HM, et al. Intensive versus conventional insulin therapy: a randomized controlled trial in medical and surgical critically ill patients. Crit Care Med 2008;36:3190–7.
84. Brunkhorst FM, Engel C, Bloos F, et al. Intensive insulin therapy and pentastarch resuscitation in severe sepsis. N Engl J Med 2008;358:125–39.
85. De La Rosa G, Donado JH, Restrepo AH, et al. Strict glycaemic control in patients hospitalised in a mixed medical and surgical intensive care unit: a randomised clinical trial. Crit Care 2008;12:R120.
86. Finfer S, Chittock DR, Su SY, et al. Intensive versus conventional glucose control in critically ill patients. N Engl J Med 2009;360:1283–97.
87. Van den Berghe G, Wilmer A, Hermans G, et al. Intensive insulin therapy in the medical ICU. N Engl J Med 2006;354:449–61.
88. Vlasselaers D, Milants I, Desmet L, et al. Intensive insulin therapy for patients in paediatric intensive care: a prospective, randomised controlled study. Lancet 2009;373:547–56.
89. Griesdale DE, de Souza RJ, van Dam RM, et al. Intensive insulin therapy and mortality among critically ill patients: a meta-analysis including NICE-SUGAR study data. CMAJ 2009;180:821–7.
90. Network TARDS. Ventilation with lower tidal volumes as compared with traditional tidal volumes for acute lung injury and the acute respiratory distress syndrome. The Acute Respiratory Distress Syndrome Network. N Engl J Med 2000;342:1301–8.
91. Gajic O, Dara SI, Mendez JL, et al. Ventilator-associated lung injury in patients without acute lung injury at the onset of mechanical ventilation. Crit Care Med 2004;32:1817–24.
92. Lionetti V, Recchia FA, Ranieri VM. Overview of ventilator-induced lung injury mechanisms. Curr Opin Crit Care 2005;11:82–6.
93. Schreiber TC, Boyle WA III. Lung injury caused by mechanical ventilation: patients with acute respiratory distress syndrome are not the only ones at risk. Contemp Crit Care 2005;3:1–11.
94. Klein Y, Blackbourne L, Barquist ES. Non-ventilatory-based strategies in the management of acute respiratory distress syndrome. J Trauma 2004;57: 915–24.
95. Behbehani NA, Al-Mane F, D'Yachkova Y, et al. Myopathy following mechanical ventilation for acute severe asthma: the role of muscle relaxants and corticosteroids. Chest 1999;115:1627–31.
96. de Jonghe B, Lacherade JC, Sharshar T, et al. Intensive care unit-acquired weakness: risk factors and prevention. Crit Care Med 2009;37:S309–15.
97. Hall JB, Schweickert W, Kress JP. Role of analgesics, sedatives, neuromuscular blockers, and delirium. Crit Care Med 2009;37:S416–21.
98. Leatherman JW, Fluegel WL, David WS, et al. Muscle weakness in mechanically ventilated patients with severe asthma. Am J Respir Crit Care Med 1996;153: 1686–90.
99. Murray MJ, Cowen J, DeBlock H, et al. Clinical practice guidelines for sustained neuromuscular blockade in the adult critically ill patient. Crit Care Med 2002;30: 142–56.

100. Dissanaike S, Pham T, Shalhub S, et al. Effect of immediate enteral feeding on trauma patients with an open abdomen: protection from nosocomial infections. J Am Coll Surg 2008;207:690–7.
101. McKibbin B, Cresci G, Hawkins M. Nutrition support for the patient with an open abdomen after major abdominal trauma. Nutrition 2003;19:563–6.
102. Moore FA, Feliciano DV, Andrassy RJ, et al. Early enteral feeding, compared with parenteral, reduces postoperative septic complications. The results of a meta-analysis. Ann Surg 1992;216:172–83.
103. Collier B, Guillamondegui O, Cotton B, et al. Feeding the open abdomen. JPEN J Parenter Enteral Nutr 2007;31:410–5.
104. Malbrain ML, Cheatham ML. Definitions and pathophysiological implications of intra-abdominal hypertension and abdominal compartment syndrome. Am Surg 2011;77:S6–11.
105. Burch JM, Moore EE, Moore FA, et al. The abdominal compartment syndrome. Surg Clin North Am 1996;76:833–42.
106. Malbrain ML, Cheatham ML, Kirkpatrick A, et al. Results from the International Conference of Experts on Intra-abdominal Hypertension and Abdominal Compartment Syndrome. I. Definitions. Intensive Care Med 2006;32: 1722–32.
107. Barnes GE, Laine GA, Giam PY, et al. Cardiovascular responses to elevation of intra-abdominal hydrostatic pressure. Am J Physiol 1985;248:R208–13.
108. Kirkpatrick AW, Brenneman FD, McLean RF, et al. Is clinical examination an accurate indicator of raised intra-abdominal pressure in critically injured patients? Can J Surg 2000;43:207–11.
109. Obeid F, Saba A, Fath J, et al. Increases in intra-abdominal pressure affect pulmonary compliance. Arch Surg 1995;130:544–7 [discussion: 547–8].
110. De Keulenaer BL, Regli A, Malbrain ML. Intra-abdominal measurement techniques: is there anything new? Am Surg 2011;77:S17–22.
111. De Keulenaer BL, De Waele JJ, Malbrain ML. Nonoperative management of intra-abdominal hypertension and abdominal compartment syndrome: evolving concepts. Am Surg 2011;77:S34–41.
112. Ouellet JF, Leppaniemi A, Ball CG, et al. Alternatives to formal abdominal decompression. Am Surg 2011;77:S51–7.
113. Schein M. Planned reoperations and open management in critical intra-abdominal infections: prospective experience in 52 cases. World J Surg 1991; 15:537–45.
114. Hau T, Ohmann C, Wolmershauser A, et al. Planned relaparotomy vs relaparotomy on demand in the treatment of intra-abdominal infections. The Peritonitis Study Group of the Surgical Infection Society—Europe. Arch Surg 1995;130: 1193–6 [discussion: 1196–7].
115. Lamme B, Boermeester MA, Belt EJT, et al. Mortality and morbidity of planned relaparotomy versus relaparotomy on demand for secondary peritonitis. Br J Surg 2004;91:1046–54.
116. Lamme B, Boermeester MA, Reitsma JB, et al. Meta-analysis of relaparotomy for secondary peritonitis. Br J Surg 2002;89:1516–24.
117. Opmeer BC, Boer KR, van Ruler O, et al. Costs of relaparotomy on-demand versus planned relaparotomy in patients with severe peritonitis: an economic evaluation within a randomized controlled trial. Crit Care 2010;14:R97.
118. van Ruler O, Mahler CW, Boer KR, et al. Comparison of on-demand vs planned relaparotomy strategy in patients with severe peritonitis: a randomized trial. JAMA 2007;298:865–72.

119. van Goor H, Hulsebos RG, Bleichrodt RP. Complications of planned relaparotomy in patients with severe general peritonitis. Eur J Surg 1997;163:61–6.

120. Bosscha K, Hulstaert PF, Visser MR, et al. Open management of the abdomen and planned reoperations in severe bacterial peritonitis. Eur J Surg 2000;166:44–9.

121. Sautner T, Gotzinger P, Redl-Wenzl EM, et al. Does reoperation for abdominal sepsis enhance the inflammatory host response? Arch Surg 1997;132:250–5.

122. Mayberry JC. Bedside open abdominal surgery. Utility and wound management. Crit Care Clin 2000;16:151–72.

123. Tsuei BJ, Skinner JC, Bernard AC, et al. The open peritoneal cavity: etiology correlates with the likelihood of fascial closure. Am Surg 2004;70:652–6.

124. Miller PR, Thompson JT, Faler BJ, et al. Late fascial closure in lieu of ventral hernia: the next step in open abdomen management. J Trauma 2002;53:843–9.

125. Jernigan TW, Fabian TC, Croce MA, et al. Staged management of giant abdominal wall defects: acute and long-term results. Ann Surg 2003;238:349–55 [discussion: 355–7].

126. Rodriguez ED, Bluebond-Langner R, Silverman RP, et al. Abdominal wall reconstruction following severe loss of domain: the R Adams Cowley Shock Trauma Center algorithm. Plast Reconstr Surg 2007;120:669–80.

127. de Vries Reilingh TS, van Goor H, Rosman C, et al. "Components separation technique" for the repair of large abdominal wall hernias. J Am Coll Surg 2003;196:32–7.

128. Ennis LS, Young JS, Gampper TJ, et al. The "open-book" variation of component separation for repair of massive midline abdominal wall hernia. Am Surg 2003; 69:733–42 [discussion: 742–3].

129. Fabian TC, Croce MA, Pritchard FE, et al. Planned ventral hernia. Staged management for acute abdominal wall defects. Ann Surg 1994;219:643–50 [discussion: 651–3].

130. Ramirez OM, Ruas E, Dellon AL. "Components separation" method for closure of abdominal-wall defects: an anatomic and clinical study. Plast Reconstr Surg 1990;86:519–26.

131. Vargo D. Component separation in the management of the difficult abdominal wall. Am J Surg 2004;188:633–7.

132. Anderson O, Putnis A, Bhardwaj R, et al. Short- and long-term outcome of laparostomy following intra-abdominal sepsis. Colorectal Dis 2011;13:e20–32.

133. Tremblay LN, Feliciano DV, Schmidt J, et al. Skin only or silo closure in the critically ill patient with an open abdomen. Am J Surg 2001;182:670–5.

134. Al-Khoury G, Kaufman D, Hirshberg A. Improved control of exposed fistula in the open abdomen. J Am Coll Surg 2008;206:397–8.

135. Cro C, George KJ, Donnelly J, et al. Vacuum assisted closure system in the management of enterocutaneous fistulae. Postgrad Med J 2002;78:364–5.

136. Erdmann D, Drye C, Heller L, et al. Abdominal wall defect and enterocutaneous fistula treatment with the Vacuum-Assisted Closure (V.A.C.) system. Plast Reconstr Surg 2001;108:2066–8.

137. Goverman J, Yelon JA, Platz JJ, et al. The "Fistula VAC," a technique for management of enterocutaneous fistulae arising within the open abdomen: report of 5 cases. J Trauma 2006;60:428–31 [discussion: 431].

138. Jamshidi R, Schecter WP. Biological dressings for the management of enteric fistulas in the open abdomen: a preliminary report. Arch Surg 2007;142:793–6.

139. Subramaniam MH, Liscum KR, Hirshberg A. The floating stoma: a new technique for controlling exposed fistulae in abdominal trauma. J Trauma 2002;53: 386–8.

140. Connolly PT, Teubner A, Lees NP, et al. Outcome of reconstructive surgery for intestinal fistula in the open abdomen. Ann Surg 2008;247:440–4.
141. Calandra T, Cohen J. International Sepsis Forum Definition of Infection in the ICUCC. The international sepsis forum consensus conference on definitions of infection in the intensive care unit. Crit Care Med 2005;33:1538–48.
142. Buijk SE, Bruining HA. Future directions in the management of tertiary peritonitis. Intensive Care Med 2002;28:1024–9.
143. Evans HL, Raymond DP, Pelletier SJ, et al. Diagnosis of intra-abdominal infection in the critically ill patient. Curr Opin Crit Care 2001;7:117–21.
144. Chromik AM, Meiser A, Holling J, et al. Identification of patients at risk for development of tertiary peritonitis on a surgical intensive care unit. J Gastrointest Surg 2009;13:1358–67.
145. Malangoni MA. Evaluation and management of tertiary peritonitis. Am Surg 2000;66:157–61.
146. Weiss G, Meyer F, Lippert H. Infectiological diagnostic problems in tertiary peritonitis. Langenbecks Arch Surg 2006;391:473–82.

Pathogenesis and Clinical and Economic Consequences of Postoperative Ileus

Michael G. Doorly, MD, MS, Anthony J. Senagore, MD, MS, MBA*

KEYWORDS

- Postoperative ileus • Abdominal surgery
- Early postoperative small bowel obstruction • Ogilvie syndrome
- Alvimopan

Postoperative ileus (POI) is perceived as an unavoidable outcome of major abdominal surgery, primarily because of poorly understood multifactorial pathophysiology.[1] Although ileus is thought to be a disease of the small intestine, the duration of POI may be primarily dependent on the return of colonic motility.[2] Physicians should understand the risk factors contributing to the development of POI to help prevent, recognize, and treat this morbid and financial problem. POI is multifactorial in origin and the causative factors include neuromuscular, inflammatory, and pharmacologic influences.[1] Understanding the various causes of POI helps to guide its prevention, diagnosis, treatment, and reduction of cost. The enhanced recovery protocol (fast-track) provides a consistent checklist that benefits all postoperative patients. Not all postoperative abdominal distention is POI. Recognizing the differences between POI, early postoperative small bowel obstruction (EPSBO), and acute colonic pseudo-obstruction can expedite care and improve survival.

FISCAL BURDEN OF POI

Although not life-threatening, POI can prolong postoperative recovery, increase the length of stay in hospital, and the use and costs of health care resources.[3–6] For example, up to 25% of colectomy patients suffer POI, which doubles the cost of their care.[7] POI may lead to other costly morbidities. The resultant abdominal distention of POI increases the risk of hernia formation and wound dehiscence, while nausea and vomiting affect the resumption of enteral nutrition and increase the risk of malnutrition

The authors have nothing to disclose.
Keck School of Medicine of USC, 1441 Eastlake Avenue, Suite 7418, Los Angeles, CA 90033-4612, USA
* Corresponding author.
E-mail address: Anthony.Senagore@med.usc.edu

and impaired wound healing. The need for nasogastric decompression and prolonged venous access inhibit ambulation, which may increase rates of pulmonary complications and thromboembolism. Prolonged fasting requires parenteral nutrition, which costs 3.5 times more per day than enteral nutrition,[8] without including the cost of central venous catheter placement or its complications. The morbidities of POI and the added care place a greater economic burden on the health care system.

The prolonged hospitalization associated with POI is an important issue at hospitals with a limited number of beds and high demand for inpatient services. Efforts to minimize POI and lengths of stay in hospital without increasing the risk of postdischarge readmission have the potential to improve the financial bottom line for hospitals, private and governmental health insurers, and society at large. Approximately 161,000 Medicare recipients undergo major intestinal or rectal resection each year, which consumes an estimated 1.8 million days in hospital at a cost of $1.75 billion.[9,10] Safely shortening this length of stay would produce significant dividends because the economic impact of POI is estimated at $750 million per year.[11–13]

Recurrence of primary (delayed) POI is the cessation of flatus or stool, with bloating and nausea or vomiting after a period of apparent resolution.[14] This process usually occurs 1 or more days after the patient has been discharged home, subsequently requiring readmission to the hospital. Readmission occurs in approximately 10% of patients who undergo major abdominal surgery, and about half of these patients are readmitted for gastrointestinal (GI) failure or some measure of recurrence of their POI.[15] This is a particularly important problem because the economic costs of readmission are exaggerated in part from tests such as computed tomography (CT) scans. The readmission cost of delayed POI is comparable to the readmission cost of more serious adverse surgical complications.[7] These formidable costs obligate the pathophysiologic understanding of this frequently preventable disease.

PATHOGENESIS OF POI

The multifactorial approach to prevention and treatment of POI is due in part to its complex pathogenesis. Studies have identified 3 major precipitating mechanisms for POI: neurogenic, inflammatory, and pharmacologic (**Fig. 1**). These mechanisms overlap to cause the disease, but the neuronal mechanism seems to disproportionately affect the early postoperative period.[14] Endogenous neuromuscular inhibitors of the bowel include norepinephrine, corticotropin-releasing hormone (CRH), nitric oxide, somatostatin, glucagon, gastric inhibitory peptide, and opioids.[16] Neurogenic bowel inhibition relates to pain-induced neural reflexes, which in turn result in sympathetic hyperactivity and inhibition of GI motility.[17,18] Another response to tissue trauma is the release of CRH from the central nervous system. CRH is recognized to contribute to the induction and duration of ileus.[19] Pain-induced reflexes also generate endogenous opioids that contribute to GI inhibition. Strategies to reduce postoperative pain and POI include the use of laparoscopic surgery and epidural local anesthetics.[17,20] POI may occur after minimally invasive surgical procedures, despite obvious reductions in surgical trauma and manipulation of the bowel, possibly because of the effects of opioid analgesics mediated by the stimulation of GI opioid receptors by exogenous opioids.[21,22]

Localized postoperative inflammation inhibits GI smooth muscle, and the duration of POI seems to correspond to the magnitude of intestinal inflammatory response.[22,23] Surgical manipulation of intestine activates quiescent macrophages and mast cells to induce several inflammatory cascades, primarily via the arachidonic acid pathway. As with pain response, these inflammatory mediators cause the release of endogenous

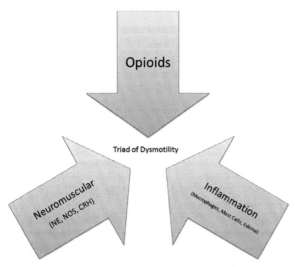

Fig. 1. Triad of dysmotility. CRH, corticotropin-releasing hormone; NE, norepinephrine; NOS, nitric oxide synthase.

opioid peptides, which further exacerbate the effects of exogenous opioid analgesics (administered for analgesia) on the inhibition of bowel function.[24–26] Bowel wall edema, from inflammation or intravenous fluid overload, is another mechanism of impairing GI motility.[18] Generalized inflammation (sepsis) causes fluid shifts that can lead to electrolyte abnormalities. Aberrations in electrolytes correlate with altered GI neuromuscular function and with prolonged POI.[27]

The pharmacologic deterrent to GI motility in postoperative patients is primarily the opioid class of medications. Opioid use for postoperative pain has been shown to correlate with the time to return of normal bowel function after surgery.[18]

The negative effect of opioids on GI motility is believed to occur because of the stimulation of μ-opioid receptors in the bowel, leading to inertia in the gut.[1,17] Opioids decrease GI secretion and profoundly inhibit peristalsis that leads to prolonged POI.[23] The opioid dose that slows peristalsis is 25% the dose of adequate analgesia.[18,28] This unfortunate mechanism is compounded in patients with analgesic tolerance because the bowel does not seem to develop tolerance.[18] Another study found no correlation between total morphine dose and incision length.[21] These results suggest that postoperative opioid management is a more important determinant of POI than the use of minimally invasive surgery.

DIAGNOSIS AND TREATMENT OF POI

POI is not life-threatening, but patients with POI typically experience substantial discomfort.[29] The current challenge of diagnosing and treating POI is the lack of an established uniform characterization of the disease. There is still dispute about the duration of normal POI. In 149 patients undergoing major abdominal surgery who were encouraged to ambulate and take oral liquids on the first postoperative day and eat solid food on the second postoperative day, more than 4 days elapsed before GI function returned to normal in half of the patients, and 25% of the patients had not regained normal GI function after more than 6 days.[29] Many surgeons have suggested that normal POI should last 3 days for laparoscopic surgery and 5 days for open surgery after bowel resection.[14] Prolonged POI lasts longer, and the symptoms are uniformly recognized: abdominal pain and distention, nausea, vomiting, lack of flatus, and intolerance to diet. POI can be further classified based on the predominance of upper versus lower of GI symptoms (**Table 1**).[14]

The diagnosis of prolonged POI is based on signs, symptoms, and abdominal imaging. Ileus reveals itself on an abdominal radiograph as a panintestinal dilatation with a spotty gas pattern throughout. However, the use of abdominal radiography in the absolute diagnosis of ileus in the immediate postoperative period is questionable. Studies report only 19% to 43% specificity and that abdominal radiography is not prognostic for reoperation.[30,31] CT is considered the gold standard for diagnosing POI because it can differentiate POI from EPSBO more than 98% of the time.[31,32] POI has been reported after up to 25% of colectomies, and EPSBO has been reported after up to 10% of colectomies.[7,33] Distinguishing POI from EPSBO is important because although they have similar presentations, EPSBO is associated with increased morbidity, reoperation, and mortality.

The treatment of prolonged POI should include bowel rest (nil by mouth), ambulation, strict electrolyte management, and minimal opioid usage. Obtaining relief of POI-related pain is a two-edged sword because the surgeon balances adequate analgesia with additional impairment of GI motility. Placement of a nondiscriminatory nasogastric tube (NGT) for POI may prolong the duration of POI and is not associated with the early return of bowel function.[16,34] Vomiting related to POI necessitates NGT placement for GI decompression. Relaparotomy for prolonged POI is rarely needed, except in situations when the diagnosis is unclear or translocation of gut flora bacteria causes a septic response (**Fig. 2**). At present, the incidence of relaparotomy for prolonged refractory POI remains unreported. Resolution of POI is signaled with the return of flatus, decreased abdominal distension, and toleration of diet.

EPSBO

In addition to symptomatic and radiographic evidence of EPSBO, some investigators include loss of POI tolerance before postoperative day 30 as the definition of EPSBO.[33,35] Although prolonged POI and EPSBO have similar presentations, the sequelae of EPSBO tend to be more serious. Understanding the incidence, etiology, and risk factors for EPSBO can expedite the diagnosis. The reported incidence of EPSBO differs, ranging from 0.7% to 10%.[33,35] The incidence of 0.7% is most likely an underestimation because it excludes conservatively managed patients.[36] Most of the literature reports an EPSBO rate between 5% and 10%. Risk factors for EPSBO do not seem to include age, body mass index, American Society of Anesthesiologists score, or blood loss.[37] Elective supracolic procedures have lower incidences of EPSBO, as does simple exploratory laparotomy (1.3%).[33,35,38,39] Laparoscopy is also associated with lower incidence of EPSBO. When compared with open resection, laparoscopic ileocolic resection for Crohn disease is associated with 69% less early/late postoperative small bowel obstruction (SBO) (35.4% vs 11.1%).[40] A multicenter French study reports that 88% of postlaparoscopic SBO is early postoperative.[41]

Table 1 Types of POI		
Type	**Location**	**Symptoms**
I	Panintestinal	Nausea, vomiting, no flatus
II	Upper GI	Nausea, vomiting, flatus present
III	Lower GI	Tolerance of diet, no flatus

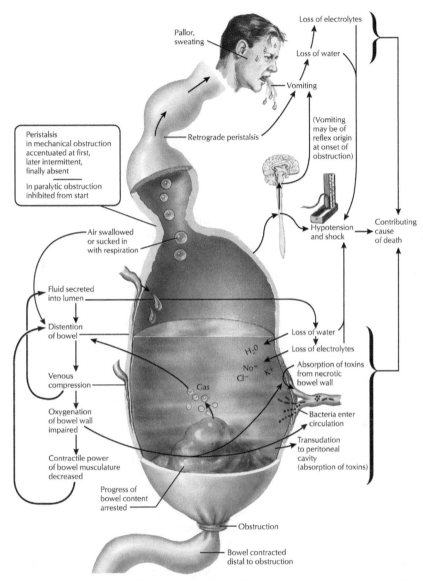

Loss of electrolytes

Loss of water

Pallor, sweating

Vomiting

(Vomiting may be of reflex origin at onset of obstruction)

Retrograde peristalsis

Peristalsis in mechanical obstruction accentuated at first, later intermittent, finally absent

In paralytic obstruction inhibited from start

Air swallowed or sucked in with respiration

Hypotension and shock

Contributing cause of death

Fluid secreted into lumen

Distention of bowel

Loss of water

Loss of electrolytes

H_2O

Na^+

Cl^- K^+

Absorption of toxins from necrotic bowel wall

Venous compression

Gas

Bacteria enter circulation

Oxygenation of bowel wall impaired

Transudation to peritoneal cavity (absorption of toxins)

Contractile power of bowel musculature decreased

Progress of bowel content arrested

Obstruction

Bowel contracted distal to obstruction

Fig. 2. Ileus versus early small bowel obstruction. (*From* www.netterimages.com. © Elsevier Inc. All rights reserved; with permission.)

Open procedures posing the highest risk of EPSBO are colectomy, omentectomy, and pelvic dissection.[37,42–44]

CT accurately distinguishes EPSBO from POI, and should be the gold standard test in the early postoperative time period because it can also identify other complications. If CT suggests EPSBO, an NGT should be placed and water-soluble contrast diatrizoic acid (Gastrografin, Hypaque) upper GI series performed. Gastrografin is safe in the GI tract or peritoneal space, accurately predicts the need for surgery, and is associated with shorter hospital stays.[45–47] Barium should be avoided because the viscous properties may exacerbate partial SBO, the prolonged half-life may confuse future imaging, and barium causes a difficult-to-treat peritonitis if the bowel perforates. The hyperosmolar property of Gastrografin may have a therapeutic effect by establishing an osmotic catharsis, thus speeding the resolution of adhesive SBO and decreasing the need for surgery.[46,48,49] Approximately 90% of early postoperative bowel obstructions treated with NGT resolve by 6 days, whereas 10% need relaparotomy.[33] The risk of bowel strangulation from EPSBO is 2% to 4%, much lower than the 17% for late adhesive SBO.[36,50]

The decision to reoperate on a patient with EPSBO can be difficult, especially if the patient is comfortable without evidence of strangulation. Operative management for EPSBO should take place between 1 and 2 weeks, although spontaneous resolution beyond 10 days is unlikely.[33,51] Adhesiolysis after 2 weeks increases the technical difficulty and the risk of inadvertent enterotomy. In cases of carcinomatosis, radiation enteritis, and frozen abdomen, conservative management of EPSBO can be used indefinitely.[36] A major problem with adhesive SBO is that the recurrence rate is the same after adhesiolysis in comparison with conservative management (about 60%).[52] Meticulous surgical technique can reduce adhesiogenesis, but the high rate of recurrence has inspired much research. Strategies to interfere with adhesiogenesis include barriers or the reduction in inflammation, fibrin, and collagen deposition.[53] Nonsteroidal anti-inflammatory drugs and corticosteroids decrease inflammation, but their safety and effectiveness is questionable.[54–56] Heparin and streptokinase decrease fibrin deposition but they cause unacceptable postoperative bleeding.[57,58] Halofuginone, a type I collagen synthase inhibitor, decreases adhesiogenesis in animals but has yet to be studied in humans because of healing and safety concerns.[59,60] The most effective inhibitor of adhesiogenesis to date is a hyaluronan carboxymethylcellulose barrier (Seprafilm).[54] Studies indicate that Seprafilm can reduce adhesiogenesis by 33% to 50%, but may increase intraperitoneal abscess and the rate of anastomotic leaks.[61,62] The clinical sequelae of using Seprafilm have recently been shown to decrease EPSBO by more than 60% with a trend toward decreasing late adhesive SBO.[63,64]

ACUTE COLONIC PSEUDO-OBSTRUCTION (OGILVIE SYNDROME)

Acute colonic pseudo-obstruction is a massive dilatation of the colon with constipation in those in whom a mechanical obstruction has been excluded. The disease commonly affects individuals with senility or neurologic disease, and those who receive drugs that affect gut motility. Acute colonic pseudo-obstruction is a serious condition because patients usually have multiple comorbidities, delayed diagnosis, inappropriate treatment, and high mortality from ischemia (25%–31%) or perforation (40%–50%).[65] Theories about the pathophysiologic cause include autonomic dysfunction, reduced colonic ganglion cells, and loss of intrinsic nitric oxide activity, but the cause remains unknown.[65] Patients are commonly critically ill, and present with a nontender distended abdomen and the inability to pass stool or flatus. They may also have nausea, vomiting, or abdominal pain. Unlike POI or EPSBO, acute colonic pseudo-obstruction has little to do with an abdominal operation. In fact, the most common procedures associated with Ogilvie syndrome are coronary artery bypass grafting, and spine and orthopedic procedures.[66]

Symptoms lead to an abdominal radiograph revealing isolated colonic dilatation. Diagnoses must exclude mechanical colonic obstruction by either CT or Gastrografin enema. The management of Ogilvie syndrome depends on the patient's condition and the risk of perforation. Realized or suspected perforation requires surgical intervention and is associated with higher mortality.[67] Perforation usually means total or segmental colectomy with ostomy, while intact colons may be proximally diverted.[68,69] Conservative management should include a risk assessment using complete blood count and serial abdominal radiographs every 12 to 24 hours, because a cecal diameter of more than14 cm is associated with a 2-fold increase in mortality.[67,70] Many surgeons agree that the risk of cecal perforation increases with a cecal diameter greater than 10 cm. Failure to improve or worsen by 48 to 72 hours indicates the need for colonic decompression, because waiting longer than 6 days has a greater risk of complication.[69,71,72] Monitored intravenous neostigmine in patients without a history of myocardial ischemia, asthma, or renal failure remains a mainstay of treatment.[73] Colonoscopic decompression is also an accepted therapy, but is technically difficult and carries at least a 2% risk of perforation.[74] Endoscopic and CT-guided percutaneous cecostomy have been described in patients intolerant to surgery, but the studies were small and with only marginal success.[75–77]

ENHANCED RECOVERY AFTER SURGERY

A multimodal approach has been developed to improve postoperative morbidity, including POI, in surgical patients.[10,78] In addition, adoption of enhanced recovery after surgery (ERAS) at teaching hospitals has been shown to decrease length of stay.[79] Preoperative counseling (patient education), intraoperative fluid restriction, use of a laparoscopic approach, immediate initiation of clear fluids after surgery, and early discontinuation of the Foley catheter are all independently associated with shortened length of stay in hospital.[79] Patient education is also an important component of fast-track protocols. The discussion should include importance of early ambulation, early enteral nutrition, and effective pain control with both narcotic and nonsteroidal combinations of oral medications. Although early ambulation does not seem to reduce the duration of POI, it may contribute to decreasing length of stay by preventing atelectasis, pneumonia, and deep vein thrombosis while preserving strength and conditioning.[23,80,81] Early enteral nutrition after bowel surgery is safe, well tolerated, and associated with a decreased length of stay, but does not change the incidence of POI.[17,23] The decreased length of stay associated with early enteral nutrition may result from an earlier recognition of postoperative tolerance translating to earlier discharge from hospital. Despite the use of a fast-track protocol, POI after abdominal surgery can still last a long time.[29,82]

Anesthesiologists are important participants in the attempt to decrease length of stay in hospital. Medications used during general anesthesia have a profound effect on the duration of POI. Inhaled anesthetics (particularly nitrous oxide), atropine, and catecholamines decrease intestinal motility, especially within the large intestine.[34] Midthoracic epidural anesthesia improves postoperative bowel function by blocking afferent autonomic pain signals, efferent catecholamines, and stress response to localized inflammation, and decreases the need for peripheral opioids.[18,83] Intraoperative fluid management affects postoperative morbidity and duration of POI. One prospective study compared restrictive and liberal intraoperative fluid administration, which resulted in no difference in duration of POI or length of stay.[84] Another prospective study showed Doppler-optimized intraoperative fluid management to decrease POI, nausea, vomiting, and wound infection rates.[85]

Other postoperative regimens to reduce duration of POI and length of stay have been met with less success. The evidence is clear that traditional prokinetic medications can neither prevent nor treat POI. Numerous prospective studies show that erythromycin simply does not have any effect, and there is a lack of evidence that cholecystokinin-like drugs, cisapride, dopamine antagonists, propranolol, or vasopressin affect the duration of POI.[86] Prospective studies on medications that block opioid receptors, such as methylnaltrexone, did not effectively show a decreased duration of POI, and use of these drugs comes at the expense of inadequate pain control.[87] The practice of sham eating (gum chewing) has been trialed, the results of which are promising yet controversial. Meta-analysis of prospective studies on sham eating revealed the practice to be well tolerated and had 25% less time to flatus, 32% less time to bowel movement, and 18% earlier discharge, with similar complication rates.[88]

POTENTIAL ROLE OF ALVIMOPAN

The newly available peripherally selective μ-opioid receptor antagonist alvimopan (Entereg) offers an adjunct to fast-track protocols with the potential to minimize POI rates.[29] A recent pooled analysis of 3 of the prospective randomized and blinded alvimopan trials confirmed that a 12-mg dose provided optimal reduction in GI morbidity and return of GI function.[89] These benefits are clinically relevant and important to clinicians when arranging discharge plans.[90] An interesting additional benefit of alvimopan was a significant decrease in the incidence of POI as a serious adverse event coupled with a reduction in the proportion of patients who had prolonged hospital stay or readmission.[88] These benefits translated into a 50% reduction in the proportion of patients defined as having prolonged hospital stay. Alvimopan has been generally well tolerated in the available trials, without producing a negative impact on narcotic analgesia as demonstrated by pain scores. All these trials included a program of early oral nutrition and ambulation, and compared with the placebo group the reduction in time to writing the discharge order confirmed the additional benefit of alvimopan even in an enhanced recovery program.

MEDICATIONS UNDER INVESTIGATION FOR POI

Promising medications to prevent and treat POI are currently under investigation. Ghrelin agonists have been shown to stimulate motilin receptors and have powerful prokinetic properties. A recent prospective study in patients undergoing major abdominal surgery reported the first-in-class ghrelin agonist TZP-101 was well tolerated and accelerated the recovery of the upper and lower GI tract, with a large proportion of patients recovering within 72 hours compared with those on placebo.[91] The perioperative intravenous administration of lidocaine has recently become an intense area of research, especially in the anesthesia literature. Although 2 studies show no difference, the preponderance of evidence suggests that perioperative intravenous lidocaine is safe, reduces postoperative pain, reduces the duration of POI, and decreases the length of stay in hospital.[92–98] Escin, a natural mixture of triterpene saponins, has been used to decrease cerebral edema (anti-inflammation) and chronic venous insufficiency (venotonic) in China. Animal studies have shown that escin may also have prokinetic properties. Universities in China are currently investigating whether escin can reduce POI. Preliminary results indicate that escin can shorten the time to recovery of GI motility in patients with cancer after colorectal surgery.[99] Escin requires central venous administration to prevent peripheral phlebitis.

SUMMARY

The clinical and economic consequences of POI are substantial. Understanding the pathogenesis contributing to POI (triad of dysmotility) will improve patient care and speed up postoperative recovery. The physician must be able to differentiate POI from EPSBO and Ogilvie syndrome. Assuming all postoperative abdominal distention to be POI is a critical mistake. The use of appropriate and timely abdominal imaging to diagnose these diseases will save lives. The goal of enhanced recovery fast-track protocols is to improve the safety of postoperative care, speed up recovery, and reduce costs. Medications such as alvimopan, ghrelin agonists, and intravenous lidocaine can help attain this goal, but it is up to physicians to implement and maintain enhanced recovery protocols. Fast-track protocols must be implemented via a multi-specialty approach with shared responsibility toward a common goal. Educating the patient preoperatively about the anticipated care regimen is also essential. The global economic importance of POI cannot be overstated. By preventing, recognizing, and treating POI, one can improve the lives of one's patients and help safeguard the financial sustainability of the health care system.

REFERENCES

1. Holte K, Kehlet H. Postoperative ileus: progress towards effective management. Drugs 2002;62:2603–15.
2. Bauer AJ, Schwarz NT, Moore BA, et al. Ileus in critical illness: mechanisms and management. Curr Opin Crit Care 2002;8:152–7.
3. Collins TC, Daley J, Henderson WH, et al. Risk factors for prolonged length of stay after major elective surgery. Ann Surg 1999;230:251–9.
4. Schuster TG, Montie JE. Postoperative ileus after abdominal surgery. Urology 2002;59:465–71.
5. Chang SS, Baumgartner RG, Wells N, et al. Causes of increased hospital stay after radical cystectomy in a clinical pathway setting. J Urol 2002;167:208–11.
6. Lauer MA, Karweit JA, Cascade EF, et al. Practice patterns and outcomes of percutaneous coronary interventions in the United States: 1995 to 1997. Am J Cardiol 2002;89:924–9.
7. Asgeirsson T, El-Badawi K, Mahmood A, et al. Postoperative ileus: it costs more than you expect. J Am Coll Surg 2010;210:228–31.
8. Braga M, Gianotti L, Gentilini O, et al. Early postoperative enteral nutrition improves gut oxygenation and reduces costs compared with total parenteral nutrition. Crit Care Med 2001;29(2):242–8.
9. Woods MS. Postoperative ileus: dogma versus data from bench to bedside. Perspect Colon Rectal Surg 2000;12:57–76.
10. Delaney CP. Clinical perspective on postoperative ileus and the effect of opiates. Neurogastroenterol Motil 2004;16(Suppl 2):61–6.
11. Senagore AJ. Pathogenesis and clinical and economic consequences of postoperative ileus. Am J Health Syst Pharm 2007;64:S3–7.
12. Livingston EH, Passaro EP Jr. Postoperative ileus. Dig Dis Sci 1990;35:121–32.
13. Postoperative Ileus Management Council. Available at: http://www.ClinicalWebcasts.com/PIMC.htm. Accessed October 2, 2009.
14. Delaney C, Kehlet H, Senagore AJ, et al. Postoperative ileus: profiles, risk factors, and definitions—a framework for optimizing surgical outcomes in patients undergoing major abdominal and colorectal surgery. In: Bosker G, editor. Clinical consensus update in general surgery. Roswell (GA): Pharmatecture; 2006. p. 1–26.
15. Kiran RP, Delaney CP, Senagore AJ, et al. Outcomes and prediction of hospital readmission after intestinal surgery. J Am Coll Surg 2004;198:877–83.
16. Kurz A, Sessler DI. Opioid-induced bowel dysfunction: pathophysiology and potential new therapies. Drugs 2003;63:649–71.
17. Kehlet H, Holte K. Review of postoperative ileus. Am J Surg 2001;182(Suppl 5A):3S–10S.

18. Holte K, Kehlet H. Postoperative ileus: a preventable event. Br J Surg 2000;87:1480–93.
19. Taché Y, Bonaz B. Corticotropin-releasing factor receptors and stress-related alterations of gut motor function. J Clin Invest 2007;117:33–40.
20. Chen HH, Wexner SD, Iroatulam AJ, et al. Laparoscopic colectomy compares favorably with colectomy by laparotomy for reduction of postoperative ileus. Dis Colon Rectum 2000;43:61–5.
21. Cali RL, Meade PG, Swanson MS, et al. Effect of morphine and incision length on bowel function after colectomy. Dis Colon Rectum 2000;43:163–8.
22. Kraft M, Erstad BL, Matuszewski K. Improving postoperative ileus outcomes. US Pharmacist; 2005. Available at: http://www.uspharmacist.com/index.asp?page=ce/10193/default.htm. Accessed March 6, 2007.
23. Bauer AJ, Boeckxstaens GE. Mechanisms of postoperative ileus. Neurogastroenterol Motil 2004;16(Suppl 2):54–60.
24. Brix-Christensen V, Tonnesen E, Sanchez RG, et al. Endogenous morphine levels increase following cardiac surgery as part of the anti-inflammatory response? Int J Cardiol 1997;62:191–7.
25. Yoshida S, Ohta J, Yamasaki K, et al. Effect of surgical stress on endogenous morphine and cytokine levels in the plasma after laparoscopic or open cholecystectomy. Surg Endosc 2000;14:137–40.
26. Kalff JC, Schraut WH, Simmons RL, et al. Surgical manipulation of the gut elicits an intestinal muscularis inflammatory response resulting in postsurgical ileus. Ann Surg 1998;228:652–63.
27. Prasad M, Matthews JB. Deflating postoperative ileus [editorial]. Gastroenterology 1999;117:489–92.
28. Sternini C, Patierno S, Selmer IS, et al. The opioid system in the gastrointestinal tract. Neurogastroenterol Motil 2004;16(Suppl 2):3–16.
29. Wolff BG, Michelassi F, Gerkin TM, et al. Alvimopan, a novel, peripherally acting mu opioid antagonist: results of a multicenter, randomized, double-blind, placebo-controlled, phase III trial of major abdominal surgery and postoperative ileus. Ann Surg 2004;240:728–35.
30. Heinberg EM, Finan MA, Chambers RB, et al. Postoperative ileus on a gynecologic oncology service–do abdominal X-rays have a role? Gynecol Oncol 2003;90(1):158–62.
31. Frager DH, Baer JW, Rothpearl A, et al. Distinction between postoperative ileus and mechanical small-bowel obstruction: value of CT compared with clinical and other radiographic findings. AJR Am J Roentgenol 1995;164:891–4.
32. Taourel PG, Fabre JM, Pradel JA, et al. Value of CT in the diagnosis and management of patients with suspected acute small-bowel obstruction. AJR Am J Roentgenol 1995;165(5):1187–92.
33. Ellozy SH, Harris MT, Bauer JJ, et al. Early postoperative small-bowel obstruction: a prospective evaluation in 242 consecutive abdominal operations. Dis Colon Rectum 2002;45(9):1214–7.
34. Miedema BW, Johnson JO. Methods for decreasing postoperative gut dysmotility. Lancet Oncol 2003;4:365–72.
35. Stewart RM, Page CP, Brender J, et al. The incidence and risk of early postoperative small bowel obstruction. A cohort study. Am J Surg 1987;154:643–7.
36. Sajja S, Schein M. Early postoperative small bowel obstruction. Br J Surg 2004;91:683–91.
37. Nakajima J, Sasaki A, Otsuka K, et al. Risk factors for early postoperative small bowel obstruction after colectomy for colorectal cancer. World J Surg 2010;34(5):1086–90.

38. Quatromoni JC, Rosoff L Sr, Halls JM, et al. Early postoperative small bowel obstruction. Ann Surg 1980;191:72–4.
39. Barmparas G, Branco BC, Schnüriger B, et al. In-hospital small bowel obstruction after exploratory laparotomy for trauma. J Trauma 2011;71(2):486–90.
40. Bergamaschi R, Pessaux P, Arnaud JP. Comparison of conventional and laparoscopic ileocolic resection for Crohn's disease. Dis Colon Rectum 2003;46:1129–33.
41. Duron JJ, Hay JM, Msika S, et al. Prevalence and mechanisms of small intestinal obstruction following laparoscopic abdominal surgery: a retrospective multicenter study. Arch Surg 2000;135:208–12.
42. Nieuwenhuijzen M, Reijnen MM, Kuijpers JH, et al. Small bowel obstruction after total or subtotal colectomy: a 10-year retrospective review. Br J Surg 1998;85:1242–5.
43. Menzies D. Postoperative adhesions: their treatment and relevance in clinical practice. Ann R Coll Surg Engl 1993;75:147–53.
44. Shin JY, Hong KH. Risk factors for early postoperative small-bowel obstruction after colectomy in colorectal cancer. World J Surg 2008;32(10):2287–92.
45. Abbas S, Bissett IP, Parry BR. Oral water soluble contrast for the management of adhesive small bowel obstruction. Cochrane Database Syst Rev 2007;3:CD004651.
46. Di Saverio S, Catena F, Ansaloni L, et al. Water-soluble contrast medium (gastrografin) value in adhesive small intestine obstruction (ASIO): a prospective, randomized, controlled, clinical trial. World J Surg 2008;32(10):2293–304.
47. Branco BC, Barmparas G, Schnüriger B, et al. Systematic review and meta-analysis of the diagnostic and therapeutic role of water-soluble contrast agent in adhesive small bowel obstruction. Br J Surg 2010;97(4):470–8.
48. Assalia A, Schein M, Kopelman D, et al. Therapeutic effect of oral Gastrografin in adhesive, partial small-bowel obstruction: a prospective randomized trial. Surgery 1994;115:433–7.
49. Choi HK, Chu KW, Law WL. Therapeutic value of Gastrografin in adhesive small bowel obstruction after unsuccessful conservative treatment: a prospective randomized trial. Ann Surg 2002;236:1–6.
50. Fevang T, Fevang J, Stangeland L, et al. Complications and death after surgical treatment of small bowel obstruction: a 35 year institutional experience. Ann Surg 2000;231(4):529–37.
51. Pickleman J, Lee RM. The management of patients with suspected early postoperative small bowel obstruction. Ann Surg 1989;210:216–9.
52. Miller G, Boman J, Shrier I, et al. Readmission for small-bowel obstruction in the early postoperative period: etiology and outcome. Can J Surg 2002;45(4):255–8.
53. Attard JP, MacLean AR. Adhesive small bowel obstruction: epidemiology, biology and prevention. Can J Surg 2007;50(4):291–300.
54. Montz FJ, Monk BJ, Lacy SM, et al. Ketorolac tromethamine, a nonsteroidal anti-inflammatory drug: ability to inhibit postradical pelvic surgery adhesions in a porcine model. Gynecol Oncol 1993;48:76–9.
55. Holtz G. Failure of a nonsteroidal anti-inflammatory agent (ibuprofen) to inhibit peritoneal adhesion reformation after lysis. Fertil Steril 1982;37:582–3.
56. Grosfeld JL, Berman IR, Schiller M, et al. Excessive morbidity resulting from the prevention of intestinal adhesions with steroids and antihistamines. J Pediatr Surg 1973;8:221–6.
57. Montz FJ, Fowler JM, Wolff AJ, et al. The ability of recombinant tissue plasminogen activator to inhibit post-radical pelvic surgery adhesions in the dog model. Am J Obstet Gynecol 1991;165:1539–42.
58. James DC, Ellis H, Hugh TB. The effect of streptokinase on experimental intraperitoneal adhesion formation. J Pathol Bacteriol 1965;90:279–87.

59. Nagler A, Genina O, Lavelin I, et al. Halofuginone, an inhibitor of collagen type I synthesis, prevents postoperative adhesion formation in the rat uterine horn model. Am J Obstet Gynecol 1999;180:558–63.
60. Nagler A, Rivkind AI, Raphael J, et al. Halofuginone—an inhibitor of collagen type I synthesis—prevents postoperative formation of abdominal adhesions. Ann Surg 1998;227:575–82.
61. Becker JM, Dayton MT, Fazio VW, et al. Prevention of postoperative abdominal adhesions by a sodium hyaluronate-based bioresorbable membrane: a prospective, randomized, double-blind multicenter study. J Am Coll Surg 1996;183:297–306.
62. Cohen Z, Senagore AJ, Dayton MT, et al. Prevention of postoperative abdominal adhesions by a novel, glycerol/sodium hyaluronate/carboxymethylcellulose-based bioresorbable membrane: a prospective, randomized, evaluator-blinded multicenter study. Dis Colon Rectum 2005;48:1130–9.
63. Mohri Y, Uchida K, Araki T, et al. Hyaluronic acid-carboxycellulose membrane (Seprafilm) reduces early postoperative small bowel obstruction in gastrointestinal surgery. Am Surg 2005;71(10):861–3.
64. Park CM, Lee WY, Cho YB, et al. Sodium hyaluronate-based bioresorbable membrane (Seprafilm) reduced early postoperative intestinal obstruction after lower abdominal surgery for colorectal cancer: the preliminary report. Int J Colorectal Dis 2009;24(3):305–10.
65. De Giorgio R, Knowles CH. Acute colonic pseudo-obstruction. Br J Surg 2009;96: 229–39.
66. Tenofsky PL, Beamer RL, Smith RS. Ogilvie syndrome as a postoperative complication. Arch Surg 2000;135:682–7.
67. Vanek VW, Al-Salti M. Acute pseudo-obstruction of the colon (Ogilvie's syndrome). An analysis of 400 cases. Dis Colon Rectum 1986;29:203–10.
68. Geelhoed GW. Colonic pseudo-obstruction in surgical patients. Am J Surg 1985; 149:258–65.
69. Williams NS. Large bowel obstruction. In: Keighley MR, Williams NS, editors. Surgery of the anus, rectum and colon. 1st edition. London: WB Saunders; 1997. p. 1823–66.
70. Sloyer AF, Panella VS, Demas BE, et al. Ogilvie's syndrome. Successful management without colonoscopy. Dig Dis Sci 1988;33:1391–6.
71. Delgado-Aros S, Camilleri M. Pseudo-obstruction in the critically ill. Best Pract Res Clin Gastroenterol 2003;17:427–44.
72. Saunders MD. Acute colonic pseudo-obstruction. Best Pract Res Clin Gastroenterol 2007;21:671–87.
73. Ponec RJ, Saunders MD, Kimmey MB. Neostigmine for the treatment of the acute colonic pseudo-obstruction. N Engl J Med 1999;341:137–41.
74. Geller A, Petersen BT, Gostout CJ. Endoscopic decompression for acute colonic pseudo-obstruction. Gastrointest Endosc 1996;44:144–50.
75. Ramage JI Jr, Baron TH. Percutaneous endoscopic cecostomy: a case series. Gastrointest Endosc 2003;57:752–5.
76. Lynch CR, Jones RG, Hilden K, et al. Percutaneous endoscopic cecostomy in adults: a case series. Gastrointest Endosc 2006;64:279–82.
77. Crass JR, Simmons RL, Frick MP, et al. Percutaneous decompression of the colon using CT guidance in Ogilvie syndrome. AJR Am J Roentgenol 1985;144:475–6.
78. Kehlet H, Dahl JB. Anaesthesia, surgery, and challenges in postoperative recovery. Lancet 2003;362:1921–8.
79. Aarts MA, Okrainec A, Glicksman A, et al. Adoption of enhanced recovery after surgery (ERAS) strategies for colorectal surgery at academic teaching hospitals and impact on total length of hospital stay. Surg Endosc 2012;26(2):442–50.

80. Ferraz AA, Cowles VE, Condon RE, et al. Nonopioid analgesics shorten the duration of postoperative ileus. Am Surg 1995;61:1079–83.
81. Waldhausen JH, Schirmer BD. The effect of ambulation on recovery from postoperative ileus. Ann Surg 1990;212:671–7.
82. Delaney CP, Fazio VW, Senagore AJ, et al. 'Fast track' postoperative management protocol for patients with high co-morbidity undergoing complex abdominal and pelvic colorectal surgery. Br J Surg 2001;88:1533–8.
83. Steinbrook RA. Epidural anesthesia and gastrointestinal motility. Anesth Analg 1998;86:837–44.
84. Holte K, Foss NB, Andersen J, et al. Liberal or restrictive fluid administration in fast-track colonic surgery: a randomized, double-blind study. Br J Anaesth 2007;99(4):500–8.
85. Pillai P, McEleavy I, Gaughan M, et al. A double-blind randomized controlled clinical trial to assess the effect of Doppler optimized intraoperative fluid management on outcome following radical cystectomy. J Urol 2011;186(6):2201–6.
86. Traut U, Brügger L, Kunz R, et al. Systemic prokinetic pharmacologic treatment for postoperative adynamic ileus following abdominal surgery in adults. Cochrane Database Syst Rev 2008;1:CD004930.
87. Yu CS, Chun HK, Stambler N, et al. Safety and efficacy of methylnaltrexone in shortening the duration of postoperative ileus following segmental colectomy: results of two randomized, placebo-controlled phase 3 trials. Dis Colon Rectum 2011;54(5):570–8.
88. Chan MK, Law WL. Use of chewing gum in reducing postoperative ileus after elective colorectal resection: a systematic review. Dis Colon Rectum 2007; 50(12):2149–57.
89. Delaney CP, Wolff BG, Viscus ER, et al. Alvimopan, for postoperative ileus following bowel resection: a pooled analysis of phase III studies. Ann Surg 2007;245(3):355–63.
90. Bungard TJ, Kale-Pradhan PB. Prokinetic agents for the treatment of postoperative ileus in adults: a review of the literature. Pharmacotherapy 1999;19:416–23.
91. Popescu I, Fleshner PR, Pezzullo JC, et al. The Ghrelin agonist TZP-101 for management of postoperative ileus after partial colectomy: a randomized, dose-ranging, placebo-controlled clinical trial. Dis Colon Rectum 2010;53(2):126–34.
92. Rimbäck G, Cassuto J, Tollesson PO. Treatment of postoperative paralytic ileus by intravenous lidocaine infusion. Anesth Analg 1990;70(4):414–9.
93. Groudine SB, Fisher HA, Kaufman RP, et al. Intravenous lidocaine speeds the return of bowel function, decreases postoperative pain, and shortens hospital stay in patients undergoing radical retropubic prostatectomy. Anesth Analg 1998; 86(2):235–9.
94. Marret E, Rolin M, Beaussier M, et al. Meta-analysis of intravenous lidocaine and postoperative recovery after abdominal surgery. Br J Surg 2008;95(11):1331–8.
95. Vigneault L, Turgeon AF, Côté D, et al. Perioperative intravenous lidocaine infusion for postoperative pain control: a meta-analysis of randomized controlled trials. Can J Anaesth 2011;58(1):22–37.
96. Swenson BR, Gottschalk A, Wells LT, et al. Intravenous lidocaine is as effective as epidural bupivacaine in reducing ileus duration, hospital stay, and pain after open colon resection: a randomized clinical trial. Reg Anesth Pain Med 2010;35(4): 370–6.
97. McCarthy GC, Megalla SA, Habib AS. Impact of intravenous lidocaine infusion on postoperative analgesia and recovery from surgery: a systematic review of randomized controlled trials. Drugs 2010;70(9):1149–63.

98. Harvey KP, Adair JD, Isho M, et al. Can intravenous lidocaine decrease postsurgical ileus and shorten hospital stay in elective bowel surgery? A pilot study and literature review. Am J Surg 2009;198(2):231–6.
99. Xie Q, Zong X, Ge B, et al. Pilot postoperative ileus study of escin in cancer patients after colorectal surgery. World J Surg 2009;33:348–54.

Perioperative Nutritional Support: Immunonutrition, Probiotics, and Anabolic Steroids

Adrian A. Maung, MD*, Kimberly A. Davis, MD

KEYWORDS

- Nutritional support • Immunonutrition • Probiotics
- Malnutrition • Anabolic steroids

Normal physiologic function requires continuous metabolism of substrates to provide energy to sustain life. This metabolism requires intake and absorption of carbohydrates, proteins, and lipids as well as water, vitamins, and trace elements. Although metabolic demands depend on physical activity and nutritional intake, the catabolic and anabolic pathways are usually balanced in a healthy adult. Surgical stress, trauma, and critical illness alter normal metabolic requirements and pathways, with a shift toward a catabolic state resulting in loss of weight, lean body mass, and fat; proteolysis; and expansion of the extracellular fluid compartment.

Perioperative nutritional support has traditionally focused on providing adequate calories in an attempt to attenuate the loss of lean body mass commonly observed after major surgery. With increasing understanding, it has become apparent that perioperative nutritional support is more complicated than just the administration of caloric support. Nutritional support can improve patient outcomes and decrease complications rates by preventing oxidative cellular injury, attenuating metabolic responses, and enhancing immune function.[1,2] Types of nutritional formulation, routes of delivery, and number of delivered calories all modulate physiologic and pathologic responses and thus affect patient outcome. In this article, the authors review the current state of nutritional support in the perioperative state and discuss the role of immunonutrition, probiotics, and anabolic steroids.

The authors have nothing to disclose.
Section of Trauma, Surgical Critical Care and Surgical Emergencies, Department of Surgery, Yale University School of Medicine, 330 Cedar Street BB310, PO Box 208062, New Haven, CT 06520-8062, USA
* Corresponding author.
E-mail address: adrian.maung@yale.edu

Surg Clin N Am 92 (2012) 273–283
doi:10.1016/j.suc.2012.01.014
0039-6109/12/$ – see front matter © 2012 Elsevier Inc. All rights reserved.

MEASUREMENT OF MALNUTRITION

Healthy well-nourished patients undergoing minor physiologic stress do not require nutritional support. However, those with preoperative protein-calorie malnutrition, especially if experiencing major physiologic stress, have increased mortality and morbidity with associated increases in hospital length of stay. It is therefore imperative to identify those at risk for the development of malnutrition, a challenging task, because currently there is neither a universally accepted definition of malnutrition nor a gold standard test for its identification. Commonly used screening parameters include a history of unintentional weight loss greater than 10% to 15% in the last 6 months or a body mass index less than 18.5 kg/m².[3] Laboratory markers frequently used in nutritional screening include albumin and prealbumin. Albumin is considered the most accurate laboratory indicator of basal protein stores, with a level less than 3.5 g/dL causing concern for malnutrition. Albumin, however, has a half-life of approximately 20 days and thus is more reflective of the nutritional status 3 weeks before the sample being drawn. Albumin levels are affected by acute inflammation and both acute and chronic diseases such as sepsis and renal and liver diseases.[4] Prealbumin, conversely, has a half-life of 1 to 3 days, and thus its levels change more rapidly with nutritional interventions. Prealbumin is commonly used as a marker of the effectiveness of nutritional support, with a level less than 15 mg/dL suggestive of malnutrition.[5] Several more sophisticated nutritional screening tools have also been developed, including the Nutritional Risk Screening, Malnutrition Universal Screening Tool, and the Mini Nutritional Assessment.[6,7]

PHYSIOLOGIC CHANGES WITH GASTROINTESTINAL TRACT DISUSE

In addition to its role in nutrient uptake and metabolism, the gastrointestinal (GI) tract is also an important part of the immune system. The GI tract is constantly exposed to and acts as a repository for multiple organisms. During the normal state, the combination of the predominant commensally anaerobic flora, the contractility of the GI tract, the production of secretory IgA (sIgA), the presence of bile salts that reduce bacterial adherence, and the action of antimicrobial secretions such as proteases and pancreatic enzymes prevent overgrowth of more pathogenic organisms. However, following a period of disuse, the GI tract demonstrates multiple structural and physiologic changes that affect its immune and metabolic functions.

Animal and human studies have demonstrated a reduction in mucosal mass and cellular proliferation as well as a decrease in villous height and brush border enzymes.[8] The production of intestinal sIgA rapidly diminishes,[9] and there is also a decrease in the production of counterinflammatory cytokines interleukin 4 and interleukin 10 with a shift toward helper T-cell subtype 1 proinflammatory cytokines.[10] Bacterial overgrowth from stasis and the altered mucosal defenses lead to bacterial translocation, which can be further exacerbated by the loss of structural integrity and increased gut permeability observed during gut disuse.[8]

DETERMINATION OF NUTRITIONAL SUPPORT

Critical illness and its treatment can profoundly alter metabolism and significantly increase resting energy expenditure (REE). Trauma, surgery, burns, brain injury, and pancreatitis have all been associated with hypermetabolism,[11,12] with reported relative metabolic rates of 116% to 158% in multiply injured patients.[12]

Accurate determination of REE is necessary in patients receiving nutritional support to ensure that their energy needs are met and to avoid the complications associated with either overfeeding or underfeeding. Several methods exist to predict patient's nutritional requirement, including the use of indirect calorimetry, as determined by a metabolic cart; several mathematical formulas; and weight-based predictors. Weight-based predictors of nutritional requirements have been proposed by 2 major consensus groups, although the recommendations differ. The American College of Chest Physicians recommends 25 kcal/kg based on the actual weight.[13] In contrast, the American Society for Parenteral and Enteral Nutrition (ASPEN) guidelines suggest that catabolic patients have caloric needs that generally fall between 25 and 30 total kcal/kg.[14] In a recent study of patients in a surgical critical care unit, indirect calorimetry correlated with 30 kcal/kg or with the predicted REE as calculated by the Harris Benedict equation adjusted with a factor of 1.5.[15]

As nutritional support is implemented, a monitoring strategy should also be implemented to assess the efficacy of nutritional replacement. Although scientific evidence is lacking, it seems that nitrogen balance provides the best assessment of nutritional support in catabolic patients.[16] However, the use of urinary urea nitrogen has been shown to lead to significant overestimation of nitrogen balance in burn patients.[17] Given these findings, multiple diagnostic tests have been proposed to monitor the response to nutritional support. By far, the most commonly assayed serum proteins used in nutritional monitoring are prealbumin, transferrin, and retinol-binding protein.[18–20] Although transferrin, which has a half-life of 8 to 10 days, is often used to assess nutritional support, the 2 studies in the literature have failed to support its use.[21,22] Prealbumin has been shown to accurately reflect changes in nitrogen balance in both burn and trauma patients.[23–25] Acute inflammation can, however, depress prealbumin levels regardless of nutritional status.[26,27] C-reactive protein (CRP) is a known indicator of inflammation with an inverse relationship to prealbumin.[26,27] Increased production of interleukin 6 with resultant stimulation of hepatic acute phase reactants has been proposed as the mechanism responsible for increased CRP levels, particularly in obese individuals.[28,29]

ENTERAL VERSUS PARENTERAL NUTRITIONAL SUPPORT

Enteral feeding is widely accepted as the preferred route of nutritional support. Compared with parenteral nutrition, enteral nutrition is cheaper, safer, and more physiologic and has less metabolic complications. Many of the changes seen with GI tract disuse are alleviated by enteral but not parenteral nutrition.[30] Significant controversy, however, exists regarding the role of parenteral nutrition in patients who are unable to tolerate enteral feeds.

Both nutritional routes have unique sets of associated complications. Enteral feeding tubes can cause sinusitis as well as nasal, pharyngeal, and upper GI trauma during their insertion. Tube feeding–related diarrhea can lead to fluid and electrolyte losses.[31] Furthermore, unrecognized or underappreciated malabsorption of enteral feeds can further compromise the nutritional status. Parenteral nutrition, which does not rely on GI tract absorption, is associated with vascular access complications, such as catheter-related blood stream infections, pneumothorax, and hemorrhage. In addition, parenteral nutrition is associated with bacterial translocation, hepatic steatosis, abnormal liver function test results, and disuse-induced changes in the GI tract. Both routes share metabolic complications such as hyperglycemia, electrolyte derangements, and refeeding syndrome, although these are often more pronounced with parenteral nutrition.[31]

Over the past 3 decades, several studies and meta-analyses have compared enteral and parenteral nutrition in varying patient populations (medical, surgical, and trauma patients). A meta-analysis performed by Braunschweig and colleagues[32] (1033 patients in 20 studies) demonstrated no difference in mortality but an increased incidence of infections in the parenteral group. Similar conclusions were drawn by Gramlich and colleagues[33] (856 patients in 13 studies), Peter and colleagues[34] (2430 patients in 30 patients), and Koretz and colleagues[35] (2005 patients in 32 studies). Conversely, Simpson and Doig[36] published a meta-analysis in 2005 (559 patients in 9 studies) that reported a lower mortality in the parenteral group despite a higher infection rate. However, concerns have also been raised that methodological weakness and heterogeneous patient populations make the conclusions of currently available meta-analyses clinically irrevelant.[31]

Parenteral nutrition has also been compared with standard therapy, that is, no artificial nutritional support. In aggregate analysis, the standard therapy group had a statistically significant reduction in infections (relative risk [RR], 0.77), with even greater reduction (RR, 0.61) seen in patients who were preoperatively well nourished,[32] as well as a reduction in hospital length of stay.[37] These findings were, however, reversed in patients with a preexisting protein-calorie malnutrition, with a reduction (RR, 0.52) in major complications in the parenteral group, thus suggesting a possible role for parenteral nutrition in malnourished patients unable to tolerate enteral feeds.[37]

The controversy regarding the use of parenteral nutrition is reflected in the current recommended guidelines; both the ASPEN and the European Society for Parenteral and Enteral Nutrition (ESPEN) recommend holding parenteral nutrition for up to 7 to 10 days in well-nourished patients who are unable to tolerate enteral nutrition but recommend starting it within 24 to 48 hours in malnourished patients.[1,38]

TIMING OF ENTERAL NUTRITION SUPPORT

Historically, postoperative patients were kept nil per os until the return of bowel function. Although there is evidence that this strategy is unnecessary,[38] many patients, especially those who are well nourished and have uncomplicated hospital course, can tolerate it. However, malnourished or critically ill patients who are expected to have a complicated hospital course require early nutritional support.

Patients who are preoperatively identified as severely malnourished and in whom surgery can be safely postponed benefit from preoperative nutritional support for 7 to 14 days.[39,40] In critically ill patients with a functioning GI tract, current practice guidelines recommend starting enteral nutrition within 48 hours of admission.[8] A 2001 meta-analysis of 738 patients in 15 studies examined early versus delayed enteral nutrition support and demonstrated that early nutrition was associated with lower risk of infection (RR, 0.45) as well as reduced hospital length of stay (mean reduction, 2.2 days).[41] A more recent systematic review of studies of early enteral nutrition (within 24 hours) in patients who underwent intestinal surgery demonstrated a significant reduction in mortality (RR, 0.42) with no effect on the anastomotic leak rate.[42] Furthermore, early enteral nutrition in patients with open abdomen has been associated with earlier abdominal closure and lower incidence of fistula formation.[43,44]

IMMUNONUTRITION

Surgery and trauma induce extensive changes in both the innate and adaptive immune systems. The initial response, which seems to be adaptive and is widely conserved across multiple species, is local inflammation. The inflammation can, however, become systemic (systemic inflammatory response syndrome) and result in multiple organ dysfunction syndrome if unchecked. Perturbations of immune function can also predispose the host to opportunistic infections.[45] Immunonutrition attempts to modulate these potentially adverse alterations in immune function through administration of specific parenteral and enteral nutrients. At present, the most extensively evaluated immunonutritients include arginine, glutamine, and ω-3 polyunsaturated long-chain fatty acids (FAs).

Arginine is normally a nonessential amino acid that can become conditionally essential during critical illness.[46] In pharmaceutical doses, arginine enhances the secretion of anabolic hormones, such as growth hormone, insulin-like growth factor, and prolactin. Arginine also supports immune function and serves as a precursor for synthesis of nitric oxide.[8,46] After trauma or major surgery, arginine deficiency syndrome can develop marked by impairment of adaptive immune response secondary to T-cell receptor abnormalities. In septic patients, arginine levels are more variable and likely depend on the stage of sepsis. These levels are lowest in early stages and then increase progressively as the severity of sepsis worsens.[47] Fish oil (ω-3) acts synergistically by inhibiting arginase 1 and thus increasing plasma arginine levels.

The clinical evidence and society guidelines supporting the use of arginine are mixed and may depend on the underlying disease. A meta-analysis published in 2001 noted adverse effects of arginine in septic patients.[48] A subsequent meta-analysis demonstrated that arginine supplementation in surgical patients had beneficial effects on the rate of infections, ventilator days, as well as intensive care unit (ICU) and total length of stay; the benefits, however, did not again extend to septic patients.[46,49] The Canadian Clinical Practice Guidelines presently do not recommend the use of arginine in any patient group and draw attention to the potential harm in septic patients. The ESPEN, the Society of Critical Care Medicine, and the ASPEN also note the potential harm in severely septic patients but also identify potential benefits in patients who underwent elective surgery and trauma patients.[46]

Humans possess only limited capacity, which is further diminished during acute illness, to synthesize ω-3 FAs, including eicosapentaenoic acid, docosahexaenoic acid, and alpha-linolenic acid. ω-3 FAs have multiple antiinflammatory properties that may be helpful in critically ill patients. These properties include reduction in the synthesis of proinflammatory eicosanoids, reduction in leukocyte and platelet-adhesive endothelial interactions, inhibition of inflammatory gene expression, and stimulation of glutathione production, which can decrease oxidative injury.[50–52]

ω-3 FAs have been most widely studied in patients with acute lung injury (ALI) and acute respiratory distress syndrome (ARDS); studies in other patient populations are limited. Three randomized clinical trials have demonstrated significant reduction in ventilator days and ICU and hospital length of stay as well as a decrease in the incidence of organ failure in mechanically ventilated patients with ALI/ARDS.[53–55] A subsequent small phase 2 trial, however, failed to show similar results.[56] A recent review concluded that there is insufficient evidence to make definitive recommendations about the routine use of ω-3 FAs in critically ill patients.[57]

Glutamine is the most abundant amino acid in the body and serves as a major fuel source for macrophages, lymphocytes, and enterocytes. As a precursor of glutathione, glutamine functions as an antioxidant. It is also involved in intracellular signaling, enhances heat shock protein expression, prevents apoptosis, and attenuates inflammation.[58] Glutamine is conditionally essential in catabolic stress states because stores of glutamine can become rapidly depleted. Deficiency may lead to impaired immunologic function and breakdown of the intestinal epithelial border function.[8]

In animal studies and clinical trials, exogenous glutamine administration has been demonstrated to restore GI mucosal integrity and decrease bacterial transloca-tion.[59] In burn patients, enteral glutamine supplementation has been shown to decrease infections and reduce the length of stay.[60,61] In 2002, Novak and col-leagues[62] reviewed all available trials of glutamine and concluded that glutamine supplementation reduced infectious complications and length of hospital stay in patients who underwent elective general surgery and possibly reduced complica-tions and mortality in critically ill patients. An updated meta-analysis published online (www.criticalcarenutrition.com) concluded that enteral glutamine should be considered in burn and trauma patients but that there were insufficient data to support its use in other critically ill patients.

PROBIOTICS

The human body exists in a commensal or symbiotic relationship with numerous colo-nizing microorganisms. These relationships may contribute to the host well-being, and therapeutic manipulation of these relationships through the use of probiotics has been attempted in several diseases, including the postoperative state. Probiotics are defined by the World Health Organization as "live organisms which provide benefit to the host when provided in an adequate quantities."[63] The term encompasses multiple organisms, including various lactobacillus species, Saccharomyces boulardii, and bifidobacteria strains.

Multiple organisms and combinations of organisms have been studied both in vitro and in vivo. Interpretation of available studies in the literature is, however, complicated by incomplete identification of used probiotic strains as well as controversy regarding the use of combination of organisms (because the organisms may act differently in isolation vs in combination).[63] The mechanisms of action likely vary with each specific organism as well as with each disease state. Proposed mechanisms include mainte-nance of appropriate host-microbe interactions, pathogen exclusion, modulation of epithelial barrier function, mucous secretion, activation of host immune system, and production of antibacterial factors.[63]

Randomized clinical trials of probiotics have demonstrated decreases in severity and duration of infectious diarrhea,[64,65] prevention of antibiotic-associated diar-rhea,[66,67] reduction in mortality in necrotizing enterocolitis,[68] and possibly prevention of Clostridium difficile infection. In a recent review article summarizing the published clinical trials of probiotics in patients with surgical, trauma, and acute pancreatitis, probiotics led to a significant reduction in bacterial infection rates in 8 of the 12 studies.[69] However, in one of the studies, patients with acute pancreatitis treated with probiotics had a significantly higher mortality rate secondary to an increased rate of bowel ischemia.[70]

Although the current evidence suggests that probiotics may have a role in postop-erative nutritional support of surgical patients, there are still many questions to be answered before their use can be widely recommended. Further studies are necessary to identify the specific agents for the specific disease states and patient populations.

ANABOLIC STEROIDS AND GROWTH FACTOR THERAPY

Anabolic steroids and other hormones have been studied as adjunctive therapies to modulate the typical catabolic state following severe injury and major surgery. The most studied agents include recombinant human growth hormone, oxandrolone, and megestrol acetate.

Growth hormone is a peptide released from the pituitary gland that stimulates the production of insulin-like growth factor 1 and thus suppresses proteolysis and increases protein synthesis, muscle growth, and lipolysis. At present, indications approved by the Food and Drug Administration for recombinant growth hormone include human immunodeficiency virus (HIV) wasting syndrome, total parenteral nutrition dependent short bowel syndrome, and pediatric chronic kidney disease. In addition, small studies have demonstrated improvement in lean body mass in malnourished patients with chronic obstructive pulmonary disease. The evidence in surgical patients is limited. A small study of 14 patients on long-term nutritional support for severe GI dysfunction published in 1993 demonstrated improvement in lean body mass and protein synthesis.[71] However, 2 subsequent prospective trials showed that administration of recombinant growth hormone in critically ill patients was associated with increased morbidity and mortality because of multiorgan failure, septic shock, and infection.[72]

Megestrol acetate, a synthetic progesterone, has been demonstrated to stimulate appetite and cause weight gain in patients with cancer.[73] The exact mechanism of action and optimal dose are unknown, but the weight gain seems to be mainly secondary to an increase in body fat and not lean body mass.[74,75] Megestrol acetate increases the risk of thromboembolic complications, especially at higher doses, and can induce transient adrenal insufficiency.[74] Data evaluating its effectiveness in surgical patients are limited.

Oxandrolone is an enterally administered synthetic derivative of testosterone that has 10 times more anabolic effects and only 10% of the adverse androgenic effects of testosterone. This anabolic steroid stimulates protein synthesis, counters the catabolic effects of cortisol through competitive inhibition of the glucocorticoid receptor, increases intracellular amino acid influx and use, and improves efficiency of skeletal muscle protein synthesis.[76] Oxandrolone has been studied in several catabolic disease states, including burn injury, trauma, HIV-related wasting, and neuromuscular disorders. In several small but prospective randomized studies in patients with severe burn injury, oxandrolone decreased weight loss and nitrogen loss and improved wound healing time without a significant difference in the rate of complications.[76] However, in trauma patients and in ventilator-dependent surgical patients, oxandrolone administration does not seem to be beneficial.[77,78] Oxandrolone was well tolerated in most studies with the most common side effect of mild increases in aspartate transaminase, alkaline transaminase, and alkaline phosphatase levels.

SUMMARY

Nutritional support in surgical patients has evolved from simple provision of adequate calories to retard loss of lean body mass to the provision of specific nutrients in an attempt to manipulate metabolic and immune responses. Although still limited, the current understanding of this complex subject indicates that the type, route, amount, and composition of nutritional support provided to patients can affect their outcome. Further studies are, however, needed to better characterize the exact nutritional support that is most beneficial for a specific disease state and a specific patient.

REFERENCES

1. Martindale RG, McClave SA, Vanek VW, et al. Guidelines for the provision and assessment of nutrition support therapy in the adult critically ill patient: society of critical care medicine and American Society for Parenteral and Enteral Nutrition: executive summary. Crit Care Med 2009;37(5):1757–61.

2. Scurlock C, Mechanick JI. Early nutrition support in the intensive care unit: a US perspective. Curr Opin Clin Nutr Metab Care 2008;11(2):152–5.

3. Cerantola Y, Grass F, Cristaudi A, et al. Perioperative nutrition in abdominal surgery: recommendations and reality. Gastroenterol Res Pract 2011;2011: 739347.

4. Delville CL. Are your patients at nutritional risk? Nurse Pract 2008;33(2):36–9.

5. Beck FK, Rosenthal TC. Prealbumin: a marker for nutritional evaluation. Am Fam Physician 2002;65(8):1575–8.

6. Kondrup J, Rasmussen HH, Hamberg O, et al. Nutritional risk screening (NRS 2002): a new method based on an analysis of controlled clinical trials. Clin Nutr 2003;22(3):321–36.

7. Neelemaat F, Meijers J, Kruizenga H, et al. Comparison of five malnutrition screening tools in one hospital inpatient sample. J Clin Nurs 2011;20(15–16): 2144–52.

8. Gerlach AT, Murphy C. An update on nutrition support in the critically ill. J Pharm Pract 2011;24(1):70–7.

9. King BK, Li J, Kudsk KA. A temporal study of TPN-induced changes in gut-associated lymphoid tissue and mucosal immunity. Arch Surg 1997;132(12): 1303–9.

10. Kudsk KA. Current aspects of mucosal immunology and its influence by nutrition. Am J Surg 2002;183(4):390–8.

11. Flancbaum L, Choban PS, Sambucco S, et al. Comparison of indirect calorimetry, the Fick method, and prediction equations in estimating the energy requirements of critically ill patients. Am J Clin Nutr 1999;69(3):461–6.

12. Frankenfield DC, Smith JS, Cooney RN, et al. Relative association of fever and injury with hypermetabolism in critically ill patients. Injury 1997;28(9–10):617–21.

13. Alexander E, Susla GM, Burstein AH, et al. Retrospective evaluation of commonly used equations to predict energy expenditure in mechanically ventilated, critically ill patients. Pharmacotherapy 2004;24(12):1659–67.

14. ASPEN Board of Directors and the Clinical Guidelines Task Force. Guidelines for the use of parenteral and enteral nutrition in adult and pediatric patients. JPEN J Parenter Enteral Nutr 2002;26(Suppl 1):1SA–138SA.

15. Davis KA, Kinn T, Esposito TJ, et al. Nutritional gain versus financial gain: the role of metabolic carts in the surgical ICU. J Trauma 2006;61(6):1436–40.

16. Manning EM, Shenkin A. Nutritional assessment in the critically ill. Crit Care Clin 1995;11(3):603–34.

17. Konstantinides FN, Radmer WJ, Becker WK, et al. Inaccuracy of nitrogen balance determinations in thermal injury with calculated total urinary nitrogen. J Burn Care Rehabil 1992;13(2 Pt 1):254–60.

18. Winkler MF, Gerrior SA, Pomp A, et al. Use of retinol-binding protein and prealbumin as indicators of the response to nutrition therapy. J Am Diet Assoc 1989; 89(5):684–7.

19. Spiekerman AM. Proteins used in nutritional assessment. Clin Lab Med 1993; 13(2):353–69.

20. Brose L. Prealbumin as a marker of nutritional status. J Burn Care Rehabil 1990; 11(4):372–5.

21. Lown D. Use and efficacy of a nutrition protocol for patients with burns in intensive care. J Burn Care Rehabil 1991;12(4):371–6.

22. Clark MA, Hentzen BT, Plank LD, et al. Sequential changes in insulin-like growth factor 1, plasma proteins, and total body protein in severe sepsis and multiple injury. JPEN J Parenter Enteral Nutr 1996;20(5):363–70.

23. Boosalis MG, Ott L, Levine AS, et al. Relationship of visceral proteins to nutritional status in chronic and acute stress. Crit Care Med 1989;17(8):741–7.
24. Erstad BL, Campbell DJ, Rollins CJ, et al. Albumin and prealbumin concentrations in patients receiving postoperative parenteral nutrition. Pharmacotherapy 1994;14(4):458–62.
25. Vehe KL, Brown RO, Kuhl DA, et al. The prognostic inflammatory and nutritional index in traumatized patients receiving enteral nutrition support. J Am Coll Nutr 1991;10(4):355–63.
26. Robinson MK, Trujillo EB, Mogensen KM, et al. Improving nutritional screening of hospitalized patients: the role of prealbumin. JPEN J Parenter Enteral Nutr 2003; 27(6):389–95 [quiz: 439].
27. Devoto G, Gallo F, Marchello C, et al. Prealbumin serum concentrations as a useful tool in the assessment of malnutrition in hospitalized patients. Clin Chem 2006;52(12):2281–5.
28. Visser M, Bouter LM, McQuillan GM, et al. Elevated C-reactive protein levels in overweight and obese adults. JAMA 1999;282(22):2131–5.
29. Greenfield JR, Samaras K, Jenkins AB, et al. Obesity is an important determinant of baseline serum C-reactive protein concentration in monozygotic twins, independent of genetic influences. Circulation 2004;109(24): 3022–8.
30. Turner P. Providing optimal nutritional support on the intensive care unit: key challenges and practical solutions. Proc Nutr Soc 2010;69(4):574–81.
31. Thomson A. The enteral vs parenteral nutrition debate revisited. JPEN J Parenter Enteral Nutr 2008;32(4):474–81.
32. Braunschweig CL, Levy P, Sheean PM, et al. Enteral compared with parenteral nutrition: a meta-analysis. Am J Clin Nutr 2001;74(4):534–42.
33. Gramlich L, Kichian K, Pinilla J, et al. Does enteral nutrition compared to parenteral nutrition result in better outcomes in critically ill adult patients? A systematic review of the literature. Nutrition 2004;20(10):843–8.
34. Peter JV, Moran JL, Phillips-Hughes J. A metaanalysis of treatment outcomes of early enteral versus early parenteral nutrition in hospitalized patients. Crit Care Med 2005;33(1):213–20 [discussion: 260–1].
35. Koretz RL, Avenell A, Lipman TO, et al. Does enteral nutrition affect clinical outcome? A systematic review of the randomized trials. Am J Gastroenterol 2007;102(2):412–29 [quiz: 468].
36. Simpson F, Doig GS. Parenteral vs. enteral nutrition in the critically ill patient: a meta-analysis of trials using the intention to treat principle. Intensive Care Med 2005;31(1):12–23.
37. Heyland DK, MacDonald S, Keefe L, et al. Total parenteral nutrition in the critically ill patient: a meta-analysis. JAMA 1998;280(23):2013–9.
38. Braga M, Ljungqvist O, Soeters P, et al. ESPEN guidelines on parenteral nutrition: surgery. Clin Nutr 2009;28(4):378–86.
39. Huhmann MB, August DA. Nutrition support in surgical oncology. Nutr Clin Pract 2009;24(4):520–6.
40. Weimann A, Braga M, Harsanyi L, et al. ESPEN guidelines on enteral nutrition: surgery including organ transplantation. Clin Nutr 2006;25(2):224–44.
41. Marik PE, Zaloga GP. Early enteral nutrition in acutely ill patients: a systematic review. Crit Care Med 2001;29(12):2264–70.
42. Lewis SJ, Andersen HK, Thomas S. Early enteral nutrition within 24 h of intestinal surgery versus later commencement of feeding: a systematic review and meta-analysis. J Gastrointest Surg 2009;13(3):569–75.

43. Collier B, Guillamondegui O, Cotton B, et al. Feeding the open abdomen. JPEN J Parenter Enteral Nutr 2007;31(5):410–5.
44. Dissanaike S, Pham T, Shalhub S, et al. Effect of immediate enteral feeding on trauma patients with an open abdomen: protection from nosocomial infections. J Am Coll Surg 2008;207(5):690–7.
45. Maung A, Fujimi S, MacConmara M, et al. Injury enhances resistance to Escherichia coli infection by boosting innate immune system function. J Immunol 2008; 180(4):2450–8.
46. Mizock BA. Immunonutrition and critical illness: an update. Nutrition 2010; 26(7–8):701–7.
47. Chiarla C, Giovannini I, Siegel JH. Plasma arginine correlations in trauma and sepsis. Amino Acids 2006;30(1):81–6.
48. Heyland DK, Novak F. Immunonutrition in the critically ill patient: more harm than good? JPEN J Parenter Enteral Nutr 2001;25(Suppl 2):S51–5 [discussion: S55–6].
49. Suchner U, Heyland DK, Peter K. Immune-modulatory actions of arginine in the critically ill. Br J Nutr 2002;87(Suppl 1):S121–32.
50. Mizock BA, DeMichele SJ. The acute respiratory distress syndrome: role of nutritional modulation of inflammation through dietary lipids. Nutr Clin Pract 2004; 19(6):563–74.
51. Serhan CN, Gotlinger K, Hong S, et al. Resolvins, docosatrienes, and neuroprotectins, novel omega-3-derived mediators, and their aspirin-triggered endogenous epimers: an overview of their protective roles in catabasis. Prostaglandins Other Lipid Mediat 2004;73(3–4):155–72.
52. Glatzle J, Kasparek MS, Mueller MH, et al. Enteral immunonutrition during sepsis prevents pulmonary dysfunction in a rat model. J Gastrointest Surg 2007;11(6): 719–24.
53. Gadek JE, DeMichele SJ, Karlstad MD, et al. Effect of enteral feeding with eicosapentaenoic acid, gamma-linolenic acid, and antioxidants in patients with acute respiratory distress syndrome. Enteral Nutrition in ARDS Study Group. Crit Care Med 1999;27(8):1409–20.
54. Singer P, Theilla M, Fisher H, et al. Benefit of an enteral diet enriched with eicosapentaenoic acid and gamma-linolenic acid in ventilated patients with acute lung injury. Crit Care Med 2006;34(4):1033–8.
55. Pontes-Arruda A, Aragão AM, Albuquerque JD. Effects of enteral feeding with eicosapentaenoic acid, gamma-linolenic acid, and antioxidants in mechanically ventilated patients with severe sepsis and septic shock. Crit Care Med 2006; 34(9):2325–33.
56. Stapleton RD, Martin TR, Weiss NS, et al. A phase II randomized placebo-controlled trial of omega-3 fatty acids for the treatment of acute lung injury. Crit Care Med 2011;39(7):1655–62.
57. Martin JM, Stapleton RD. Omega-3 fatty acids in critical illness. Nutr Rev 2010; 68(9):531–41.
58. Avenell A. Hot topics in parenteral nutrition. Current evidence and ongoing trials on the use of glutamine in critically-ill patients and patients undergoing surgery. Proc Nutr Soc 2009;68(3):261–8.
59. Marik PE, Zaloga GP. Immunonutrition in critically ill patients: a systematic review and analysis of the literature. Intensive Care Med 2008;34(11):1980–90.
60. Garrel D, Patenaude J, Nedelec B, et al. Decreased mortality and infectious morbidity in adult burn patients given enteral glutamine supplements: a prospective, controlled, randomized clinical trial. Crit Care Med 2003;31(10): 2444–9.

61. Zhou YP, Jiang ZM, Sun YH, et al. The effect of supplemental enteral glutamine on plasma levels, gut function, and outcome in severe burns: a randomized, double-blind, controlled clinical trial. JPEN J Parenter Enteral Nutr 2003;27(4):241–5.
62. Novak F, Heyland DK, Avenell A, et al. Glutamine supplementation in serious illness: a systematic review of the evidence. Crit Care Med 2002;30(9):2022–9.
63. Gareau MG, Sherman PM, Walker WA. Probiotics and the gut microbiota in intestinal health and disease. England. Nat Rev Gastroenterol Hepatol 2010;7:503–14.
64. Chen CC, Kong MS, Lai MW, et al. Probiotics have clinical, microbiologic, and immunologic efficacy in acute infectious diarrhea. Pediatr Infect Dis J 2010; 29(2):135–8.
65. Pedone CA, Bernabeu AO, Postaire ER, et al. The effect of supplementation with milk fermented by Lactobacillus casei (strain DN-114 001) on acute diarrhoea in children attending day care centres. Int J Clin Pract 1999;53(3):179–84.
66. Szajewska H, Ruszczynski M, Radzikowski A. Probiotics in the prevention of antibiotic-associated diarrhea in children: a meta-analysis of randomized controlled trials. United States. J Pediatr 2006;149:367–72.
67. Ruszczynski M, Radzikowski A, Szajewska H. Clinical trial: effectiveness of Lactobacillus rhamnosus (strains E/N, Oxy and Pen) in the prevention of antibiotic-associated diarrhoea in children. England. Aliment Pharmacol Ther 2008;28: 154–61.
68. Alfaleh K, Anabrees J, Bassler D. Probiotics reduce the risk of necrotizing enterocolitis in preterm infants: a meta-analysis. Neonatology 2009;97(2):93–9.
69. Rayes N, Soeters PB. Probiotics in surgical and critically ill patients. Ann Nutr Metab 2010;57(Suppl):29–31.
70. Besselink MG, van Santvoort HC, Buskens E, et al. Probiotic prophylaxis in predicted severe acute pancreatitis: a randomised, double-blind, placebo-controlled trial. Lancet 2008;371(9613):651–9.
71. Byrne TA, Morrissey TB, Gatzen C, et al. Anabolic therapy with growth hormone accelerates protein gain in surgical patients requiring nutritional rehabilitation. Ann Surg 1993;218(4):400–16 [discussion: 416–8].
72. Takala J, Ruokonen E, Webster NR, et al. Increased mortality associated with growth hormone treatment in critically ill adults. N Engl J Med 1999;341(11): 785–92.
73. Berenstein EG, Ortiz Z. Megestrol acetate for the treatment of anorexia-cachexia syndrome. Cochrane Database Syst Rev 2005;2:CD004310.
74. Gullett NP, Hebbar G, Ziegler TR. Update on clinical trials of growth factors and anabolic steroids in cachexia and wasting. Am J Clin Nutr 2010;91(4):1143S–7S.
75. Madeddu C, Mantovani G. An update on promising agents for the treatment of cancer cachexia. Curr Opin Support Palliat Care 2009;3(4):258–62.
76. Miller JT, Btaiche IF. Oxandrolone treatment in adults with severe thermal injury. Pharmacotherapy 2009;29(2):213–26.
77. Gervasio JM, Dickerson RN, Swearingen J, et al. Oxandrolone in trauma patients. Pharmacotherapy 2000;20(11):1328–34.
78. Bulger EM, Jurkovich GJ, Farver CL, et al. Oxandrolone does not improve outcome of ventilator dependent surgical patients. Ann Surg 2004;240(3): 472–8 [discussion: 478–80].

Surgical Prophylaxis and Other Complication Avoidance Care Bundles

Steven J. Schwulst, MD[a], John E. Mazuski, MD, PhD[b],*

KEYWORDS

• Bundle • Standardization • Quality • Surgical site infection

Care bundles are a collection of standardized clinical practices that have been individually shown to improve patient outcome. When implemented together, they are believed to result in a superior outcome compared with implementation of individual measures by themselves. The concept of care bundles was developed by the Institute for Healthcare Improvement (IHI) to improve the reliability of delivery of essential health care processes.[1] Their expressed purpose was to reduce practice variation and simultaneously improve overall quality of care and outcomes.[2]

Consistent application of strict hand hygiene and use of rounding checklists are 2 examples of practices that can individually decrease patient morbidity and mortality, as well as overall health care expenditures.[3,4] However, the concept of bundled care is relatively new. The groundwork for the concept was initially laid by Berenholtz and colleagues,[5] who identified 6 evidence-based interventions that could together improve the outcome of patients in intensive care units. The IHI combined several of these interventions into what became described as a "ventilator bundle."[6] The success of these and other care bundles led to their proliferation and use for a variety of indications.

However, the data surrounding the effectiveness of care bundles are mixed. It is important, then, that the clinician is able to assess the usefulness of a given care bundle for their specific health care setting before implementing it. To do so, the clinician must understand why the given components of the bundle were chosen, how these individual components are to be implemented together, and what is the expected result of implementation of the bundle; preferably, the last of these will have been evaluated through a methodologically sound research study.

The authors have nothing to disclose.
[a] Division of Trauma and Critical Care, Department of Surgery, Northwestern University Feinberg School of Medicine, 676 North Saint Clair Street, Suite 650, Chicago, IL 60611, USA
[b] Section of Acute and Critical Care Surgery, Department of Surgery, Washington University School of Medicine, Campus Box 8109, 660 South Euclid Avenue, St Louis, MO 63110, USA
* Corresponding author.
E-mail address: mazuskij@wudosis.wustl.edu

Surg Clin N Am 92 (2012) 285–305
doi:10.1016/j.suc.2012.01.011   surgical.theclinics.com

Currently, there are imperatives that make implementation of certain care bundles mandatory or nearly so. Payers, such as the Centers for Medicare and Medicaid Services, are increasingly monitoring compliance with bundles, both as a publicly reportable quality measure and as a tool to determine remuneration for certain medical services. Thus, use of care bundles is likely to increase in coming years, whether or not the efficacy of an individual bundle has been thoroughly tested in appropriate clinical settings.

DEVELOPMENT AND IMPLEMENTATION OF CARE BUNDLES

The development of a new care bundle is theoretically uncomplicated. As described by Fulbrook and colleagues,[7] the 6 essential steps are:

1. Identify a care theme
2. Identify a cluster of practices within a theme
3. Identify the relevant research supporting the practices
4. Categorize the research by quality
5. Delete practices for which there is inadequate evidence
6. Group the adequately evidence-based practices into a bundle.

Once a new care bundle has been developed, it is recommended that the bundle be introduced into clinical practice in carefully managed plan-do-study-act (PDSA) cycles, such that the change in practice is accepted.[8] It is critical that a multidisciplinary care team be involved in the PDSA cycles, such that all professional groups not only have an understanding of what the individual care bundle components are but also have a stake in promoting their comprehensive adoption.[9]

In the remainder of this article, the development, implementation, and usefulness of 4 different care bundles used in surgical patients are examined. These bundles relate to prevention of ventilator-associated pneumonia (VAP), prevention of central venous catheter (CVC)-related bloodstream infection, treatment of severe sepsis and septic shock, and prevention of surgical site infection (SSI).

VAP BUNDLE

VAP is the leading cause of death caused by nosocomial infection in critically ill patients, and is a particular problem for critically ill surgical patients.[10] Patients with VAP have increased mortality, longer lengths of stay, and higher costs. It is estimated that a single episode of VAP increases costs by approximately $40,000.[11] Care bundles have therefore been developed that target VAP as a preventable nosocomial infection.

As mentioned earlier, the IHI developed a ventilator bundle consisting of 4 evidence-based practices that had been shown to improve outcomes in patients undergoing mechanical ventilation.[6] The ventilator bundle consisted of the following:

1) Elevation of the head of the bed to 30° to 45°
2) Daily assessment of sedation and readiness for extubation
3) Prophylaxis against bleeding from gastric stress ulceration
4) Deep vein thrombosis (DVT) prophylaxis.

The use of this bundle by hospitals seemed to result in a significant reduction in rates of VAP. The 4 original components of the ventilator bundle were then modified and incorporated into what is now referred to as the "VAP bundle."[12]

Head of Bed Elevation

Elevation of the head of the bed is one of the cornerstones of the VAP bundle. It had been hypothesized that a semirecumbent position would decrease aspiration of gastrointestinal and oropharyngeal secretions, thereby decreasing the incidence of VAP.[13] By monitoring the appearance of radiolabeled gastric contents in endobronchial secretions of intubated patients, Torres and colleagues[14] showed significantly less aspiration of gastric contents in patients maintained in the semirecumbent position compared with patients maintained in the supine position. Drakulovic and colleagues[15] found lower rates of VAP in patients randomized to the semirecumbent position compared with patients randomized to the supine position. However, the optimal degree of elevation has not yet been determined. A recent prospective trial by van Nieuwenhoven and colleagues[16] reported no difference in VAP rates when a target semirecumbent position of 45° was used compared with an observed elevation of 10° to 30°.

Daily Assessment of Sedation and Readiness for Extubation

The number of days of mechanical ventilation is directly related to the risk of developing VAP.[10] Dries and colleagues[17] showed that standardizing use of daily sedation vacations and daily assessment of readiness to extubate into a single daily weaning protocol decreased the duration of mechanical ventilation and resulted in a nearly 2-fold decrease in the rate of VAP. Similarly, in the Awakening and Breathing Controlled Trial,[18] intervention patients managed with a standardized spontaneous awakening trial paired with a spontaneous breathing trial had an average of 3 ventilator-free days more than control patients. This finding was associated with a significant improvement in mortality; it was calculated that 1 life was saved for every 7 patients placed on the protocol. In practice, implementation of weaning protocols has not necessarily resulted in similar outcomes. In a multicenter observational study, the implementation of a daily weaning protocol in 10 different intensive care units resulted in only 55% of eligible patients being liberated from mechanical ventilation when they first passed a spontaneous breathing trial.[19] Thus, many patients were left intubated and remained at increased risk for VAP.

Prophylaxis Against Bleeding from Gastric Stress Ulceration and DVT

Prophylactic measures to prevent bleeding from stress ulceration and to prevent thromboembolic disease are commonly used in patients in the intensive care unit. Mechanical ventilation is recognized as a strong independent risk factor for bleeding from gastric stress ulceration.[20] However, controversy remains as to whether or not the type of pharmacologic therapy used as prophylaxis to prevent this bleeding influences rates of VAP. A recent meta-analysis[21] did suggest that stress ulcer prophylaxis using histamine-2-receptor antagonists resulted in higher rates of gastric colonization and VAP compared with prophylaxis using sucralfate. Likewise, mechanical ventilation is a strong predictor of venous thromboembolic disease.[22,23] The increased risk of DVT may be caused by decreased venous return to the heart during mechanical ventilation, although the patient's underlying disease process that prompted the need for mechanical ventilation is likely an important confounding factor.[24] As with prophylaxis against bleeding from stress ulceration, it is uncertain if prophylactic measures to prevent DVT have any direct impact on rates of VAP.[22,23] Nonetheless, it is likely that both of these prophylactic measures will be retained in VAP bundles for the foreseeable future, because they may lead to decreased complications associated with prolonged mechanical ventilation, even if they do not directly influence rates of VAP.[25]

Potential VAP Bundle Components

Although the VAP bundle included only the 4 components outlined earlier, there are other evidence-based practices that might also be considered for prevention of VAP. Two adjunctive practices for which some evidence exists are (1) oropharyngeal decontamination with chlorhexidine and (2) continuous aspiration of subglottic secretions. In prospective, randomized, controlled studies, oropharyngeal decontamination in general, and oropharyngeal decontamination with chlorhexidine in particular, were found to reduce rates of VAP.[26,27] Similarly, in randomized trials in cardiac surgical patients, continuous aspiration of subglottic secretions was noted to reduce the incidence of VAP.[28,29] These adjunctive measures might be included in VAP bundles in the future, as more evidence accumulates regarding their efficacy.

CVC BUNDLE

CVCs are commonly used in the care of critically ill surgical patients. CVCs allow estimation of intravascular volume by the measurement of central venous pressure (CVP), allow delivery of parenteral nutrition, vasoactive agents, and other pharmaceuticals that should not be administered through a peripheral intravenous line, and provide a route for intravenous access in patients whose peripheral veins have been exhausted. However, they are also a source of significant morbidity and mortality, the most important being CVC-related bloodstream infection (CRBSI). It has been estimated that there are as many as 250,000 such infections per year.[30] Conservative estimates of attributable mortality are 14,000 deaths per year, and the estimated cost per infection may be as high as $55,000.[31–33] There have been several published recommendations from professional societies pertaining to the prevention of CRBSI. In particular, the IHI recommends the following as part of a CVC bundle[34]:

1. Hand hygiene
2. Maximal barrier precautions on insertion
3. Chlorhexidine skin antisepsis
4. Optimal catheter site selection
5. Daily review of catheter necessity.

Use of various components of the IHI CVC bundle has led to substantial decreases in the rate of CRBSI; in various reports this reduction has ranged from 47% to 84%.[35]

Hand Hygiene

The importance of hand hygiene in American health care can be traced back to William Stewart Halsted, who was the first American surgeon to require use of strict hand hygiene and use of sterile gloves by all personnel in the operating theater.[36] Hand hygiene is equally important as the first step in preventing CRBSI.[37] Numerous studies[38,39] have documented that poor hand hygiene is a risk factor for the development of CRBSI. Rosenthal and colleagues[40] reported a 77% reduction in CRBSI with a hand hygiene intervention even although compliance with the intervention was noted only 64% of the time. Despite the convincing data on the importance of hand hygiene, it has been observed that physicians perform appropriate hand hygiene only half the time, which is significantly less often than that performed by other health care professionals.[41]

Maximal Barrier Precautions on Insertion

Halsted was also the first American surgeon to mandate full barrier precautions with sterile drapes, gowns, caps, and gloves in the American operating theater.[42] When applied to CVC insertion, use of full barrier precautions has also been shown to reduce rates of CRBSI. In 1 randomized trial comparing CVC insertion using full barrier precautions with CVC insertion using sterile gloves and a small sterile drape only, the rate of CRBSI was 6 times higher in patients who had catheters inserted using less than full barrier precautions.[43] Mermel and colleagues[44] showed a 2-fold decrease in the CRBSI rate in patients who had full barrier precautions used during CVC insertion compared with a control patient population. From an economic perspective, Hu and colleagues[45] estimated that at a cost of $40 per CVC insertion, full barrier precautions would save $252 per CVC placed by decreasing the rate of CRBSI.

Chlorhexidine Skin Antisepsis

The use of skin antisepsis followed use of diligent hand hygiene, sterile gloves, and full barrier precautions as an accepted practice to reduce the risk infection in the operating theater.[46] However, the optimal agent for skin antisepsis continues to be debated. Chlorhexidine has theoretic advantages over iodine-based skin antiseptics because of its longer duration of action as well as its ability to resist inactivation by blood and serum.[47] These theoretic advantages were supported by a meta-analysis[48] that reported that rates of CRBSI were reduced by half when chlorhexidine rather than an iodine-based skin antiseptic was used for site preparation. The investigators concluded that routine chlorhexidine use could prevent 11 CRBSIs for every 1000 CVCs placed. Even although chlorhexidine is more expensive than iodine-based skin antiseptics, it was estimated that an overall saving of $113 per CVC placed would accrue because of the decreased incidence of CRBSI associated with use of chlorhexidine.

Optimal Catheter Site Selection

The IHI CVC bundle indicates that femoral venous access should be avoided, and that the subclavian vein is the preferred site for venous cannulation.[34] As pointed out by Goede and Coopersmith,[49] there are no prospective, randomized trials to support this component of the bundle. However, 2 prospective, nonrandomized trials comparing femoral, internal jugular, and subclavian CVC positioning reported significantly higher rates of CRBSI at the femoral site; 1 of the 2 studies also showed a trend toward higher CRBSI rates with use of the internal jugular, compared with the subclavian site.[50,51] There are other studies that found no significant differences in CRBSI between the femoral, internal jugular, or subclavian sites.[52,53] However, despite these conflicting data, the IHI consensus opinion remains that the subclavian vein is the preferred first site for CVC insertion.[30]

Daily Review of Catheter Necessity

The final component of the IHI CVC bundle is a daily review of CVC necessity. This process was included in the CVC bundle because the risk of CRBSI is directly related to the amount of time the CVC is in place.[54] Because of this relationship, CVCs should be discontinued as soon as they are no longer clinically indicated. The daily assessment of the need for a CVC requires institution of an active intervention program. The impact of this type of preventative program was illustrated by the team at Johns Hopkins University, who were able to virtually eliminate CRBSI after implementation.[55] Although CVCs should be definitively removed when no longer clinically indicated, it is also important to note that there is no benefit to routine rotation of CVCs to other sites or to guidewire exchange of CVCs.[56,57]

SEPSIS BUNDLES

Over the past decade, there has been strong interest in the use of bundles for the treatment of septic patients, including those with surgical sepsis, in order to decrease the lethality associated with this disorder. The benefits of sepsis bundles were reported in a trial by Rivers and colleagues, in which a striking absolute reduction in mortality was realized from implementation of early goal-directed therapy (EGDT) in the emergency department.[58] EGDT has been a key component of the Surviving Sepsis Campaign, which first developed guidelines in 2004 aimed at improving outcomes in patients with severe sepsis and septic shock.[59] These guidelines were revised and updated in 2008.[60] Based on these guidelines, 2 sets of sepsis bundles have been created by the Surviving Sepsis Campaign: the Sepsis Resuscitation Bundle and the Sepsis Management Bundle. The Sepsis Resuscitation Bundle includes components that should be implemented and achieved within the first 6 hours of admission to the hospital, whereas the Sepsis Management Bundle relates to interventions that should take place within the first 24 hours of admission. The bundles identify specific physiologic or operational targets, such that compliance can be easily measured (**Box 1**).[61] Since these sepsis bundles have been developed, several studies have found a significant survival benefit associated with their implementation.[62–64]

Box 1
Sepsis bundles

Sepsis Resuscitation Bundle (6 hours):

1. Measure serum lactate concentration

2. Obtain blood cultures before antibiotic administration

3. Administer appropriate broad-spectrum antibiotic early

4. If there is hypotension or a serum lactate level >4 mmol/L:

   a. Initially treat with 20 mL/kg of crystalloid fluids

   b. Administer a vasopressor if a mean arterial pressure (MAP) of 65 mm Hg is not achieved after initial fluid resuscitation

5. If hypotension or an increased serum lactate level persists:

   a. Achieve a CVP of 8 mm Hg

   b. Achieve a central venous oxygen saturation (ScVo$_2$) of 70% or a mixed venous oxygen saturation of 65%

Sepsis Management Bundle (24 hours):

1. Maintain adequate glycemic control (blood glucose <180 mg/dL)

2. In mechanically ventilated patients, prevent excessive inspiratory plateau pressures of ≥30 cm H$_2$0

3. Administer low-dose corticosteroids according to the local protocol

4. Administer recombinant human activated protein C (rhAPC) according to the local protocol

Data from Marshall JC, Dellinger RP, Levy M. The Surviving Sepsis Campaign: a history and a perspective. Surg Infect (Larchmt) 2010;11:275–81; and Surviving Sepsis Campaign. Available at: http://www.survivingsepsis.org/Bundles/Pages/default.aspx. Accessed September 26, 2011.

The Sepsis Resuscitation Bundle (6-hour Bundle)

It is recommended that the Sepsis Resuscitation Bundle be initiated as soon as signs and symptoms of hypoperfusion in the septic patient are recognized. The first component of this bundle is the measurement of the serum lactic acid level as a relatively simple and rapid way of determining which patients need EGDT. Additional goals of this bundle include diagnosis using appropriate microbiologic cultures before antibiotic administration, administration of antibiotics as soon as possible after recognition that severe sepsis or septic shock exists, and EGDT with attainment of CVP, MAP, and ScVo$_2$ targets within 6 hours.[61]

Measurement of serum lactic acid concentrations

In the Sepsis Resuscitation Bundle, serum lactic acid levels are used to assess the need for and the response to EGDT.[60] Hyperlactic acidemia often accompanies severe sepsis and septic shock. Lactate levels more than 4 mmol/L, and the failure to clear lactate with resuscitation, are associated with worse outcomes.[65] A serum lactate level of 4 mmol/L or greater was used in the prospective trial of Rivers and colleagues[58] to identify patients for whom EGDT would be used.

Obtain microbiologic cultures before antimicrobial administration

The Surviving Sepsis Campaign guidelines from 2008 recommend obtaining appropriate microbiologic cultures before the initiation of antimicrobial therapy, provided that this does not unduly delay the administration of appropriate antibiotics.[60] This strategy is included as a component of the Sepsis Resuscitation Bundle. The rationale behind obtaining cultures before antibiotic therapy is that sterilization of cultures can occur within a few hours of giving antibiotics; this may in turn delay or preclude optimization and eventual de-escalation of antibiotic therapy.[66] The guidelines state that the cultures should consist of at least 2 blood cultures (with at least one coming from a peripheral puncture site), and quantitative cultures of respiratory tract secretions as well as other body fluids that may be a source of infection, such as urine, cerebrospinal fluid, or wounds.[67,68] If the patient is stable enough to undergo imaging studies, it is recommended that these studies be performed promptly so that a source of infection potentially amenable to an appropriate source control procedure can be identified.

Early initiation of appropriate antimicrobial therapy

A delay in the initiation of appropriate antimicrobial therapy in patients with sepsis is associated with an increase in mortality.[69,70] One study documented a measurable increase in mortality for every hour of delay in administering appropriate antibiotics in patients with septic shock.[71] The Surviving Sepsis Campaign guidelines also recommend that the choice of initial antimicrobial therapy include at least 1 agent effective against all likely pathogens. Therefore, in most cases of severe sepsis or septic shock, broad-spectrum therapy should be initiated until the causative organisms are identified. Adjustments to the antimicrobial regiment can be made at 48 to 72 hours, with the therapy being de-escalated if clinically indicated.[72] The target goal for this component of the Sepsis Resuscitation Bundle is administration of appropriate antimicrobial therapy within 3 hours of presentation to the emergency department, or within 1 hour of admission to an intensive care unit from somewhere other than the emergency department.[61]

EGDT

The remainder of the Sepsis Resuscitation Bundle focuses on goal-directed resuscitation of the septic patient. Use of intravenous fluids to resuscitate the patient is an important component of the early therapy for severe sepsis and septic shock. The

Surviving Sepsis Campaign guidelines recommend using the CVP to guide initial resuscitation. A goal CVP of 8 mm Hg or greater is recommended in nonmechanically ventilated patients, and a goal CVP of 12 mm Hg or greater in patients undergoing positive pressure ventilation. Fluid challenges using either natural colloid or crystalloid fluids are acceptable to meet this goal.[60] The Saline versus Albumin Fluid Evaluation (SAFE) trial published in 2004 reported no difference in mortality between patients resuscitated with natural colloid and those resuscitated with crystalloid fluids.[73] However, administration of synthetic colloids, such as hydroxyethyl starch, has been associated with an increased risk of renal failure in patients with sepsis.[74] The measurement target for this component of the Sepsis Resuscitation Bundle is an initial crystalloid fluid challenge of 20 mL/kg for patients who have either hypotension or a serum lactate 4.0 mmol/L or greater. If hypotension or an increased lactic acid level persists, a second goal is to achieve a CVP of 8 mm Hg or greater through further fluid resuscitation by the end of the initial 6-hour period.[61]

Another component of early EGDT is the use of vasopressors to attain a MAP of 65 mm Hg or greater in the event of systemic hypotension unresponsive to initial fluid resuscitation. In septic patients, it is believed that blood flow to the tissues becomes dependent on blood pressure if the MAP is less than 65 mm Hg.[75] Nonetheless, MAP goals should be adjusted based on individual patient requirements and comorbidities. For example, an elderly patient with severe long-standing hypertension may require a significantly higher MAP to maintain adequate blood flow, whereas an otherwise healthy young patient may tolerate a lower MAP. The initial vasopressor used should be norepinephrine or dopamine, according to the Surviving Sepsis Campaign guidelines; there is no high-level evidence to recommend one over the other. Vasopressin may be added in patients with shock refractory to catecholamines, although a large trial[76] reported no significant difference in mortality between patients receiving norepinephrine plus vasopressin compared with those receiving norepinephrine alone. The benchmark for this component of the Sepsis Resuscitation Bundle is use of vasopressors in patients who remain hypotensive (MAP <65 mm Hg) after initial administration of 20 mL/kg of crystalloid fluid.

The Surviving Sepsis Campaign guidelines recommend attempting to achieve an ScVo$_2$ of 70% or greater in patients with persistent hypotension or increased lactate levels; if a mixed venous oxygen saturation is measured, the target is 65%.[60] This end point is again one of the measurement targets of the Sepsis Resuscitation Bundle.[61] An ScVo$_2$ goal of 70% was included as a component of EGDT in the trial reported by Rivers and colleagues.[58] These data were further supported by a large meta-analysis, which suggested a 2-fold increase in survival in patients in whom the end point of resuscitation was an ScVo$_2$ of 70%.[77] When the target ScVo$_2$ of 70% cannot be achieved with fluid resuscitation alone, further recommended therapies include red blood cell transfusion to achieve a hematocrit of 30% or greater or the addition of a dobutamine infusion. However, the former suggestion must be weighed against other reported data, in which a trend toward increased survival was seen in critically ill patients who were transfused with packed red blood cells only if the hemoglobin concentration was less than 7 g/dL.[78]

Sepsis Management Bundle (24-hour Bundle)

The Sepsis Management Bundle, based on the Surviving Sepsis Campaign guidelines, should be implemented within the first 24 hours of admission.[60,61] This bundle consists of 4 main components: maintenance of adequate glycemic control, maintenance of lower ventilator plateau pressures, and administration of low-dose corticosteroids or rhAPC when appropriate. The data linking improved survival with use of this bundle are not as strong as they are with the Sepsis Resuscitation Bundle, although an initial large meta-analysis suggested that implementation of the Sepsis Management Bundle could lead to improved survival.[77] However, rhAPC has recently been withdrawn from the market by the manufacturer because of lack of efficacy, and is not included in current versions of the Sepsis Management Bundle.

Maintenance of adequate glycemic control

The goal for this component of the Sepsis Management Bundle is a blood glucose value greater than the upper limit of the normal range, but less than or equal to 180 mg/dL.[61] This goal has been modified from initial, stricter recommendations for glycemic control, which were based on studies by Van den Berghe and colleagues.[79,80] In those studies, critically ill patients randomized to receive intensive insulin treatment to maintain the blood glucose in the range of 80 to 110 mg/dL had improved overall survival compared with control patients receiving less intensive insulin regimens. However, high rates of hypoglycemia and adverse events were noted with use of such regimens outside the study environment. In the Normoglycemia in Intensive Care Evaluation and Survival Using Glucose Algorithm Regulation trial, critically ill patients were randomly assigned to a glucose target of 80 to 110 mg/dL versus 180 mg/dL or less; in this trial, patients randomized to the target glucose range of 80 to 110 mg/dL had a higher 90-day mortality compared with those randomized to the glucose target of 180 mg/dL or less.[81] These data prompted revision of the Surviving Sepsis Campaign guidelines, which now suggest that until more data are available, a more conservative blood glucose concentration target should be used for most septic patients. A meta-analysis based on an earlier blood glucose target did show that patients whose blood glucose concentrations were maintained in the 120 to 150 mg/dL range were 2.5 times more likely to survive than those who were not, confirming that some degree of glycemic control is likely beneficial for septic patients.[77]

Prevent excessive inspiratory plateau airway pressures in mechanically ventilated patients

Sepsis-induced acute lung injury/acute respiratory distress syndrome (ALI/ARDS) develops in nearly 50% of patients with severe sepsis or septic shock.[82] In patients with ALI/ARDS, inappropriate mechanical ventilation strategies may worsen lung inflammation and lead to further systemic inflammation and nonpulmonary organ dysfunction. The Sepsis Management Bundle includes maintenance of inspiratory plateau airway pressures of less than 30 cm H_2O as a target.[61] The rationale behind this component of the bundle derives from the Acute Respiratory Distress Syndrome Network (ARDSNet) trial, which reported a 9% decrease in all-cause mortality by using a pressure-limited ventilation strategy, with a target inspiratory plateau pressure of <30 cm H_2O.[83] In order to achieve this end point, the ARDSNet guidelines suggest ventilation with 6 mL/kg based on predicted body weight (PBW). However, even lower tidal volumes, as low as 4 mL/kg PBW, may be required in selected patients to achieve this lower pressure.

Administration of low-dose corticosteroids

The utilization of low-dose corticosteroids for sepsis remains controversial. The Surviving Sepsis Campaign guidelines now recommend their use in the setting of fluid and vasopressor-refractory septic shock.[60] Conflicting data have been published regarding the efficacy of these agents. A multicenter randomized controlled trial reported a significant decrease in mortality in patients with septic shock who received 50 mg of intravenous hydrocortisone 4 times daily and 50 μg of oral fludrocortisones once daily for 7 days compared with those receiving placebos, although the benefit seemed to be restricted to patients who failed to respond to adrenocorticotropin stimulation.[84] However, in a subsequent multicenter randomized controlled trial, use of hydrocortisone did not improve overall survival in patients with severe sepsis, although it did hasten the reversal of shock.[85] The Sepsis Management Bundle indicates that low-dose corticosteroid use should be based on a locally developed protocol, and that documentation should be provided as to why these agents were not used if local criteria for use were met.[61]

Administration of rhAPC (drotrecogin alfa activated)

As with the use of low-dose corticosteroids, there was considerable controversy regarding the use of rhAPC. The Surviving Sepsis Campaign guidelines suggested its use in patients who have associated multiple organ dysfunction or an Acute Physiology and Chronic Health Evaluation (APACHE) II score of 25 or greater, provided there were no contraindications to its use. Use of rhAPC was not recommended in patients with severe sepsis and a low risk of death, usually associated with an APACHE II score of 20 or less.[60] These recommendations were based on 2 large randomized controlled trials. The Recombinant Human Protein C Worldwide Evaluation in Severe Sepsis (PROWESS) study reported a 6.1% absolute reduction and a 19.4% relative reduction in the risk of death with administration of rhAPC in patients with severe sepsis and septic shock. However, several methodological concerns were expressed with respect to this trial. Further, the results suggested that the observed reduction in the risk of death was largely confined to subgroups of patients with APACHE II scores of 25 or greater or 2 or more organ failures.[86] The Administration of Drotrecogin Alfa in Early Stage Severe Sepsis (ADDRESS) trial included patients with severe sepsis but with a lower risk of death (APACHE II ≤20). This study reported higher mortality in the rhAPC group compared with the control group and was terminated early for futility.[87] Based on these data, the Sepsis Management Bundle indicates that rhAPC use should be according to a locally derived protocol, and that documentation should be provided as to why patients did not qualify for treatment with rhAPC.[61] As discussed earlier, this product is no longer available, but readers should be aware of the historical derivations of recommendations and trial data that preceded the product withdrawal.

SSI PREVENTION BUNDLES

A variety of approaches, including use of prophylactic antibiotics, have been shown to reduce the risk that a patient develops a postoperative SSI. Increasingly, use of these measures is being monitored as an indicator of the quality of surgical practice. Although not labeled as a bundle per se, the combination of these measures certainly constitutes a group of practices that would be expected to improve patient outcomes, and thus could be considered a bundle.

Several of these measures relate to the use of prophylactic antibiotics. Timing, appropriateness, and duration of prophylactic antibiotics were first monitored as part of an effort to decrease the incidence of SSI known as the Surgical Infection Prevention (SIP) project. These measures and additional ones are now included as part of the Surgical Care Improvement Project (SCIP). SCIP was developed jointly by several surgical and other organizations to reduce the rates of both infectious and noninfectious complications developing after surgical procedures.[88,89] However, there has been some debate as to the usefulness of the SCIP measures in reducing rates of SSI.

The SCIP components related to the prevention of surgical infections are listed in **Box 2**. Three components (SCIP INF 1, 2, and 3) are related to prophylactic antibiotics,

---

Box 2
SCIP: measures related to prevention of perioperative infections

SCIP INF 1: prophylactic antibiotics were administered within 1 hour before making the surgical incision (2 hours if using vancomycin or a fluoroquinolone)

SCIP INF 2: prophylactic antibiotics used were agents recommended for the specific surgical procedure

SCIP INF 3: prophylactic antibiotics were discontinued within 24 hours of the surgery end time (48 hours for cardiac surgical procedures)

SCIP INF 4: cardiac surgery patients had a controlled postoperative glucose value ($\leq$200 mg/dL) at 6:00 AM on the first 2 postoperative days

SCIP INF 6: surgery patients had appropriate hair removal with clippers or depilatories or did not have hair removal

SCIP INF 7[a]: colorectal surgery patients had perioperative temperature management, with a first recorded temperature $\geq$36.0°C within 15 minutes of leaving the operating room

SCIP INF 9: urinary catheter was removed on postoperative day 1 or day 2

SCIP INF 10: surgery patients had perioperative temperature management, with either active intraoperative warming or a first recorded temperature $\geq$36.0°C within 30 minutes before or 15 minutes after anesthesia end time

[a] Supplanted by SCIP INF 10.
  Data from Rosenberger LH, Politano AD, Sawyer RG. The Surgical Care Improvement Project and prevention of post-operative infection, including surgical site infection. Surg Infect (Larchmt) 2011;12:163–8; and Stulberg JJ, Delaney CP, Neuhauser DV, et al. Adherence to Surgical Care Improvement Project measures and the association with postoperative infections. JAMA 2010;303:2479–85.

---

and were part of the original SIP project. SCIP INF 1 relates to the timeliness of prophylactic antibiotic administration, SCIP INF 2 monitors the appropriateness of the antibiotic used for prophylaxis, and SCIP INF 3 examines timely discontinuation of prophylactic antibiotics.[90,91] These measures are applied to patients undergoing colorectal operations, total hip and knee replacements, open heart operations, peripheral vascular procedures, and abdominal or vaginal hysterectomy. As the SIP project evolved into SCIP, 3 additional measures have been added: SCIP INF 4 monitors the management of perioperative glucose levels in cardiac surgery patients, SCIP INF 6 examines appropriate hair removal in all surgery patients, and SCIP INF 7 looks at maintenance of normothermia in patients undergoing colorectal procedures; SCIP INF 7 has been modified and now applies to all surgery patients as SCIP INF 10.[92] An additional measure, SCIP INF 9 relates to the prevention of perioperative urinary tract infection and checks for early removal of urinary catheters as a goal toward preventing those infections.[93]

Optimal Use of Prophylactic Antibiotics

SCIP INF 1 defines the optimal timing of prophylactic antibiotics to be within 1 hour of incision, or within 2 hours of incision if vancomycin or a fluoroquinolone is administered.[90,91] The importance of timely administration of prophylactic antibiotics was identified in a large prospective observational study that showed that rates of SSI were lowest if patients received prophylactic antibiotics within 2 hours of the incision time.[94] Most subsequent observational data have supported these findings, including the narrower SCIP window.[95–97] However, another study was not able to find an association between adherence to the SCIP INF 1 and incidence of SSI.[98] This was believed to be potentially caused by the narrowness of the SCIP window, because patients who received antibiotics more than 60 minutes before incision did not seem to have an increased number of infections. There have also been conflicting findings as to whether or not the timing of antibiotic administration within the SCIP window (0–30 minutes or 31–60 minutes before incision) makes any difference in outcome.[99,100]

The SCIP INF 2 measure relates to the appropriateness of antibiotic selection for SSI prophylaxis.[90,91] Because the SCIP INF 2 measure applies only to select operations, appropriate use of antibiotic prophylaxis for other procedures and, perhaps more importantly, avoidance of antibiotic prophylaxis when there is no indication for such is not followed as part of the SCIP initiative. For monitored procedures, the general principle is to use antimicrobial agents from the pathogens that would likely be responsible for a postoperative SSI.[99,100] Typically, the recommended agents are first-generation and second-generation cephalosporins, although alternatives are suggested for patients with β-lactam allergies. For colorectal procedures and hysterectomy, additional anaerobic coverage is recommended, either through use of an antianaerobic second-generation cephalosporin or with administration of a supplemental antianaerobic agent.[99,101]

The SCIP INF 3 measure monitors duration of antibiotic use for SSI prophylaxis. For this measure, prophylactic antibiotic therapy should be discontinued within 24 hours (48 hours for cardiovascular procedures). Many authorities believe that giving prophylactic antibiotics for even 24 hours is excessive[100,102]; several studies have shown that there is no benefit to the continuation of prophylactic antibiotics after the incision is closed.[103,104] Nonetheless, it has proved more difficult to achieve compliance with this measure than any of the other SCIP INF measures.[90,105] This situation may be because of the perception that compliance with this measure is unlikely to have an impact on patient outcome. With respect to reducing SSI rates, this suggestion is probably true, as Dellinger[106] has observed. However, the principal goal of limiting the duration of prophylactic antibiotic is to avoid the selection of resistant or superinfecting bacteria such as *Clostridium difficile*, and thereby reduce risks of infection caused by resistant organisms for both the individual patient as well as all hospitalized patients.[99,105,106]

Other SCIP Measures

The goal of the SCIP INF 4 measure is a 6:00 AM blood glucose value of less than 200 mg/dL in cardiac surgery patients on the first and second postoperative days.[90,91] This value is used as a marker of the adequacy of glucose control during the perioperative period. Hyperglycemia has been associated with an increased risk of SSIs, including deep SSIs and mediastinitis in cardiac surgery patients. A large number of clinical studies have reported that control of hyperglycemia in the perioperative period decreases the risk of such infections in both diabetic and nondiabetic patients.[107–111]

The SCIP INF 6 measure monitors the appropriateness of hair removal in surgical patients.[90,91,93] Removal of hair by shaving, especially when performed the day before the operative procedure, has been associated with increased rates of SSI.[101,112] This SCIP measure monitors the number of patients undergoing a surgical procedure who either have no hair removal or, if needed, appropriate hair removal, which is defined as being performed with clippers or depilatories. Dellinger[106] has argued that this measure may be the least relevant of the SCIP measures, because compliance is usually high and does not necessarily correlate with compliance with other SCIP measures.

The SCIP INF 7 measure followed maintenance of perioperative normothermia in patients undergoing colorectal procedures.[90,91] This measure was subsequently modified and extended in 2009 to all surgical patients as the SCIP INF 10 measure[92,93]; however, most of the available literature regarding perioperative normothermia used the SCIP INF 7 measure. For this SCIP component, what was monitored was the number of patients who had an initial postoperative temperature of 36.0°C within 15 minutes of leaving the operating room. The use of active warming to maintain perioperative normothermia was studied by Kurz and colleagues.[113] In this prospective randomized controlled trial of patients undergoing colorectal operations, patients randomized to receive active warming to maintain normothermia during the perioperative period had a substantially lower rate of SSI than did patients randomized to receive standard cares, which did not generally include active warming. Nonetheless, additional observational studies have questioned whether the immediate postoperative temperature correlates with an increased risk of SSI.[114–116] It has also been pointed out that the experimental intervention in the study of Kurz and colleagues was a specific protocol to maintain intraoperative normothermia, and not simply a measurement of postoperative temperature.[93]

Efficacy of the SCIP Measures in Preventing SSI

The goal of the SCIP INF measures is to decrease perioperative infection, chiefly SSI, in surgical patients. However, there has been some controversy as to whether or not these measures achieve that goal and lead to measurable decreases in rates of SSI.

There is little doubt that focused efforts to improve compliance with the SCIP INF measures have led to improvements in process end points, both at the individual institution level and at a national level.[88,117,118] In 1 multi-institutional study, statistically significant improvement in compliance with all measures was noted over a 12-month period; during that same period, there was a decrease in infection rates from 2.28% to 1.65%.[117] A single-center study looking at rates of SSI in colorectal surgery patients also documented a decrease in the observed/expected ratio of SSI from 1.39 to 0.81, because compliance with SCIP measures increased from 38% to 92% during 2 periods 1 year apart.[119]

However, other investigators have not been able to document similar benefits associated with improved compliance with the SCIP measures. In a single-center study, compliance with all SCIP INF measures combined improved from 40% to 68% for patients undergoing colorectal surgery in 2 consecutive 14-month periods, but SSI rates were unchanged (18.9% and 19.4% in the 2 periods).[118] Another single-center study[120] of colorectal surgery patients found no sustained improvement in compliance with SCIP INF measures over a 54-month period, and likewise no change in SSI rates. However, these investigators speculated that compliance with SCIP measures was already high in their setting, and that most instances of noncompliance were failures of documentation and not failures to comply with the established principles of SSI prophylaxis.

Two studies of large databases have been reported that provide additional information with regard to the effectiveness of the SCIP measures in reducing SSI. As part of a study by Ingraham and colleagues,[121] compliance with SCIP INF measures 1, 2, 3, and 6 were correlated with risk-adjusted SSI rates. A total of 81,524 patients were included from 200 hospitals participating in both an American College of Surgeons National Surgical Quality Improvement Project and the SCIP initiative. Average compliance with these different measures was high (92%–98% for all hospitals combined); however, compliance with certain measures at specific hospitals could be substantially lower. Risk-adjusted SSI rates decreased in association with all the individual SCIP INF measures, but this was significant only for compliance with SCIP INF 2 (use of appropriate antibiotics). The correlation did approach significance for SCIP INF 1 (appropriate timing of antibiotic administration).

Another large database study was reported by Stulberg and colleagues.[122] These investigators reported on 405,720 patients from 398 hospitals who developed 3996 infections related to an operation. Associations were determined between the rates of postoperative infections and compliance with individual SCIP INF measures 1, 2, 3, 4, 6, and 7 and with a composite measure of compliance with the SCIP INF measures 1, 2, and 3 (all related to appropriate use of prophylactic antibiotics), or a composite measure of compliance with any 2 of the 6 SCIP measures. Compliance with the individual SCIP INF measures was 80% to 94%. The adjusted odds ratios for development of a postoperative infection appeared to be lower for SCIP INF measures 1, 2, 3, and 4, and the composite measures, but not for SCIP INF measures 6 and 7. However, with the exception of the composite measure of compliance with at least 2 SCIP measures, none of these decreases was statistically significant. The odds ratios for the reduction of postoperative infection and compliance with either the SCIP core measures (1, 2, and 3) or with the SCIP INF 2 measure alone nearly reached significance.

The results of these studies have called into question whether or not compliance with all of the SCIP measures necessarily results in measurable decreases in rates of SSI. However, there are several reasons why the SCIP measures, particularly those related to prophylactic antibiotic use, should still be considered valid. Dellinger has argued that overall compliance with these measures has increased greatly; thus, it may be difficult to detect changes in SSI rates when widespread compliance has been achieved. Further, he argues that compliance with multiple measures may be more important than compliance with individual measures, as the study by Stulberg and colleagues seems to show. As noted earlier, Dellinger notes that certain measures, such as SCIP INF 3 (duration of prophylactic antibiotics) are unlikely to have a direct impact on SSI rates, but are still important in preventing infectious morbidity related to resistant organisms.[106] Thus, the SCIP bundle may have already had a significant impact on the incidence of SSI, even although it cannot easily be measured.

However, equally important is the need to recognize that modifications of the SCIP bundle can and should be made. It seems clear that not all the SCIP INF measures are equally efficacious. Alternative measures that would ultimately be incorporated into an SSI prevention bundle, particularly those not related to use of prophylactic antibiotics, should be rigorously studied before being adopted as standards of care. A recent prospective randomized controlled trial examining use of a bundle of several other preventative measures shows the importance of this strategy. In this trial, patients undergoing colorectal operations were randomized to receive 5 evidence-based measures that were believed to reduce rates of SSI; only one of these was an SCIP INF measure (maintenance of normothermia). However, patients randomized to be treated according to the bundle had higher SSI rates than did control patients.[123] Although this was a negative study, data such as these are essential in ensuring that SSI prevention bundles lead to meaningful impacts on rates of SSI, and not just to a need to document processes that have little or no benefit to the patient.

SUMMARY

The gap between evidence-based medicine and clinical practice is often wide. The concept of bringing together several individual evidence-based practices into standardized care bundles has the potential to narrow this gap. The federal government and independent organizations, such as the IHI, have promoted the use of bundles with the hope that this improves the overall quality of health care delivery throughout all layers of the health care system. The use of care bundles clearly holds promise for decreasing morbidity and mortality in critically ill surgical patients. As indicated earlier, the CVC and VAP bundles have led to substantial decreases in rates of CRBSI and VAP in these patients, and the use of sepsis bundles has led to improved survival of these critically ill patients.

Bundles to prevent SSI have an impact on the care of all surgical patients, not just those who are critically ill. The SCIP INF measures have become a de facto SSI prevention bundle. In many institutions, considerable effort has been expended to monitor compliance with the various SCIP INF measures. Nevertheless, many of the data suggest that widespread adoption of SCIP measures is not producing the expected decrease in SSI rates, distinct from the benefits observed after implementation of VAP, CVC, and sepsis bundles. Whether this situation represents a failure of the bundle or an inability to measure an effect of the bundle on outcome remains an important issue for debate.

Notwithstanding the question as to whether or not the SCIP INF measures have resulted in improved outcome, institutions and individual practitioners are increasingly being graded according to their compliance with these measurements as well as overall rates of SSI. The results are being publicly reported, such that the public at large has access to these data. Further, payers are applying both financial rewards for following best practices in preventing SSI and financial penalties when such infections occur. It is reasonable to expect that reimbursement to institutions and individuals will be further tied to these measurements in the future.[124] A worthwhile goal, then, is to develop robust tools to rigorously analyze the components and the overall usefulness of bundles, such that their implementation, in many cases mandated by regulatory agencies, does not simply result in a need for further documentation but produces a real improvement in patient outcome.

REFERENCES

1. Marwick C, Davey P. Care bundles: the holy grail of infectious risk management in hospital? Curr Opin Infect Dis 2009;22:364–9.
2. Medicare program: changes to the hospital inpatient prospective payment systems and fiscal year 2008 rates. Fed Regist 2007;72:47379–428.
3. Hansen S, Schwab F, Asensio A, et al. Methicillin-resistant *Staphylococcus aureus* (MRSA) in Europe: which infection control measures are taken? Infection 2010;38:159–64.
4. Byrnes M, Schuerer D, Schallom M, et al. Implementation of a mandatory checklist of protocols and objectives improves compliance with a wide range of evidence-based intensive care unit procedures. Crit Care Med 2009;37: 2775–81.
5. Berenholtz S, Dorman T, Ngo K, et al. Qualitative review of intensive care unit quality indicators. J Crit Care 2002;17:1–12.
6. Dodek P, Keenan S, Cook D, et al. Evidence-based clinical practice guideline for the prevention of ventilator-associated pneumonia. Ann Intern Med 2004; 141:305–13.
7. Fulbrook P, Mooney S. Care bundles in critical care: a practical approach to evidence-based practice. Nurs Crit Care 2003;8:249–55.
8. Berwick D. Continuous improvement as an ideal in health care. N Engl J Med 1989;320:53–6.

9. Sundin-Huard D. Subject positions theory: its application to understanding collaboration (and confrontation) in critical care. J Adv Nurs 2001;34:376–82.
10. Rello J, Ollendorf D, Oster G, et al. Epidemiology and outcomes of ventilator-associated pneumonia in a large US database. Chest 2002;122:2115–21.
11. Warren D, Shukla S, Oslen M, et al. Outcome and attributable cost of ventilator-associated pneumonia among intensive care unit patients in a suburban medical center. Crit Care Med 2003;31:1312–7.
12. Wip C, Napolitano L. Bundles to prevent ventilator-associated pneumonia: how valuable are they? Curr Opin Infect Dis 2009;22:159–66.
13. Metheny N, Clouse R, Chang Y, et al. Tracheobronchial aspiration of gastric contents in critically-ill tube fed patients: frequency, outcomes, and risk factors. Crit Care Med 2006;34:1007–15.
14. Torres A, Serra-Batlles J, Ros E, et al. Pulmonary aspiration of gastric contents in patients receiving mechanical ventilation: the effect of body position. Ann Intern Med 1992;116:540–3.
15. Drakulovic M, Torres A, Bauer T, et al. Supine body position as a risk factor for nosocomial pneumonia in mechanically ventilated patients: a randomized trial. Lancet 1999;354(9193):1851–8.
16. van Nieuwenhoven C, Vandenbroucke-Grauls C, van Tiel F, et al. Feasibility and effects of the semirecumbent position to prevent ventilator-associated pneumonia: a randomized study. Crit Care Med 2006;34:396–402.
17. Dries D, McGonigal M, Malian M, et al. Protocol-driven ventilator weaning reduces use of mechanical ventilation, rate of early reintubation, and ventilator-associated pneumonia. J Trauma 2004;56:943–51.
18. Girard T, Kress J, Fuchs B, et al. Efficacy and safety of a paired sedation and ventilator weaning protocol for mechanically ventilated patients in intensive care (Awakening and Breathing Controlled Trial): a randomized controlled trial. Lancet 2008;371(9607):126–34.
19. Robertson T, Mann H, Hyzy R, et al. Multicenter implementation of a consensus-developed, evidence-based, spontaneous breathing trial protocol. Crit Care Med 2008;36:2753–62.
20. Cook D, Fuller H, Guyatt G, et al. Risk factors for gastrointestinal bleeding in critically ill patients. Canadian Critical Care Trials Group. N Engl J Med 1994;330:377–81.
21. Huang J, Cao Y, Liao C, et al. Effect of histamine-2-receptor antagonists versus sucralfate on stress ulcer prophylaxis in mechanically ventilated patients: a meta-analysis of 10 randomized controlled trials. Crit Care 2010;14:R145.
22. Hirsch D, Ingenito E, Goldhaber S, et al. Prevalence of deep venous thrombosis among patients in medical intensive care. JAMA 1995;274:335–7.
23. Cook D, Attia J, Weaver B, et al. Venous thromboembolic disease: an observational study in medical-surgical intensive care unit patients. J Crit Care 2000;15:127–32.
24. Jellinek H, Krenn H, Oczenski W, et al. Influence of positive airway pressure on the pressure gradient for venous return in humans. J Appl Physiol 2000;88:926–32.
25. Geerts W, Heit J, Clagett G, et al. Prevention of venous thromboembolism. Chest 2001;119(Suppl 1):132S–75S.
26. Bergmans D, Bonten M, Gaillard C, et al. Prevention of ventilator-associated pneumonia by oral decontamination: a prospective, randomized, double-blind, placebo-controlled study. Am J Respir Crit Care Med 2001;164:382–8.
27. Koeman M, van der Ven A, Hak E, et al. Oral decontamination with chlorhexidine reduces the incidence of ventilator-associated pneumonia. Am J Respir Crit Care Med 2006;173:1348–55.

28. Kollef M, Skubas N, Sundt T, et al. A randomized clinical trial of continuous aspiration of subglottic secretions in cardiac surgery patients. Chest 1999;116:1339–46.

29. Bouza E, Perez M, Munoz P, et al. Continuous aspiration of subglottic secretions in the prevention of ventilator-associated pneumonia in the postoperative period of major heart surgery. Chest 2008;134:938–46.

30. O'Grady NP, Alexander M, Dellinger EP, et al. Guidelines for the prevention of intravascular catheter-related infections. Healthcare Infection Control Practices Advisory Committee. Infect Control Hosp Epidemiol 2002;23:759–69.

31. Pittet D, Tarara D, Wenzel RP. Nosocomial bloodstream infection in critically ill patients. Excess length of stay, extra costs, and attributable mortality. JAMA 1994;271:1598–601.

32. Dimick JB, Pelz RK, Consunji R, et al. Increased resource use associated with catheter-related bloodstream infection in the surgical intensive care unit. Arch Surg 2001;136:229–34.

33. Digiovine B, Chenoweth C, Watts C, et al. The attributable mortality and costs of primary nosocomial bloodstream infections in the intensive care unit. Am J Respir Crit Care Med 1999;160:976–81.

34. Implement the central line bundle. Institute for Healthcare Improvement. Available at: http://www.ihi.org/IHI/Topics/CriticalCare/IntensiveCare/Changes/ImplementtheCentralLineBundle.htm. Accessed May 10, 2011.

35. Chittick P, Sherertz RJ. Recognition and prevention of nosocomial vascular device and related bloodstream infections in the intensive care unit. Crit Care Med 2010;38(Suppl 8):S363–72.

36. Earle AS. The germ theory in America: antisepsis and asepsis (1867-1900). Surgery 1969;65:508–22.

37. Goldmann D. System failure versus personal accountability–the case for clean hands. N Engl J Med 2006;355:121–3.

38. Albert RK, Condie F. Hand-washing patterns in medical intensive-care units. N Engl J Med 1981;304:1465–6.

39. Yilmaz G, Koksal I, Aydin K, et al. Risk factors of catheter-related bloodstream infections in parenteral nutrition catheterization. JPEN J Parenter Enteral Nutr 2007;31:284–7.

40. Rosenthal VD, Guzman S, Safdar N. Reduction in nosocomial infection with improved hand hygiene in intensive care units of a tertiary care hospital in Argentina. Am J Infect Control 2005;33:392–7.

41. Jenner EA, Fletcher BC, Watson P, et al. Discrepancy between self-reported and observed hand hygiene behaviour in healthcare professionals. J Hosp Infect 2006;63:418–22.

42. Doberneck RC, Kleinman R. The surgical garb. Surgery 1984;95:694–8.

43. Raad II, Hohn DC, Gilbreath BJ, et al. Prevention of central venous catheter-related infections by using maximal sterile barrier precautions during insertion. Infect Control Hosp Epidemiol 1994;15:231–8.

44. Mermel LA, McCormick RD, Springman SR, et al. The pathogenesis and epidemiology of catheter-related infection with pulmonary artery Swan-Ganz catheters: a prospective study utilizing molecular subtyping. Am J Med 1991; 91(3B):197S–205S.

45. Hu KK, Veenstra DL, Lipsky BA, et al. Use of maximal sterile barriers during central venous catheter insertion: clinical and economic outcomes. Clin Infect Dis 2004;39:1441–5.

46. Toledo-Pereyra LH, Toledo MM. A critical study of Lister's work on antiseptic surgery. Am J Surg 1976;131:736–44.

47. Maki DG, Ringer M, Alvarado CJ. Prospective randomised trial of povidone-iodine, alcohol, and chlorhexidine for prevention of infection associated with central venous and arterial catheters. Lancet 1991;338(8763):339–43.

48. Chaiyakunapruk N, Veenstra DL, Lipsky BA, et al. Chlorhexidine compared with povidone-iodine solution for vascular catheter-site care: a meta-analysis. Ann Intern Med 2002;136:792–801.

49. Goede MR, Coopersmith CM. Catheter-related bloodstream infection. Surg Clin North Am 2009;89:463–74.

50. Goetz AM, Wagener MM, Miller JM, et al. Risk of infection due to central venous catheters: effect of site of placement and catheter type. Infect Control Hosp Epidemiol 1998;19:842–5.

51. Lorente L, Henry C, Martín MM, et al. Central venous catheter-related infection in a prospective and observational study of 2,595 catheters. Crit Care 2005;9:R631–5.

52. Deshpande KS, Hatem C, Ulrich HL, et al. The incidence of infectious complications of central venous catheters at the subclavian, internal jugular, and femoral sites in an intensive care unit population. Crit Care Med 2005;33:13–20.

53. Parienti JJ, Thirion M, Mégarbane B, et al. Femoral vs jugular venous catheterization and risk of nosocomial events in adults requiring acute renal replacement therapy: a randomized controlled trial. JAMA 2008;299:2413–22.

54. Pronovost P, Needham D, Berenholtz S, et al. An intervention to decrease catheter-related bloodstream infections in the ICU. N Engl J Med 2006;355:2725–32.

55. Berenholtz SM, Pronovost PJ, Lipsett PA, et al. Eliminating catheter-related bloodstream infections in the intensive care unit. Crit Care Med 2004;32:2014–20.

56. Cook D, Randolph A, Kernerman P, et al. Central venous catheter replacement strategies: a systematic review of the literature. Crit Care Med 1997;25:1417–24.

57. Cobb DK, High KP, Sawyer RG, et al. A controlled trial of scheduled replacement of central venous and pulmonary-artery catheters. N Engl J Med 1992;327:1062–8.

58. Rivers E, Nguyen B, Havstad S, et al. Early goal-directed therapy in the treatment of severe sepsis and septic shock. N Engl J Med 2001;345:1368–77.

59. Dellinger RP, Carlet JM, Masur H, et al. Surviving Sepsis Campaign guidelines for management of severe sepsis and septic shock. Crit Care Med 2004;32:858–73.

60. Dellinger RP, Levy MM, Carlet JM, et al. Surviving Sepsis Campaign: international guidelines for management of severe sepsis and septic shock: 2008. Crit Care Med 2008;36:296–327.

61. Marshall JC, Dellinger RP, Levy M. The Surviving Sepsis Campaign: a history and a perspective. Surg Infect (Larchmt) 2010;11:275–81.

62. Jones AE, Focht A, Horton JM, et al. Prospective external validation of the clinical effectiveness of an emergency department-based early goal-directed therapy protocol for severe sepsis and septic shock. Chest 2007;132:425–32.

63. Kortgen A, Niederprüm P, Bauer M, et al. Implementation of an evidence-based "standard operating procedure" and outcome in septic shock. Crit Care Med 2006;34:943–9.

64. Ferrer R, Artigas A, Levy MM, et al. Improvement in process of care and outcome after a multicenter severe sepsis educational program in Spain. JAMA 2008;299:2294–303.

65. Bakker J, Coffernils M, Leon M, et al. Blood lactate levels are superior to oxygen-derived variables in predicting outcome in human septic shock. Chest 1991;99:956–62.

66. Weinstein MP, Murphy JR, Reller LB, et al. The clinical significance of positive blood cultures: a comprehensive analysis of 500 episodes of bacteremia and fungemia in adults. II. Clinical observations, with special reference to factors influencing prognosis. Rev Infect Dis 1983;5:54–70.

67. Blot F, Schmidt E, Nitenberg G, et al. Earlier positivity of central-venous- versus peripheral-blood cultures is highly predictive of catheter-related sepsis. J Clin Microbiol 1998;36:105–9.

68. American Thoracic Society, Infectious Diseases Society of America. Guidelines for the management of adults with hospital-acquired, ventilator-associated, and healthcare-associated pneumonia. Am J Respir Crit Care Med 2005;171:388–416.

69. Ibrahim EH, Sherman G, Ward S, et al. The influence of inadequate antimicrobial treatment of bloodstream infections on patient outcomes in the ICU setting. Chest 2000;118:146–55.

70. Iregui M, Ward S, Sherman G, et al. Clinical importance of delays in the initiation of appropriate antibiotic treatment for ventilator-associated pneumonia. Chest 2002;122:262–8.

71. Kumar A, Roberts D, Wood KE, et al. Duration of hypotension before initiation of effective antimicrobial therapy is the critical determinant of survival in human septic shock. Crit Care Med 2006;34:1589–96.

72. Kollef MH, Sherman G, Ward S, et al. Inadequate antimicrobial treatment of infections: a risk factor for hospital mortality among critically ill patients. Chest 1999;115:462–74.

73. Finfer S, Bellomo R, Boyce N, et al. A comparison of albumin and saline for fluid resuscitation in the intensive care unit. N Engl J Med 2004;350:2247–456.

74. Schortgen F, Lacherade JC, Bruneel F, et al. Effects of hydroxyethylstarch and gelatin on renal function in severe sepsis: a multicentre randomised study. Lancet 2001;357(9260):911–6.

75. LeDoux D, Astiz ME, Carpati CM, et al. Effects of perfusion pressure on tissue perfusion in septic shock. Crit Care Med 2000;28:2729–32.

76. Russell JA, Walley KR, Singer J, et al. Vasopressin versus norepinephrine infusion in patients with septic shock. N Engl J Med 2008;358:877–87.

77. Chamberlain DJ, Willis EM, Bersten AB. The severe sepsis bundles as processes of care: a meta-analysis. Aust Crit Care 2011;24(4):229–43.

78. Hébert PC, Wells G, Blajchman MA, et al. A multicenter, randomized, controlled clinical trial of transfusion requirements in critical care. N Engl J Med 1999;340:409–17.

79. Van den Berghe G, Wouters P, Weekers F, et al. Intensive insulin therapy in the critically ill patients. N Engl J Med 2001;345:1359–67.

80. Van den Berghe G, Wilmer A, Hermans G, et al. Intensive insulin therapy in the medical ICU. N Engl J Med 2006;354:449–61.

81. Finfer S, Chittock DR, Su SY, et al. Intensive versus conventional glucose control in critically ill patients. N Engl J Med 2009;360:1283–97.

82. Sevransky JE, Levy MM, Marini JJ, et al. Mechanical ventilation in sepsis-induced acute lung injury/acute respiratory distress syndrome: an evidence-based review. Crit Care Med 2004;32(Suppl 11):S548–53.

83. The Acute Respiratory Distress Syndrome Network. Ventilation with lower tidal volumes as compared with traditional tidal volumes for acute lung injury and the acute respiratory distress syndrome. N Engl J Med 2000;342:1301–8.

84. Annane D, Sébille V, Charpentier C, et al. Effect of treatment with low doses of hydrocortisone and fludrocortisone on mortality in patients with septic shock. JAMA 2002;288:862–71.

85. Sprung CL, Annane D, Keh D, et al. Hydrocortisone therapy for patients with septic shock. N Engl J Med 2008;358:111–24.

86. Bernard GR, Vincent JL, Laterre PF, et al. Efficacy and safety of recombinant human activated protein C for severe sepsis. N Engl J Med 2001;344:699–709.

87. Abraham E, Laterre PF, Garg R, et al. Drotrecogin alfa (activated) for adults with severe sepsis and a low risk of death. N Engl J Med 2005;353:1332–41.

88. Bratzler DW. The surgical infection prevention and surgical care improvement projects: promises and pitfalls. Am Surg 2006;72:1010–6.

89. Fry DE. Surgical site infections and the surgical care improvement project (SCIP): evolution of national quality measures. Surg Infect (Larchmt) 2008;9: 579–84.

90. Bratzler DW, Hunt DR. The Surgical Infection Prevention and Surgical Care Improvement Projects: national initiatives to improve outcomes for patients having surgery. Clin Infect Dis 2006;43:322–30.

91. Anderson DJ, Kaye KS, Classen D, et al. Strategies to prevent surgical site infections in acute care hospitals. Infect Control Hosp Epidemiol 2008; 29(Suppl 1):S51–61.

92. National Quality Measures Clearinghouse. Surgical care improvement project: percent of surgery patients with perioperative temperature management. Available at: http://www.qualitymeasures.ahrq.gov/content.aspx?id=27417&search= scip+10. Accessed September 23, 2011.

93. Rosenberger LH, Politano AD, Sawyer RG. The Surgical Care Improvement Project and prevention of post-operative infection, including surgical site infection. Surg Infect (Larchmt) 2011;12:163–8.

94. Classen DC, Evans RS, Pestotnik SL, et al. The timing of prophylactic administration of antibiotics and the risk of surgical-wound infection. N Engl J Med 1992; 326:281–6.

95. Weber WP, Marti WR, Zwahlen M, et al. The timing of surgical antimicrobial prophylaxis. Ann Surg 2008;247:918–26.

96. Steinberg JP, Braun BI, Hellinger WC, et al. Timing of antimicrobial prophylaxis and the risk of surgical site infections: results from the trial to reduce antimicrobial prophylaxis errors. Ann Surg 2009;250:10–6.

97. Nguyen N, Yegiyants S, Kaloostian C, et al. The Surgical Care Improvement Project (SCIP) initiative to reduce infection in elective colorectal surgery: which performance measures affect outcome? Am Surg 2008;74:1012–6.

98. Hawn MT, Itani KM, Gray SH, et al. Association of timely administration of prophylactic antibiotics for major surgical procedures and surgical site infection. J Am Coll Surg 2008;206:814–21.

99. ASHP Therapeutic Guidelines on Antimicrobial Prophylaxis in Surgery. Am J Health Syst Pharm 1999;56:1839–88.

100. Nichols RL, Condon RE, Barie PS. Antibiotic prophylaxis in surgery–2005 and beyond. Surg Infect (Larchmt) 2005;6:349–61.

101. Mangram AJ, Horan TC, Pearson ML, et al. Guideline for prevention of surgical site infection, 1999. Infect Control Hosp Epidemiol 1999;20:250–78.

102. Barie PS. Modern surgical antibiotic prophylaxis and therapy–less is more. Surg Infect (Larchmt) 2000;1:23–9.

103. DiPiro JT, Cheung RP, Bowden TA Jr, et al. Single dose systemic antibiotic prophylaxis of surgical wound infections. Am J Surg 1986;152:552–9.

104. McDonald M, Grabsch E, Marshall C, et al. Single- versus multiple-dose antimicrobial prophylaxis for major surgery: a systematic review. Aust N Z J Surg 1998;68:388–96.

105. Bratzler DW, Houck PM. Surgical Infection Prevention Guidelines Writers Workgroup. Antimicrobial prophylaxis for surgery: an advisory statement from the National Surgical Infection Prevention Project. Clin Infect Dis 2004;38:1706–15.
106. Dellinger EP. Adherence to Surgical Care Improvement Project measures: the whole is greater than the parts. Future Microbiol 2010;5:1781–5.
107. Zerr KJ, Furnary AP, Grunkemeier GL, et al. Glucose control lowers the risk of wound infection in diabetics after open heart operations. Ann Thorac Surg 1997;63:356–61.
108. Furnary AP, Zerr KJ, Grunkemeier GL, et al. Continuous intravenous insulin infusion reduces the incidence of deep sternal wound infection in diabetic patients after cardiac surgical procedures. Ann Thorac Surg 1999;67:352–62.
109. Lazar HL, Chipkin SR, Fitzgerald CA, et al. Tight glycemic control in diabetic coronary artery bypass graft patients improves perioperative outcomes and decreases recurrent ischemic events. Circulation 2004;109:1497–502.
110. Carr JM, Sellke FW, Fey M, et al. Implementing tight glucose control after coronary artery bypass surgery. Ann Thorac Surg 2005;80:902–9.
111. Leibowitz G, Raizman E, Brezis M, et al. Effects of moderate intensity glycemic control after cardiac surgery. Ann Thorac Surg 2010;90:1825–32.
112. Kjønniksen I, Andersen BM, Søndenaa VG, et al. Preoperative hair removal–a systematic literature review. AORN J 2002;75:928–38.
113. Kurz A, Sessler DI, Lenhardt R. Perioperative normothermia to reduce the incidence of surgical-wound infection and shorten hospitalization. N Engl J Med 1996;334:1209–15.
114. Barone JE, Tucker JB, Cecere J, et al. Hypothermia does not result in more complications after colon surgery. Am Surg 1999;65:356–9.
115. Walz JM, Paterson CA, Seligowski JM, et al. Surgical site infection following bowel surgery: a retrospective analysis of 1446 patients. Arch Surg 2006;141:1014–8.
116. Lehtinen SJ, Onicescu G, Kuhn KM, et al. Normothermia to prevent surgical site infections after gastrointestinal surgery: holy grail or false idol? Ann Surg 2010; 252:696–704.
117. Dellinger EP, Hausmann SM, Bratzler DW, et al. Hospitals collaborate to decrease surgical site infections. Am J Surg 2005;190:9–15.
118. Pastor C, Artinyan A, Varma MG, et al. An increase in compliance with the Surgical Care Improvement Project measures does not prevent surgical site infection in colorectal surgery. Dis Colon Rectum 2010;53:24–30.
119. Berenguer CM, Oschsner MG Jr, Lord SA, et al. Improving surgical site infections: using national surgical quality improvement program data to institute surgical care improvement project protocols in improving surgical outcomes. J Am Coll Surg 2010;210:737–43.
120. Larochelle M, Hyman N, Gruppi L, et al. Diminishing surgical site infections after colorectal surgery with surgical care improvement project: is it time to move on? Dis Colon Rectum 2011;54:394–400.
121. Ingraham AM, Cohen ME, Bilimoria KY, et al. Association of Surgical Care Improvement Project infection-related process measure compliance with risk-adjusted outcomes: implications for quality measurement. J Am Coll Surg 2010;211:705–14.
122. Stulberg JJ, Delaney CP, Neuhauser DV, et al. Adherence to Surgical Care Improvement Project measures and the association with postoperative infections. JAMA 2010;303:2479–85.
123. Anthony T, Murray BW, Sun-Ping JT, et al. Evaluating an evidence-based bundle for preventing surgical site infection. A randomized trial. Arch Surg 2011;146:263–9.
124. Snyder L, Neubauer RL. Pay-for-performance principles that promote patient-centered care: an ethics manifesto. Ann Intern Med 2007;147:792–4.

Organ Failure Avoidance and Mitigation Strategies in Surgery

Kevin W. McConnell, MD[a], Craig M. Coopersmith, MD[b],*

KEYWORDS

• Organ failure • Sepsis • Resuscitation • Critical care

ORGAN FAILURE AND MULTIORGAN DYSFUNCTION SYNDROME

The ability of physicians to treat failing organs is a recent development in the history of medicine. For most of human history, the development of organ failure resulted in the quick demise of the patient. It was not until the second half of the twentieth century, around the same time as the initial description of multiple organ failure, that the ability to support failing organs evolved from the realm of theory into a host of interventions that could be used at the bedside.[1,2]

The initial description of multiorgan dysfunction syndrome (MODS) came in a 1991 consensus conference between the American College of Chest Physicians and the Society of Critical Care Medicine, which produced definitions of the systemic inflammatory response syndrome (SIRS), sepsis, and MODS.[3] SIRS is defined as the presence of at least 2 of the following 4 criteria: (1) body temperature greater than 38°C or less than 36°C; (2) heart rate greater than 90 beats per minute; (3) respiratory rate greater than 20 breaths per minute or hyperventilation with $Paco_2$ less than 32 mm Hg; or (4) white blood cell count greater than $12,000/mm^3$, less than $4000/mm^3$, or greater than 10% immature neutrophils. If these changes occur in the setting of an infectious source, then the process is defined as sepsis. MODS is defined as an acutely ill patient with altered organ function in whom homeostasis cannot be maintained without intervention.

Studies now indicate that MODS is the leading cause of death in noncoronary intensive care units (ICUs), accounting for 50% to 81% of deaths,[4–7] and its incidence is increasing.[8] Surgical patients represent a subpopulation at significant risk for MODS because of the increased risk associated with sepsis, polytrauma, burns, pancreatitis,

The authors have nothing to disclose.
[a] Acute and Critical Care Surgery, Emory University School of Medicine, Atlanta, GA, USA
[b] Emory Center for Critical Care, Emory University School of Medicine and Emory Healthcare, Atlanta, GA, USA
* Corresponding author. 101 Woodruff Circle, Suite WMB 5105, Atlanta, GA 30322.
E-mail address: cmcoop3@emory.edu

aspiration, severe hemorrhage, massive transfusion, ischemia-reperfusion, and other complications.[7,9,10]

Although the number of organs failing and the severity of failure correlate strongly with patient outcomes,[6,11,12] defining the pathophysiology of MODS continues to be challenging. Most agree that alterations in systemic inflammation lead, at least in part, to the development of MODS. However, the severity, balance between hyperin-flammation/hypoinflammation, and time course of inflammation are all incompletely understood and therefore represent topics of intense research interest.[13] The initial definition of MODS served to capture individuals with systemic inflammation and organ dysfunction for clinical trials, but may have contributed to the failure of these trials by including a broad distribution of patients with different ages, severities, sources, and genetics.[14–16] Although further efforts were made to update the definitions of sepsis, severe sepsis, and septic shock, they remain nonspecific.[17]

Several scoring systems have been developed to characterize the degree of MODS and predict mortality. Of these, Multiorgan Dysfunction Score, Sequential Organ Failure Assessment (SOFA), Acute Physiology and Chronic Health Evaluation (APACHE II and III), and Simplified Acute Physiology Score (SAPS) are some of the most commonly used.[18] The individual strengths and weaknesses of each scoring system are beyond the scope of this article, but many are used without a clearly accepted gold standard, which implies variable usefulness and a lack of consensus on which might best identify patients for potential new interventions.

CURRENT STRATEGIES FOR PREVENTION AND MITIGATION

Developing strategies to prevent or treat MODS has proved to be challenging. The reasons behind this are complex. On a cellular/subcellular level, there are many mechanisms known to contribute to MODS. Microvascular thrombosis, apoptosis, neutrophil-induced damage, bacterial translocation, cytokine release, endothelial dysfunction, enteric barrier dysfunction, and other mechanisms have been implicated in the process.[19–28] Each of these (and multiple other) mechanisms have been shown to be important in animal models, but none has translated into targeted therapy for MODS that is useful at the bedside. On a whole-body level, each patient with critical illness is subjected to the injury or infection causing SIRS, which can frequently cause dysfunction or failure in 1 or multiple organs. The health care team responds to this with supportive care and/or potentially therapeutic interventions. However, these interventions may cause inadvertent harm to the patient, exacerbating the underlying insult.[29] For instance, mechanical ventilation can be lifesaving but, depending on the settings on the ventilator, it may also injure the lung and adversely affect host defense mechanisms, secondarily affecting the function of other organs, and ultimately leading to a preventable increase in mortality.[30,31]

GENERALIZED PREVENTION

As with any disease, the best treatment of MODS is preventing it from occurring in the first place. In the surgical patient, MODS prevention can occur by identifying high-risk groups before elective surgery, and weighing the risk/benefit ratio of proceeding with an operation. There are numerous scoring systems that identify a patient's risk for postoperative cardiac or respiratory complications. Surgeons and anesthesiologists (as well as medical specialty consultants, if indicated) are ultimately responsible for ensuring that surgery is being performed only on candidates who have an acceptable risk profile. In addition, preoperative status may need to be optimized before agreeing to operate on a patient. This optimization may take the form of improved nutrition, weight loss, respiratory rehabilitation, quitting smoking, and so forth.

Once an operation has occurred (either elective or emergent), a certain number of patients have organ dysfunction, which progresses to MODS in a subset of them. However, this risk is modifiable by adherence to best practice, which can prevent development of further complications. For floor (and at times ICU) patients, this means rapid ambulation and deep breathing/incentive spirometer. For high-risk patients (studied most notably in vascular patients), perioperative β-blockade may prevent cardiovascular complications.[32] Initiating appropriate prophylaxis against deep venous thrombosis and (if indicated) stress ulceration may also prevent complications that can lead to MODS. Removing central venous catheters, arterial lines, Foley catheters, and endotracheal tubes as soon as possible can prevent development of central line–associated bloodstream infection, catheter-associated urinary tract infection, and ventilator-associated pneumonia (VAP), respectively.

ONCE MODS SETS IN, WHAT THERAPIES ARE AVAILABLE TO THE PATIENT?

The mainstays of prevention of MODS include early recognition/resuscitation, removal of the inciting source, and prevention of iatrogenic injury. Once organ failure sets in, most treatment is supportive, allowing the host to heal without causing additional iatrogenic injury. In a global view, most care provided in the ICU is not intended to cure but to support. Pressors do not cure shock, but instead potentially prevent inadequate tissue perfusion until the body is able to maintain its own blood pressure. Mechanical ventilation does not cure respiratory failure but instead supports the lungs until the body is able to regulate ventilation and oxygenation on its own. Similarly, renal replacement therapy does not cure acute renal failure but supports the body until the kidneys recover to the point that they are able to clear both toxins and volume. As such, the best that can be offered to many patients is to effectively support them, with the hope that prevention of further decompensation will allow their bodies to have sufficient time to heal from the initial insults.

STRATEGIES BY ORGAN SYSTEM

Despite most treatment in MODS being supportive rather than curative, it is helpful to be fully versed in strategies that may result in positive outcomes for critically ill patients. Because the most common cause of organ failure is sepsis, the Surviving Sepsis guidelines are an excellent resource for an evidence-based approach that identifies key interventions to improve survival in patients with this complex process.[33,34]

Neurologic Conditions

Effective management centers on maintaining patient comfort (generally, although not always, with narcotics or an epidural, when appropriate) while minimizing common sequelae of MODS including delirium and agitation. Although sedation may be necessary to safely ventilate a subset of patients, unchecked sedative use can lead to iatrogenic harm. This harm can be broken down into direct neurologic complications and indirect complications caused by an inability to liberate patients from mechanical ventilation.

Delirium is an important measure of organ dysfunction and has been shown to be a predictor of mortality in the ICU.[35] However, studies indicate that delirium is under-recognized in the ICU, especially hypoactive delirium. Patient should be screened for delirium each day using a validated screen such as the Confusion Assessment Method for the ICU (CAM-ICU).[36] Minimization of benzodiazepines by either avoidance or using other agents may reduce delirium and ICU length of stay.[37,38] If patients do develop delirium, initial treatment should be nonpharmacologic, using frequent re-orientation of the patient and attempts to correct sleep-wake cycle deficits. If unsuccessful, antipsychotic agents such as haloperidol or newer atypical agents may be beneficial. Delirium is best treated with a protocol using evidence-based standards and adopted for local usage.

The use of excessive sedation medicines can have secondary effects outside the neurologic system. Patients who do not wake up once their sedatives are stopped have continued need for mechanical ventilation, with the concordant risk of VAP. For this reason, sedation protocols are recommended because they have been shown to conclusively reduce duration of mechanical ventilation, ICU length of stay, and need for tracheostomy.[39,40] In addition, a daily sedation holiday, allowing the patient to wake, is also strongly supported.[39,41,42] Although historically there have been concerns about daily awakening in surgical patients, all patients in the ICU, including postoperative patients, should have a sedation holiday assuming they are physiologically able to have one.

Surgeons also need to be cognizant of the potential for the development of neuropathy/myopathy of critical illness. Use of neuromuscular blocking agents is generally discouraged because they exacerbate neuropathy and require additional sedation. This problem is further exacerbated in patients receiving steroids.[43] This concern should not prevent steroid usage in patients who may potentially benefit from them, such as patients with acute respiratory distress syndrome (ARDS)[44] or septic shock; however, a careful weighing of available literature and the risk/benefit ratio should be undertaken before their initiation.

Cardiovascular Conditions

Cardiovascular organ failure support primarily consists of hemodynamic stabilization and fluid resuscitation. Surgical patients often have significant blood loss or dehydration reducing their intravascular fluid volume, ultimately leading to hypovolemic shock. This condition may be further complicated by the inflammatory response, which can cause worsened capillary permeability and decreased vascular resistance (distributive shock).

The treatment of cardiovascular failure depends on the underlying cause. The treatment of hypovolemia is volume. The treatment of bleeding is resuscitation with blood and/or blood products.

The treatment of distributive shock is multifactorial as described in early goal-directed therapy.[45] Although additional studies are ongoing to further optimize early goal-directed therapy, current guidelines for septic shock recommend resuscitation to a central venous pressure of 8 to 12 mm Hg (12–15 mm Hg in mechanically ventilated patients) with desired end points of a mean arterial pressure greater than 65 mm Hg, urine output 0.5 mL/kg/h, and central venous oxygen saturation greater than 70%.[33,45] If patients are not volume responsive and are intravascularly resuscitated, vasopressors are recommended to keep a mean arterial pressure greater than 65 mm Hg, although the goal pressure needed for adequate perfusion may vary with individual patients and data to support this number are limited.[46] Norepinephrine and dopamine have traditionally been the vasopressors of choice, but norepinephrine has become the preferred agent at many centers because of fewer adverse events.[47] If patients continue to have a low central venous oxygen saturation despite adequate volume status and mean arterial pressure, the next step is to transfuse to a hemoglobin greater than 10 mg/dL. If, despite all these steps, the patient continues to have a low central venous oxygen saturation, consideration should be given to the addition of an inotrope.

Myocardial function may be decreased in the perioperative period as a result of either myocardial infarction or a globally decreased left ventricular function that is mediated by an inflammatory response. High-risk vascular patients and those on preoperative β-blockers should have β-blockers continued in the perioperative period. Patients with perioperative myocardial infarctions should receive rapid cardiology consults. Therapy includes aspirin, β-blockade, oxygen, adequate oxygen-carrying capacity with transfusion if indicated, and statin therapy.[32] The determination of whether to begin anticoagulation and/or to send the patient for a cardiac catheterization is an individualized decision. Right ventricular dysfunction is more rare but is frequently seen in the setting of a physiologically significant pulmonary embolism. Treatment includes anticoagulation or lytics if indicated or an inferior vena cava filter if the risk for bleeding is too high to safely anticoagulate the patient. The myocardium should be supported with inotropic support if needed, with minimization of fluid resuscitation.

Another common cause of shock in the patient with trauma is spinal cord injury. Pressors to maintain vascular tone are appropriate in this setting. Clinicians must be concerned about obstructive shock secondary to tension pneumothorax, pericardial tamponade, or pulmonary embolism. Treatment includes a high index of suspicion when clinically indicated, followed by needle decompression, pericardiocentesis, and/or window and anticoagulation or inferior vena cava filter, respectively.

Respiratory Conditions

The key aspects of organ failure prevention involve minimization of volutrauma and barotrauma to the lung, minimization of VAP, and minimization of volume overload. There are strong data to support the use of a lung-protective, low-tidal-volume (starting at 6 mL/kg ideal body weight) ventilation strategy in patients with acute lung injury, maintaining a plateau pressure less than 30 mm Hg, because higher tidal volumes worsen organ failure and mortality.[34,48–50] The use of positive end-expiratory pressure to prevent atelectasis and recruit closed alveoli in patients with ARDS is also well supported.[51,52]

All ventilated patients are at risk for VAP. Elevating the head of the bed to 30 to 45°, oral care, and early liberation from the ventilator decreases the incidence of VAP.[53] Several studies show that patients who are given a daily spontaneous breathing trial have a reduction in the duration of mechanical ventilation.[54–56] Recent studies show that a positive fluid balance is associated with longer mechanical ventilation and increased mortality,[57,58] which can be especially challenging in postoperative patients who have significant third spacing, especially when they are critically ill. Although it is difficult to have a single rule of thumb for these patients, the best practice is to ensure that patients have adequate intravascular volume without excessive volume resuscitation. Assaying volume status in surgical patients can be difficult. In patients who are less sick, noninvasive methods such as following urine output are adequate. In more critically ill patients, additional monitoring may be appropriate. The simplest method is the use of central venous pressure; however, there are multiple studies indicating that this correlates poorly with intravascular volume status, despite its common usage. Newer technologies, such as those assessing stroke volume variance from an arterial line tracing and esophageal Dopplers, may play a role in assessing volume status. Bedside echocardiography is also being increasingly used for this purpose. Historically, pulmonary artery catheters have been used to aid in management of volume status, but several trials suggest that these should not be used on a routine basis for this indication.[59–61]

Renal Conditions

Protection of the kidneys in the surgical patient can be challenging. Acute kidney injury still occurs in up to 65% of septic shock and is an independent risk factor for death in patients with MODS.[62] The mainstay of therapy involves ensuring adequate hemodynamic resuscitation and, if possible, avoidance of iodinated contrast and nephrotoxic drugs. Although several agents have been proposed, there are no proven therapies that improve renal function in patients with MODS. However, there are unequivocal data that renal-dose dopamine is not effective in preventing acute renal failure, and its use cannot be supported.[33]

A certain subset of patients with MODS require an intravenous dye load in the setting of a computed tomography scan or angiography. Prevention of contrast-induced nephropathy has received significant attention recently. As with other causes of renal failure in MODS, the most important factor in protecting kidney function is adequate hydration. In addition, there are some data that suggest that bicarbonate may be useful in preventing contrast-induced nephropathy, although the largest trial to date suggests that there is no benefit to n-acetylcysteine, an agent commonly used for this purpose.[63]

In general, there is no advantage to using crystalloids or colloids in preventing perioperative renal failure. The SAFE (Saline vs Albumin Fluid Evaluation) study suggests that the choice of crystalloid versus albumin as the resuscitation fluid in patients in the ICU makes no difference except in patients with head injury, for whom albumin may be worse.[64] There are some patient population–specific data to suggest that albumin may be beneficial in patients with liver failure, acute lung injury (when given with furosemide), and sepsis.[65,66] Unless a patient is in a specific subcategory in which albumin has been shown to have benefit compared with crystalloid, it should be avoided if possible because it is significantly more expensive. When using crystalloids for resuscitation, it is important to choose a balanced solution. For this reason, it is important that practitioners be aware that normal saline is associated with a significant incidence of hyperchloremic metabolic acidosis.[67]

Despite optimal medical therapy, some surgical patients progress to anuric renal failure and require dialysis. Hypotensive patients who require dialysis are generally placed on continuous renal replacement therapy rather than intermittent hemodialysis because it causes less hemodynamic instability. However, the optimal timing and rate of renal replacement therapy continues to be controversial and is therefore a topic of active research.[68,69] In addition, there are experimental protocols to use alternative hemofiltration to remove inflammatory mediators, a technique that is commonly used in select ICUs outside the United States.[70]

Gastrointestinal Conditions

The intestine is often described as the motor of the systemic inflammatory response.[71] The most well-supported intervention associated with the gut and prevention of organ failure in the postoperative setting is early enteral nutrition. There have been several randomized trials, including enteral feeding versus total parenteral nutrition, that show improved outcomes and decreased organ failure in patients given early enteral nutrition.[72–75] In contrast, there does not seem to be a benefit of early parenteral nutrition in critically ill patients.[76]

Immunonutrition is an evolving field. Although an exhaustive review of the literature is beyond the scope of this article, there is strong evidence that supplemental enteral glutamine should be considered in patients with burns and trauma, and supplemental glutamine is recommended for critically ill patients receiving parental nutrition.[77] Supplemental combined vitamins, trace elements, and selenium supplementation should also be considered in critically ill patients. In contrast, diets supplemented with arginine should not be used in critically ill patients based on current data.

Although many surgical patients receive stress ulcer prophylaxis, data support their use only in patients with significant risk factors. These risk factors include mechanical ventilation for longer than 48 hours and coagulopathy. Other relative indications include acute kidney injury, sepsis, burn, and head injury. For patients who meet these indications, there is more evidence to support the usage of H2 blockers than proton pump inhibitors. Both classes of agents are associated with complications including development of *Clostridium difficile* infections and pneumonia and should be avoided unless a clear indication is present.

Endocrine Conditions

Although panendocrine dysfunction can occur in critical illness, the most well-studied abnormalities include those involving glucose control and adrenocorticoid secretion.[78] Although a single-center study in 2001 showed a significant mortality improvement in critically ill patients after cardiac surgery with tight glucose control (80–110 mg/dL),[79] multiple large-scale trials have failed to reproduce this benefit.[80–82] In addition, tight glucose control has been associated with a marked increase in hypoglycemia. Current recommendations suggest keeping blood glucose levels at less than 150 mg/dL.

Steroid use in critically ill patients remains controversial. A multicenter randomized trial showed improvement of shock and mortality in patients with relative adrenal insufficiency.[83] However, a subsequent larger trial did not show a mortality benefit, but did have a more rapid resolution of shock in patients treated with steroids.[84] Thus, current recommendations suggest supplementing patients with refractory septic shock with hydrocortisone.[33] However, the definition of refractory shock is unclear, so the appropriate trigger for initiating steroid therapy in patients with septic shock is not known. Obtaining an adrenocorticotropic hormone stimulation test is not indicated in patients with septic shock.

Hematology

The treatment of bleeding is transfusion of blood and blood products. When a surgical patient or a patient with trauma is bleeding, transfusion should be initiated immediately and can be a lifesaving therapy. However, although blood has historically been transfused to improve oxygen-carrying capacity in nonbleeding patients, there are significant data in critically ill patients that transfusing patients to a hemoglobin of 10 mg/dL is not beneficial and is potentially harmful.[85,86] Patients should generally have a hemoglobin of 7 mg/dL before transfusion, likely because of the immunosuppressive effects of blood and the underrecognized complication of transfusion-associated acute lung injury. Although most patients can safely be anemic, higher hemoglobin levels should be targeted in patients having an acute myocardial infarction, those with unstable angina, and those with class 3 or 4 congestive heart failure. In addition, the protocol for early goal-directed therapy for sepsis includes transfusion to a hemoglobin of 10 mg/dL if the patient has a central venous oxygen saturation less than 70% despite adequate fluid resuscitation and pressors. Although this is controversial and is the topic of a current study funded by the National Institutes of Health,[87] following this protocol is a reasonable evidenced-based approach.

Infectious Disease

The one organ system that is unequivocally amenable to curative (as opposed to supportive) care is infectious disease. This care involves appropriate source control when appropriate via surgery, interventional radiology drainage, or removal of an infected catheter. Source control should occur in the least invasive manner possible.

Administration of appropriate antibiotics can be lifesaving. In the setting of septic shock, a delay in the administration of appropriate antibiotics results in an 8% per hour increase in mortality.[88,89] Patients should initially receive broad-spectrum antibiotics targeted to suspected microorganisms (this varies based on the anatomic site of infection). Antibiotics should then be narrowed, based on culture results, to prevent generation of resistant organisms.

Apart from antibiotics, there are no biological adjuncts that are known to be beneficial for the treatment of MODS. Previously, drotrecogin α (Xigris) had US Food and Drug Administration approval for the treatment of septic shock. However, follow-up studies showed a lack of efficacy for this agent and it was recently withdrawn from the market worldwide.[90,91]

THE FUTURE

In the last decade, there has been increasing interest in studying homogenous subgroups of critically ill patients, rather than looking at a large heterogeneous population, in which important differences may be masked by the diversity of the group as a whole. A commonly used analogy is that no oncologist would enroll patients with stage I melanoma and stage IV pancreatic cancer in the same trial independently of disease state; however, to some degree, this is what has historically be done in critical care research. As a framework for future studies, the PIRO system has been advocated as a method for developing more patient-based therapies. In this acronym, P stands for predisposition (including age, genetic factors, and baseline comorbidities), I refers to the insult or infection that brought on the organ dysfunction (including site, whether hospital or community acquired, and microbiology), R is the response (evaluated by laboratory values and vital signs), and O is organ dysfunction (with evaluation of number of organs failing).[14,92,93] The hope is that this new approach will help stage patients with organ failure so that trials can be more effectively designed and more effective therapies can be designed to mitigate or treat MODS.

SUMMARY

Postoperative organ failure is a challenging disease process that is better prevented than treated. Providers should use close observation and clinical judgment, and checklists of best practices to minimize the risk of organ failure in their patients. The treatment of MODS generally remains supportive, outside of rapid initiation of source control (when appropriate) and targeted antibiotic therapy. More specific treatments may be developed as the complex pathophysiology of MODS is better understood and more homogenous patient populations are selected for study.

REFERENCES

1. Skillman JJ, Bushnell LS, Goldman H, et al. Respiratory failure, hypotension, sepsis, and jaundice. A clinical syndrome associated with lethal hemorrhage from acute stress ulceration of the stomach. Am J Surg 1969;117(4):523–30.
2. Baue AE. Multiple, progressive, or sequential systems failure. A syndrome of the 1970s. Arch Surg 1975;110(7):779–81.

3. American College of Chest Physicians/Society of Critical Care Medicine Consensus Conference: definitions for sepsis and organ failure and guidelines for the use of innovative therapies in sepsis. Crit Care Med 1992;20(6):864–74.
4. Barie PS, Hydo LJ. Epidemiology of multiple organ dysfunction syndrome in critical surgical illness. Surg Infect 2000;1(3):173–85 [discussion: 185–6].
5. Martin CM, Hill AD, Burns K, et al. Characteristics and outcomes for critically ill patients with prolonged intensive care unit stays. Crit Care Med 2005;33(9): 1922–7 [quiz: 1936].
6. Vincent JL, Sakr Y, Sprung CL, et al. Sepsis in European intensive care units: results of the SOAP study. Crit Care Med 2006;34(2):344–53.
7. Dewar D, Moore FA, Moore EE, et al. Postinjury multiple organ failure. Injury 2009; 40(9):912–8.
8. Martin GS, Mannino DM, Eaton S, et al. The epidemiology of sepsis in the United States from 1979 through 2000. N Engl J Med 2003;348(16):1546–54.
9. Barie PS, Hydo LJ, Pieracci FM, et al. Multiple organ dysfunction syndrome in critical surgical illness. Surg Infect 2009;10(5):369–77.
10. Kallinen O, Maisniemi K, Bohling T, et al. Multiple organ failure as a cause of death in patients with severe burns. J Burn Care Res 2011. [Epub ahead of print].
11. Marshall JC, Cook DJ, Christou NV, et al. Multiple organ dysfunction score: a reliable descriptor of a complex clinical outcome. Crit Care Med 1995;23(10):1638–52.
12. Le Gall JR, Klar J, Lemeshow S, et al. The Logistic Organ Dysfunction System. A new way to assess organ dysfunction in the intensive care unit. ICU Scoring Group. JAMA 1996;276(10):802–10.
13. Hotchkiss RS, Opal S. Immunotherapy for sepsis–a new approach against an ancient foe. N Engl J Med 2010;363(1):87–9.
14. Vincent JL, Martinez EO, Silva E. Evolving concepts in sepsis definitions. Crit Care Nurs Clin North Am 2011;23(1):29–39.
15. Marshall JC. Sepsis research: where have we gone wrong? Crit Care Resusc 2006;8(3):241–3.
16. Carlet J, Cohen J, Calandra T, et al. Sepsis: time to reconsider the concept. Crit Care Med 2008;36(3):964–6.
17. Levy MM, Fink MP, Marshall JC, et al. 2001 SCCM/ESICM/ACCP/ATS/SIS International Sepsis Definitions Conference. Crit Care Med 2003;31(4):1250–6.
18. Ferreira AM, Sakr Y. Organ dysfunction: general approach, epidemiology, and organ failure scores. Semin Respir Crit Care Med 2011;32(5):543–51.
19. Coopersmith CM, Stromberg PE, Dunne WM, et al. Inhibition of intestinal epithelial apoptosis and survival in a murine model of pneumonia-induced sepsis. JAMA 2002;287(13):1716–21.
20. Marshall JC. Modeling MODS: what can be learned from animal models of the multiple-organ dysfunction syndrome? Intensive Care Med 2005;31(5):605–8.
21. Dorinsky PM, Gadek JE. Mechanisms of multiple nonpulmonary organ failure in ARDS. Chest 1989;96(4):885–92.
22. Hotchkiss RS, Karl IE. The pathophysiology and treatment of sepsis. N Engl J Med 2003;348(2):138–50.
23. Paulus P, Jennewein C, Zacharowski K. Biomarkers of endothelial dysfunction: can they help us deciphering systemic inflammation and sepsis? Biomarkers 2011;16(Suppl 1):S11–21.
24. Fink MP. Gastrointestinal mucosal injury in experimental models of shock, trauma, and sepsis. Crit Care Med 1991;19(5):627–41.
25. Marshall JC. Neutrophils in the pathogenesis of sepsis. Crit Care Med 2005; 33(Suppl 12):S502–5.

26. Patel KN, Soubra SH, Lam FW, et al. Polymicrobial sepsis and endotoxemia promote microvascular thrombosis via distinct mechanisms. J Thromb Haemostasis 2010;8(6):1403–9.

27. Dixon B. The role of microvascular thrombosis in sepsis. Anaesth Intensive Care 2004;32(5):619–29.

28. Suliburk J, Helmer K, Moore F, et al. The gut in systemic inflammatory response syndrome and sepsis. Enzyme systems fighting multiple organ failure. Eur Surg Res 2008;40(2):184–9.

29. Marshall JC. Critical illness is an iatrogenic disorder. Crit Care Med 2010; 38(Suppl 10):S582–9.

30. Ranieri VM, Suter PM, Tortorella C, et al. Effect of mechanical ventilation on inflammatory mediators in patients with acute respiratory distress syndrome: a randomized controlled trial. JAMA 1999;282(1):54–61.

31. Imai Y, Parodo J, Kajikawa O, et al. Injurious mechanical ventilation and end-organ epithelial cell apoptosis and organ dysfunction in an experimental model of acute respiratory distress syndrome. JAMA 2003;289(16):2104–12.

32. Fleisher LA, Beckman JA, Brown KA, et al. ACC/AHA 2007 guidelines on perioperative cardiovascular evaluation and care for noncardiac surgery: a report of the American College of Cardiology/American Heart Association Task Force on Practice Guidelines (Writing Committee to Revise the 2002 Guidelines on Perioperative Cardiovascular Evaluation for Noncardiac Surgery): developed in collaboration with the American Society of Echocardiography, American Society of Nuclear Cardiology, Heart Rhythm Society, Society of Cardiovascular Anesthesiologists, Society for Cardiovascular Angiography and Interventions, Society for Vascular Medicine and Biology, and Society for Vascular Surgery. Circulation 2007;116(17):e418–99.

33. Dellinger RP, Levy MM, Carlet JM, et al. Surviving Sepsis Campaign: international guidelines for management of severe sepsis and septic shock: 2008. Crit Care Med 2008;36(1):296–327.

34. Ventilation with lower tidal volumes as compared with traditional tidal volumes for acute lung injury and the acute respiratory distress syndrome. The Acute Respiratory Distress Syndrome Network. N Engl J Med 2000;342(18):1301–8.

35. Ely EW, Shintani A, Truman B, et al. Delirium as a predictor of mortality in mechanically ventilated patients in the intensive care unit. JAMA 2004;291(14):1753–62.

36. Ely EW, Inouye SK, Bernard GR, et al. Delirium in mechanically ventilated patients: validity and reliability of the confusion assessment method for the intensive care unit (CAM-ICU). JAMA 2001;286(21):2703–10.

37. Riker RR, Shehabi Y, Bokesch PM, et al. Dexmedetomidine vs midazolam for sedation of critically ill patients: a randomized trial. JAMA 2009;301(5):489–99.

38. Pichot C, Ghignone M, Quintin L. Dexmedetomidine and clonidine: from second-to-first-line sedative agents in the critical care setting? J Intensive Care Med 2011. [Epub ahead of print].

39. Brook AD, Ahrens TS, Schaiff R, et al. Effect of a nursing-implemented sedation protocol on the duration of mechanical ventilation. Crit Care Med 1999;27(12):2609–15.

40. MacLaren R, Plamondon JM, Ramsay KB, et al. A prospective evaluation of empiric versus protocol-based sedation and analgesia. Pharmacotherapy 2000;20(6):662–72.

41. Girard TD, Kress JP, Fuchs BD, et al. Efficacy and safety of a paired sedation and ventilator weaning protocol for mechanically ventilated patients in intensive care (Awakening and Breathing Controlled Trial): a randomised controlled trial. Lancet 2008;371(9607):126–34.

42. Devlin JW, Boleski G, Mlynarek M, et al. Motor Activity Assessment Scale: a valid and reliable sedation scale for use with mechanically ventilated patients in an adult surgical intensive care unit. Crit Care Med 1999;27(7):1271–5.
43. De Jonghe B, Sharshar T, Lefaucheur JP, et al. Paresis acquired in the intensive care unit: a prospective multicenter study. JAMA 2002;288(22):2859–67.
44. Papazian L, Forel JM, Gacouin A, et al. Neuromuscular blockers in early acute respiratory distress syndrome. N Engl J Med 2010;363(12):1107–16.
45. Rivers E, Nguyen B, Havstad S, et al. Early goal-directed therapy in the treatment of severe sepsis and septic shock. N Engl J Med 2001;345(19):1368–77.
46. Bourgoin A, Leone M, Delmas A, et al. Increasing mean arterial pressure in patients with septic shock: effects on oxygen variables and renal function. Crit Care Med 2005;33(4):780–6.
47. De Backer D, Biston P, Devriendt J, et al. Comparison of dopamine and norepinephrine in the treatment of shock. N Engl J Med 2010;362(9):779–89.
48. Stewart TE, Meade MO, Cook DJ, et al. Evaluation of a ventilation strategy to prevent barotrauma in patients at high risk for acute respiratory distress syndrome. Pressure- and Volume-Limited Ventilation Strategy Group. N Engl J Med 1998;338(6):355–61.
49. Tobin MJ. Culmination of an era in research on the acute respiratory distress syndrome. N Engl J Med 2000;342(18):1360–1.
50. Marini JJ, Gattinoni L. Ventilatory management of acute respiratory distress syndrome: a consensus of two. Crit Care Med 2004;32(1):250–5.
51. Brower RG, Lanken PN, MacIntyre N, et al. Higher versus lower positive end-expiratory pressures in patients with the acute respiratory distress syndrome. N Engl J Med 2004;351(4):327–36.
52. Amato MB, Barbas CS, Medeiros DM, et al. Beneficial effects of the "open lung approach" with low distending pressures in acute respiratory distress syndrome. A prospective randomized study on mechanical ventilation. Am J Respir Crit Care Med 1995;152(6 Pt 1):1835–46.
53. Kollef MH. Prevention of hospital-associated pneumonia and ventilator-associated pneumonia. Crit Care Med 2004;32(6):1396–405.
54. Ely EW, Baker AM, Dunagan DP, et al. Effect on the duration of mechanical ventilation of identifying patients capable of breathing spontaneously. N Engl J Med 1996;335(25):1864–9.
55. Esteban A, Alia I, Tobin MJ, et al. Effect of spontaneous breathing trial duration on outcome of attempts to discontinue mechanical ventilation. Spanish Lung Failure Collaborative Group. Am J Respir Crit Care Med 1999;159(2):512–8.
56. Esteban A, Alia I, Gordo F, et al. Extubation outcome after spontaneous breathing trials with T-tube or pressure support ventilation. The Spanish Lung Failure Collaborative Group. Am J Respir Crit Care Med 1997;156(2 Pt 1):459–65.
57. Flori HR, Church G, Liu KD, et al. Positive fluid balance is associated with higher mortality and prolonged mechanical ventilation in pediatric patients with acute lung injury. Crit Care Res Pract 2011;2011:854142.
58. Wiedemann HP, Wheeler AP, Bernard GR, et al. Comparison of two fluid-management strategies in acute lung injury. N Engl J Med 2006;354(24):2564–75.
59. Wheeler AP, Bernard GR, Thompson BT, et al. Pulmonary-artery versus central venous catheter to guide treatment of acute lung injury. N Engl J Med 2006;354(21):2213–24.
60. Sandham JD, Hull RD, Brant RF, et al. A randomized, controlled trial of the use of pulmonary-artery catheters in high-risk surgical patients. N Engl J Med 2003;348(1):5–14.

61. Richard C, Warszawski J, Anguel N, et al. Early use of the pulmonary artery catheter and outcomes in patients with shock and acute respiratory distress syndrome: a randomized controlled trial. JAMA 2003;290(20):2713–20.
62. Bagshaw SM, Lapinsky S, Dial S, et al. Acute kidney injury in septic shock: clinical outcomes and impact of duration of hypotension prior to initiation of antimicrobial therapy. Intensive Care Med 2009;35(5):871–81.
63. ACT Investigators. Acetylcysteine for prevention of renal outcomes in patients undergoing coronary and peripheral vascular angiography: main results from the randomized Acetylcysteine for Contrast-induced nephropathy Trial (ACT). Circulation 2011;124(11):1250–9.
64. Myburgh J, Cooper DJ, Finfer S, et al. Saline or albumin for fluid resuscitation in patients with traumatic brain injury. N Engl J Med 2007;357(9):874–84.
65. Martin GS, Mangialardi RJ, Wheeler AP, et al. Albumin and furosemide therapy in hypoproteinemic patients with acute lung injury. Crit Care Med 2002;30(10): 2175–82.
66. Delaney AP, Dan A, McCaffroy J, et al. The role of albumin as a resuscitation fluid for patients with sepsis: a systematic review and meta-analysis. Crit Care Med 2011;39(2):386–91.
67. Yunos NM, Kim IB, Bellomo R, et al. The biochemical effects of restricting chloride-rich fluids in intensive care. Crit Care Med 2011;39(11):2419–24.
68. Ricci Z, Polito A, Ronco C. The implications and management of septic acute kidney injury. Nat Rev Nephrol 2011;7(4):218–25.
69. Honore PM, Jacobs R, Joannes-Boyau O, et al. Septic AKI in ICU patients. diagnosis, pathophysiology, and treatment type, dosing, and timing: a comprehensive review of recent and future developments. Ann Intensive Care 2011;1(1):32.
70. Oda S, Sadahiro T, Hirayama Y, et al. Non-renal indications for continuous renal replacement therapy: current status in Japan. Contrib Nephrol 2010;166: 47–53.
71. Clark JA, Coopersmith CM. Intestinal crosstalk: a new paradigm for understanding the gut as the "motor" of critical illness. Shock 2007;28(4):384–93.
72. Moore FA, Moore EE, Kudsk KA, et al. Clinical benefits of an immune-enhancing diet for early postinjury enteral feeding. J Trauma 1994;37(4):607–15.
73. Moore FA, Feliciano DV, Andrassy RJ, et al. Early enteral feeding, compared with parenteral, reduces postoperative septic complications. The results of a meta-analysis. Ann Surg 1992;216(2):172–83.
74. Moore FA, Moore EE, Jones TN, et al. TEN versus TPN following major abdominal trauma–reduced septic morbidity. J Trauma 1989;29(7):916–22 [discussion: 922–3].
75. Kudsk KA, Croce MA, Fabian TC, et al. Enteral versus parenteral feeding. Effects on septic morbidity after blunt and penetrating abdominal trauma. Ann Surg 1992;215(5):503–11 [discussion: 511–3].
76. Casaer MP, Mesotten D, Hermans G, et al. Early versus late parenteral nutrition in critically ill adults. N Engl J Med 2011;365(6):506–17.
77. Available at: http://www.criticalcarenutrition.com/docs/cpg/srrev.pdf. Accessed August 1, 2011.
78. Vanhorebeek I, Langouche L, Van den Berghe G. Endocrine aspects of acute and prolonged critical illness. Nat Clin Pract Endocrinol Metab 2006;2(1):20–31.
79. van den Berghe G, Wouters P, Weekers F, et al. Intensive insulin therapy in the critically ill patients. N Engl J Med 2001;345(19):1359–67.
80. Finfer S, Chittock DR, Su SY, et al. Intensive versus conventional glucose control in critically ill patients. N Engl J Med 2009;360(13):1283–97.

81. Griesdale DE, de Souza RJ, van Dam RM, et al. Intensive insulin therapy and mortality among critically ill patients: a meta-analysis including NICE-SUGAR study data. CMAJ 2009;180(8):821–7.

82. Marik PE, Preiser JC. Toward understanding tight glycemic control in the ICU: a systematic review and metaanalysis. Chest 2010;137(3):544–51.

83. Annane D, Sebille V, Charpentier C, et al. Effect of treatment with low doses of hydrocortisone and fludrocortisone on mortality in patients with septic shock. JAMA 2002;288(7):862–71.

84. Sprung CL, Annane D, Keh D, et al. Hydrocortisone therapy for patients with septic shock. N Engl J Med 2008;358(2):111–24.

85. Hebert PC, Wells G, Blajchman MA, et al. A multicenter, randomized, controlled clinical trial of transfusion requirements in critical care. Transfusion Requirements in Critical Care Investigators, Canadian Critical Care Trials Group. N Engl J Med 1999;340(6):409–17.

86. Napolitano LM, Kurek S, Luchette FA, et al. Clinical practice guideline: red blood cell transfusion in adult trauma and critical care. Crit Care Med 2009;37(12): 3124–57.

87. Available at: http://clinicaltrials.gov/ct2/show/NCT00510835?term=process&rank=1. Accessed August 1, 2011.

88. Iregui M, Ward S, Sherman G, et al. Clinical importance of delays in the initiation of appropriate antibiotic treatment for ventilator-associated pneumonia. Chest 2002;122(1):262–8.

89. Dickinson JD, Kollef MH. Early and adequate antibiotic therapy in the treatment of severe sepsis and septic shock. Curr Infect Dis Rep 2011;13(5):399–405.

90. Laterre PF, Abraham E, Janes JM, et al. ADDRESS (ADministration of DRotrecogin alfa [activated] in Early stage Severe Sepsis) long-term follow-up: one-year safety and efficacy evaluation. Crit Care Med 2007;35(6):1457–63.

91. Dhainaut JF, Laterre PF, Janes JM, et al. Drotrecogin alfa (activated) in the treatment of severe sepsis patients with multiple-organ dysfunction: data from the PROWESS trial. Intensive Care Med 2003;29(6):894–903.

92. Rubulotta F, Marshall JC, Ramsay G, et al. Predisposition, insult/infection, response, and organ dysfunction: a new model for staging severe sepsis. Crit Care Med 2009;37(4):1329–35.

93. Moreno RP, Metnitz B, Adler L, et al. Sepsis mortality prediction based on predisposition, infection and response. Intensive Care Med 2008;34(3):496–504.

Postoperative Pulmonary Complications: Pneumonia and Acute Respiratory Failure

Gaurav Sachdev, MD[a], Lena M. Napolitano, MD[b],*

KEYWORDS

- Pulmonary complications • Pneumonia • Respiratory failure
- Ventilator-associated pneumonia

POSTOPERATIVE PULMONARY COMPLICATIONS

Pulmonary complications in the postoperative period are a significant cause of morbidity and mortality.[1] Examples of these complications include atelectasis, bronchospasm, bronchitis, pneumonia, exacerbation of chronic obstructive pulmonary disease (COPD), pulmonary edema, and various forms of upper airway obstruction. The incidence of these complications varies among hospitals and by the procedure performed.

Thoracic surgery impairs postoperative respiratory function, resulting in a higher incidence (19%–59%) of pulmonary complications compared with upper (16%–20%) or lower (0%–5%) abdominal surgery. In patients undergoing thoracic surgery for lung resection, postoperative pulmonary complications occurred in 14.5% of patients and were associated with increased hospital length of stay, intensive care unit (ICU) admission, and increased mortality. Multivariate analysis confirmed that age older than 75 years, body mass index greater than 30 kg/m^2, American Society of Anesthesiology (ASA) score greater than 3, smoking history, and COPD were significant independent risk factors for the development of postoperative pulmonary complications.[2]

In a recent Medicare study of 22,752 patients (aged 65 years and older) with diverticulitis who underwent elective left colon resection, it was identified that surgical

[a] Division of Acute Care Surgery [Trauma, Burns, Critical Care, Emergency Surgery], Department of Surgery, University of Michigan, 1500 East Medical Drive, Ann Arbor, MI 48109–0033, USA
[b] Division of Acute Care Surgery [Trauma, Burns, Critical Care, Emergency Surgery], Department of Surgery, University of Michigan Health System, Room 1C421, University Hospital, 1500 East Medical Drive, Ann Arbor, MI 48109-0033, USA
* Corresponding author.
E-mail address: lenan@umich.edu

Surg Clin N Am 92 (2012) 321–344
doi:10.1016/j.suc.2012.01.013
0039-6109/12/$ – see front matter © 2012 Published by Elsevier Inc.

surgical.theclinics.com

patients with comorbidities of congestive heart failure (CHF) and COPD had a significantly greater risk for postoperative pulmonary complications (CHF, odds ratio [OR] 4.2, 95% confidence interval [CI] 3.59–4.85; COPD, OR 2.2, 95% CI 1.94–2.50), which were associated with increased morbidity and mortality.[3] These studies provide data to support careful assessment of risk factors for postoperative pulmonary complications in the preoperative period, and additional assessment to determine how best to optimize the patient preoperatively to prevent these complications.

A comprehensive systematic review of risk factors for postoperative pulmonary complications after noncardiothoracic surgery separated them into (1) patient-related and (2) procedure-related risk factors (**Table 1**).[4] Among patient-related risk factors, good evidence supports advanced age, ASA class II or greater, functional dependence, COPD, and CHF. Fair evidence, based on fewer studies or a lower odds ratio, supports impaired sensorium, abnormal findings on chest examination, cigarette use, alcohol use, and weight loss. A recent study of elective surgical patients (n = 393,794) from the Veterans Administration Surgical Quality Improvement Program, with 6225 postoperative pneumonias reported, confirmed that current smokers had significantly more postoperative pneumonia and that there was a dose-dependent increase in pulmonary complications based on pack-year exposure.[5] Good evidence suggests that obesity and well-controlled asthma are not risk factors. Fair evidence suggests that poorly controlled asthma confers an increased risk. Evidence is insufficient to estimate risk due to corticosteroid use or poor exercise capacity. Most recently, a study of the National Inpatient Sample data from 1998 to 2007 confirmed that patients with sleep apnea developed pulmonary complications significantly more frequently than matched controls after both orthopedic and general surgical procedures.[6] The major procedure-related risk factors (thoracic surgery, open aortic surgery, abdominal surgery) confer higher risk for pulmonary complications than patient-related risk factors.

PREVENTION OF POSTOPERATIVE PULMONARY COMPLICATIONS

Given the increased morbidity and mortality associated with postoperative pulmonary complications, all efforts to prevent these complications should be implemented in surgical patients. A systematic review of strategies to reduce postoperative pulmonary complications after noncardiothoracic surgery identified that few interventions have been shown to definitively reduce postoperative pulmonary complications (**Table 2**).[7,8]

These prevention strategies should begin before surgery with smoking cessation and management of lung disease (COPD, asthma). Preoperative smoking cessation at least 8 weeks before surgery has shown benefit. A shorter period of cessation has actually been shown to increase postoperative complications. One blinded prospective study among elective coronary artery bypass patients compared pulmonary complication rates, and reported that those who stopped smoking for 2 months or less had a pulmonary complication rate almost 4 times higher than those who had stopped smoking for longer than 2 months (57.1% vs 14.5%). Also, patients who had stopped smoking for more than 6 months had the same rates as those who never smoked (11.1% vs 11.9%).[9]

Patients with a diagnosis of COPD already have a high risk for postoperative pulmonary complications. However, patients who undergo preoperative optimization of pulmonary function (various combinations of bronchodilators, antibiotics, systemic glucocorticoids) have a lower incidence of postoperative pulmonary complications than those who receive no preoperative optimization.[10,11]

Table 1
Patient-related, procedure-related, and laboratory risk factors for postoperative pulmonary complications

Factor	Strength of Recommendation[a]	Odds Ratio[b]
Potential Patient-Related Risk Factor		
Advanced age	A	2.09–3.04
ASA class ≥II	A	2.55–4.87
CHF	A	2.93
Functionally dependent	A	1.65–2.51
COPD	A	1.79
Weight loss	B	1.62
Impaired sensorium	B	1.39
Cigarette use	B	1.26
Alcohol use	B	1.21
Abnormal findings on chest examination	B	NA
Diabetes	C	—
Obesity	D	—
Asthma	D	—
Obstructive sleep apnea	I	—
Corticosteroid use	I	—
HIV infection	I	—
Arrhythmia	I	—
Poor exercise capacity	I	—
Potential Procedure-Related Risk Factor		
Aortic aneurysm repair	A	6.90
Thoracic surgery	A	4.24
Abdominal surgery	A	3.01
Upper abdominal surgery	A	2.91
Neurosurgery	A	2.53
Prolonged surgery	A	2.26
Head and neck surgery	A	2.21
Emergency surgery	A	2.21
Vascular surgery	A	2.10
General anesthesia	A	1.83
Perioperative transfusion	B	1.47
Hip surgery	D	—
Gynecologic or urologic surgery	D	—
Esophageal surgery	I	—
Laboratory Tests		
Albumin level <35 g/L	A	2.53
Chest radiography	B	4.81
BUN level >7.5 mmol/L (>21 mg/dL)	B	NA
Spirometry	I	—

Abbreviations: BUN, blood urea nitrogen; HIV, human immunodeficiency virus; NA, not available.

[a] Recommendations: A = good evidence to support the particular risk factor or laboratory predictor; B = at least fair evidence to support the particular risk factor or laboratory predictor; C = at least fair evidence to suggest that the particular factor is not a risk factor or that the laboratory test does not predict risk; D = good evidence to suggest that the particular factor is not a risk factor or that the laboratory test does not predict risk; I = insufficient evidence to determine whether the factor increases risk or whether the laboratory test predicts risk, and evidence is lacking, is of poor quality, or is conflicting.

[b] For factors with A or B ratings, odds ratios are trim-and-fill estimates. When these estimates were not possible, the pooled estimate is provided.

Data from Smetana GW, Lawrence VA, Cornell JE. Preoperative pulmonary risk stratification for noncardiothoracic surgery: systematic review for the American College of Physicians. Ann Intern Med 2006;144:581–95.

Table 2
Specific interventions to reduce the risk for postoperative pulmonary complications

Risk-Reduction Strategy	Strength of Evidence[a]	Type of Complication Studied
Postoperative lung expansion modalities	A	Atelectasis, pneumonia, bronchitis, severe hypoxemia
Selective postoperative nasogastric decompression	B	Atelectasis, pneumonia, aspiration
Short-acting neuromuscular blockade	B	Atelectasis, pneumonia
Laparoscopic (vs open) operation	C	Spirometry, atelectasis, pneumonia, overall respiratory complications
Smoking cessation	I	Postoperative ventilator support
Intraoperative neuraxial blockade	I	Pneumonia, postoperative hypoxia, respiratory failure
Postoperative epidural analgesia	I	Atelectasis, pneumonia, respiratory failure
Immunonutrition	I	Overall infectious complications, pneumonia, respiratory failure
Routine total parenteral or enteral nutrition[b]	D	Atelectasis, pneumonia, empyema, respiratory failure
Right-heart catheterization	D	Pneumonia

[a] Definitions for categories of strength of evidence, modified from the US Preventive Services Task Force categories (11). A = good evidence that the strategy reduces postoperative pulmonary complications and benefit outweighs harm; B = at least fair evidence that the strategy reduces postoperative pulmonary complications and benefit outweighs harm; C = at least fair evidence that the strategy may reduce postoperative pulmonary complications, but the balance between benefit and harm is too close to justify a general recommendation; D = at least fair evidence that the strategy does not reduce postoperative pulmonary complications or harm outweighs benefit; I = evidence of effectiveness of the strategy to reduce postoperative pulmonary complications is conflicting, of poor quality, lacking, or insufficient, or the balance between benefit and harm cannot be determined.

[b] Evidence remains uncertain (strength of evidence I) on total parenteral or enteral nutrition for severely malnourished patients or when a protracted time of inadequate nutritional intake is anticipated.

Data from Lawrence VA, Cornell JE, Smetana GW. Strategies to reduce postoperative pulmonary complications after noncardiothoracic surgery: systematic review for the American College of Physicians. Ann Intern Med 2006;144:596–608.

Patients with poorly controlled asthma have an increased risk for postoperative pulmonary complications. Patients with asthma should undergo a preoperative evaluation to assess whether they need a step-up in their therapy.[12] The use of preoperative systemic glucocorticoid administration has been recommended by some investigators, but has not shown benefit in all studies. Steroids are best reserved for patients with poorly controlled severe asthma.[13]

Intraoperative strategies to reduce the incidence of postoperative pneumonia include choice in the type of anesthesia, length of neuromuscular blockade, and duration of surgery. There is some evidence suggesting that using epidural anesthesia, when both general and epidural anesthesia are safe and appropriate for the procedure, may potentially reduce the risk of pulmonary complications.[14] However, the evidence is not conclusive.

The choice of neuromuscular blockade has a significant influence on postoperative pulmonary complications. In one prospective nonrandomized study, the difference in postoperative pneumonia between pancuronium and atracurium was 13% versus 5%.[15] Evidence suggested that using short-acting or intermediate-acting neuromuscular blockers is preferred to reduce postoperative pulmonary complications. A prospective randomized study showed that patients treated with longer-acting neuromuscular blockers were 4 times as likely to develop postoperative pulmonary complications.[16]

Postoperative strategies to prevent pneumonia focus on increasing lung volume, pulmonary toilet, pain control, and preventing aspiration. Lung expansion interventions via deep-breathing exercises and incentive spirometry have shown some benefit in reducing postoperative pulmonary complications.[17] However, a recent Cochrane Database review found no evidence in the effectiveness of incentive spirometry for the prevention of postoperative pulmonary complications.[18,19]

The use of nasal continuous positive airway pressure (nCPAP) may show some benefit. In a prospectively randomized trial in cardiac surgery patients, use of long-term prophylactic nCPAP improved oxygenation and reduced the incidence of postoperative pneumonia.[20] The use of intermittent positive pressure breathing (IPPB) was a popular method thought to prevent postoperative pneumonia. However, there is no difference between patients who use incentive spirometry, deep-breathing exercises, or IPPB. Similarly, inconclusive results have also been reported for continuous positive airway pressure (CPAP).[21] The overall benefit from deep-breathing exercises, incentive spirometry, IPPB, and different forms of CPAP is still in question. For CPAP, the danger of gastric distention in patients undergoing abdominal surgery is one prohibitive factor to take into consideration, in addition to the cost of administration.

Postoperative pain control has a significant contribution to efficient pulmonary toilet. If a patient cannot take deep breaths or ambulate secondary to pain, their risk of postoperative pneumonia increases. Several studies have shown the benefit of adequate pain control in improving pneumonia.[22] This improvement can be achieved either by patient-controlled analgesia or by epidural block when appropriate. Some studies have shown improved postoperative cardiac and pulmonary complications in patients with abdominal aneurysm and those who received epidural analgesia.[23]

Selective, rather than routine, use of nasogastric tubes is recommended to reduce postoperative pulmonary complications. Several studies, meta-analyses, and Cochrane Database systematic reviews have clearly demonstrated increased risk of pulmonary complications, particularly pneumonia, with the presence of a nasogastric tube.[24,25] It is important to consider the reason for use of a nasogastric tube, and consideration for removal as soon as possible, in a vigilant effort to reduce the incidence of pneumonia.

PNEUMONIA

The incidence of postoperative pneumonia varies depending on risk factors, ranging from an incidence of 1.5% to as high as 15.3% in high-risk groups. The 30-day postoperative mortality for all groups can be as high as 21%, depending on the severity of illness, comorbidities, and causative pathogens.[26,27] In a recent study of 48,247 adults who underwent colectomy with data available in the American College of Surgeons NSQIP program (2005–2008), postoperative pneumonia was significantly more common in patients undergoing emergent compared with elective surgery (11.1% vs 2.9%) and decreased in the overall cohort over time (4.60% in 2005 to 3.97% in 2008).[28] In 2005, the American Thoracic Society (ATS)/Infectious Diseases Society of America (IDSA) provided guidelines to further categorize pneumonia into hospital-acquired pneumonia (HAP), ventilator-associated pneumonia (VAP), and health care–associated pneumonia (HCAP).[29] In this article, the authors discuss the definition, diagnosis, and management of perioperative pneumonia.

Pathophysiology

Under normal circumstances, the lower respiratory tract is sterile. Both HAP and VAP are generally associated with introduction of bacteria to the sterile lower respiratory tract; this can be exacerbated by impaired host defenses. The introduction of bacteria to the lower airways occurs through 2 important mechanisms: bacterial colonization of the aerodigestive tract and aspiration of contaminated secretions into the lower airway.[30–33] Several factors promote these mechanisms, including the presence of invasive devices, medications altering gastric emptying and pH, contaminated water, medications, and respiratory therapy equipment. In VAP, the colonization pathway occurs according to the steps illustrated in **Fig. 1**.

Definitions

Pneumonia is an acute infection of the pulmonary parenchyma. It is important to distinguish between community-acquired pneumonia and HAP, because the causative pathogens are different. In the postoperative period, HAP is of more relevance, and can be further classified (**Fig. 2**). HAP is defined as pneumonia occurring more than 48 hours after hospital admission. VAP is a type of HAP that develops more than 48 hours after endotracheal intubation. HCAP is pneumonia that occurs in a patient with health care contact as defined by 1 or more of the following criteria: a patient hospitalized for 2 days or more in an acute care facility within 90 days of infection; a patient residing in a nursing home or long-term care facility; a patient who has attended a hospital or hemodialysis center; a patient who has received intravenous antibiotic therapy, chemotherapy, or wound care within 30 days of the current

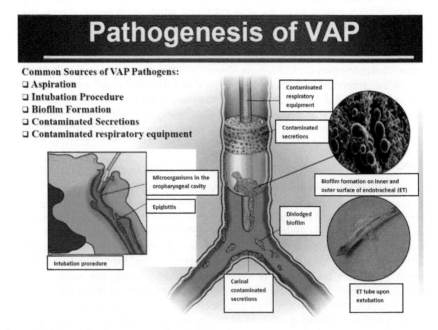

Fig. 1. Pathway of colonization of airway in VAP.

Definitions: The ATS/IDSA Guidelines

Hospital-acquired pneumonia (HAP)

- Pneumonia occurring ≥ 48 hours post-hospital admission

Ventilator-associated pneumonia (VAP)

- Pneumonia occurring > 48-72 hours post-intubation

Healthcare-associated pneumonia (HCAP)

- Includes HAP and VAP
- Pneumonia in patients
  - Hospitalized for ≥2 days in an acute care facility within 90 days of infection
  - Resided in a NH or LTC facility
  - Attended a hospital or hemodialysis center
  - Received IV antibiotic therapy, chemotherapy or wound care within 30 days of current infection
  - Family member of patient with MDR pathogens

Fig. 2. ATS/IDSA guideline: definitions of pneumonia. IV, intravenous; LTC, long-term care; MDR, multidrug-resistant; NH, nursing home. (*Data from* American Thoracic Society. Guidelines for the management of adults with hospital-acquired, ventilator-associated, and healthcare-associated pneumonia. Am J Respir Crit Care Med 2005;171(4):388–416.)

infection; and any patient who is a family member of a patient with a multidrug-resistant (MDR) pathogen.[3]

Reports from the National Healthcare Safety Network (NHSN) in the United States have documented a recent decline in VAP rates related to the implementation of prevention strategies. However, the highest rates of VAP remain in surgical ICUs, particularly in burn and trauma ICUs (**Table 3**).[34] It is therefore very important to implement VAP-preventive strategies in all postsurgical patients.

Diagnosis

The diagnosis of pneumonia is difficult because the clinical findings are nonspecific. Pneumonia should be suspected in a patient with new or progressive infiltrate on chest radiographs as well as clinical characteristics such as fever, purulent sputum, leukocytosis, and hypoxia.[3] When findings at autopsy are used as a reference, the combination of radiographic infiltrate plus 2 of 3 clinical features (fever >38°C, leukocytosis/leukopenia, purulent secretions) resulted in 69% sensitivity and 75% specificity for pneumonia.[35]

The diagnosis of VAP is suspected when a patient on mechanical ventilation develops new pulmonary infiltrate with fever, leukocytosis, and purulent secretions. Further signs of increased ventilator support or oxygen requirements also raise this suspicion. However, the differential diagnosis for these findings can be broad (atelectasis, acute respiratory distress syndrome [ARDS], chemical pneumonitis, contusion, pulmonary embolism, drug reaction, infiltrative tumor).[36] Radiographic and clinical abnormalities occur frequently in patients without a true diagnosis of VAP. Only 43% of patients with radiographic evidence were found to have VAP by postmortem examination.[37]

At present, the Centers for Disease Control and Prevention (CDC) define VAP using a combination of radiologic, clinical, and laboratory criteria, in patients who are

Table 3
Decline in VAP cases per 1000 ventilator days in ICUs in the United States

Type of ICU	2004 Pooled Means[a]	2006 Pooled Means[b]	2007 Pooled Means[c]	2007 Pooled Means[d]	2009 Pooled Means[e]
Burn	12.0	12.3	10.7	10.7	7.4
Cardiothoracic	7.2	5.7	4.7	3.9	2.1
Coronary	4.4	2.8	2.5	2.1	1.5
Medical	4.9	3.1	2.5	2.4	1.4
Medical/surgical: major teaching	5.4	3.6	3.3	2.9	2.0
Medical/surgical: all others	5.1	2.7	2.3	2.2	1.4
Neurosurgical	11.2	7.0	6.5	5.3	3.8
Pediatric	2.9	2.5	2.1	2.3	1.1
Surgical	9.3	5.2	5.3	4.9	3.8
Trauma	15.2	10.2	9.3	8.1	6.5

Note the higher VAP rates in surgical and neurosurgical ICUs and highest rates in burn and trauma ICUs.

[a] National Nosocomial Infections Surveillance System. National Nosocomial Infections Surveillance (NNIS) System Report, data summary from January 1992 through June 2004, issued October 2004. Am J Infect Control 2004;32:470–85.

[b] Edwards JR, Peterson KD, Andrus ML, et al. NHSN Facilities. National Healthcare Safety Network (NHSN) Report, data summary for 2006, issued June 2007. Am J Infect Control 2007;35:290–301.

[c] Edwards JR, Peterson KD, Andrus ML, et al. National Healthcare Safety Network Facilities. National Healthcare Safety Network (NHSN) Report, data summary for 2006 through 2007, issued November 2008. Am J Infect Control 2008;36:609–26. Erratum in: Am J Infect Control 2009;37:425.

[d] Edwards JR, Peterson KD, Mu Y, et al. National Healthcare Safety Network (NHSN) report: data summary for 2006 through 2008, issued December 2009. Am J Infect Control 2009;37(10):783–805.

[e] Dudeck MA, Horan TC, Peterson KD, et al. National Healthcare Safety Network (NHSN) report, data summary for 2009, device-associated module. Am J Infect Control 2011;39(5):349–67.

ventilated for longer than 48 hours. Pneumonia is classified into 3 types as illustrated in **Fig. 3**. These types are clinically defined (PNEU-1), common bacterial, fungal, or atypical pneumonia (PNEU-2), and pneumonia in immunocompromised patients (PNEU-3). The diagnosis requires new or progressive and persistent infiltrate/consolidation/cavitation on 2 or more serial chest radiographs. In addition, it must meet minimum criteria in 2 separate clinical categories (**Fig. 4**). Furthermore, it must meet minimum criteria in 3 separate laboratory categories (**Fig. 5**).

Diagnostic testing is often required when VAP is suspected because radiologic and clinical findings are nonspecific. It is therefore recommended that all patients with possible VAP undergo lower respiratory tract sampling with microscopic evaluation and culture. This procedure can be done using bronchoscopic sampling of the lower respiratory tract (bronchoalveolar lavage [BAL]) or without the use of a bronchoscope (mini-BAL) with similar safety and diagnostic accuracy.[38] In patients with left lower lobe infiltrates and possible VAP, bronchoscopic BAL is preferred to obtain a sample from this area because mini-BAL sampling catheters most commonly advance into the bronchus of the right lower lobe. Bronchoscopic sampling is not associated with improved mortality or reduced duration of ventilation, ICU stay, or hospital stay. However, it does influence antibiotic selection and de-escalation of antibiotics.[39]

Given the severity of VAP and the frequency of serious conditions that can mimic VAP, additional tests that provide further evidence for VAP are clearly warranted.[40]

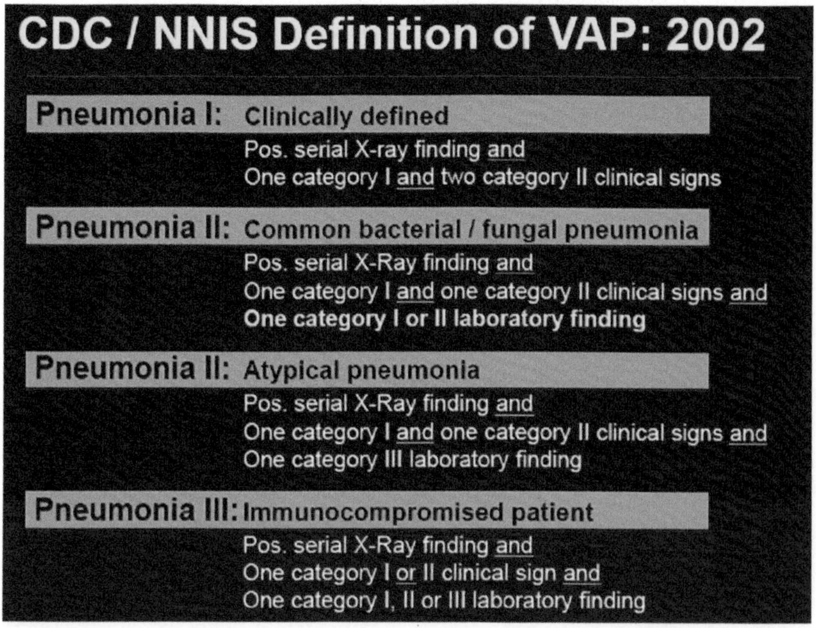

CDC / NNIS Definition of VAP: 2002

Pneumonia I: Clinically defined

Pos. serial X-ray finding and
One category I and two category II clinical signs

Pneumonia II: Common bacterial / fungal pneumonia

Pos. serial X-Ray finding and
One category I and one category II clinical signs and
One category I or II laboratory finding

Pneumonia II: Atypical pneumonia

Pos. serial X-Ray finding and
One category I and one category II clinical signs and
One category III laboratory finding

Pneumonia III: Immunocompromised patient

Pos. serial X-Ray finding and
One category I or II clinical sign and
One category I, II or III laboratory finding

Fig. 3. CDC definition of VAP. NNIS, National Nosocomial Infections Surveillance.

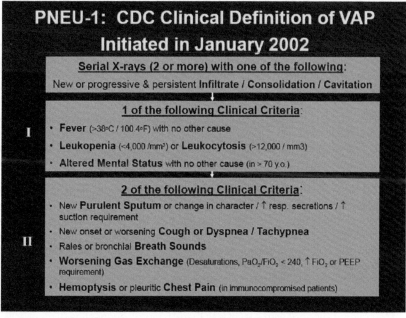

PNEU-1: CDC Clinical Definition of VAP
Initiated in January 2002

Serial X-rays (2 or more) with one of the following:

New or progressive & persistent Infiltrate / Consolidation / Cavitation

↓

1 of the following Clinical Criteria:

I

- **Fever** (>38°C / 100.4°F) with no other cause
- **Leukopenia** (<4,000 /mm^2) or **Leukocytosis** (>12,000 / mm3)
- **Altered Mental Status** with no other cause (in > 70 y.o.)

↓

2 of the following Clinical Criteria:

- New **Purulent Sputum** or change in character / ↑ resp. secretions / ↑ suction requirement
- New onset or worsening **Cough or Dyspnea / Tachypnea**

II
- Rales or bronchial **Breath Sounds**
- **Worsening Gas Exchange** (Desaturations, PaO$_2$/FiO$_2$ < 240, ↑ FiO$_2$ or PEEP requirement)
- **Hemoptysis** or pleuritic **Chest Pain** (in immunocompromised patients)

Fig. 4. CDC clinical definition of VAP. PEEP, positive end-expiratory pressure.

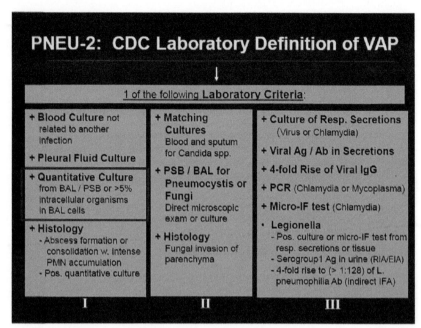

Fig. 5. CDC definition of VAP. Ab, antibody; BAL, bronchoalveolar lavage; EIA, enzyme immunoassay; IF, immunofluorescence; IFA, immunofluorescence assay; IgG, immunoglobulin G; PCR, polymerase chain reaction; PMN, polymorphonuclear leukocytes; PSB, protected specimen brush; RIA, radioimmunoassay.

No sensitive and specific biomarker is currently available to confirm a diagnosis of VAP. C-reactive protein, procalcitonin, and soluble triggering receptor expressed on myeloid cells (sTREM-1, a member of the immunoglobulin superfamily whose expression on phagocytes is specifically upregulated by microbial products) have been evaluated as biomarkers for diagnosing VAP. Multiple studies have confirmed that C-reactive protein and procalcitonin have poor diagnostic value for VAP.[41–43] Additional studies have confirmed conflicting results for sTREM-1.[44–47]

Treatment

When HAP or HCAP is suspected based on clinical findings and chest radiography, it can be very difficult to obtain a lower respiratory tract sample because these patients are usually not intubated. In these circumstances, initiation of empiric antibiotics is recommended based on the patient's risk factors for possible MDR pathogens, and local microbiologic data should also be considered.

When VAP is suspected based on clinical and radiographic findings, it is important first to obtain lower respiratory tract samples for cultures and microscopy. Early empiric antimicrobial therapy for VAP is then initiated. In the next 48 hours, an assessment of clinical response and cultures should be performed. If there is clinical improvement and culture results are negative, consider stopping antibiotics. If culture results are positive, consider de-escalating or narrowing the antibiotics. If there is no clinical response, consider searching for other causes. If cultures are negative, assess for other pathogens, complications, or other sources of infection. If cultures are positive, adjust antibiotic therapy and search for other sources as well. The ATS/IDSA 2005 guidelines provide an algorithm for diagnosis and treatment of pneumonia (**Fig. 6**).

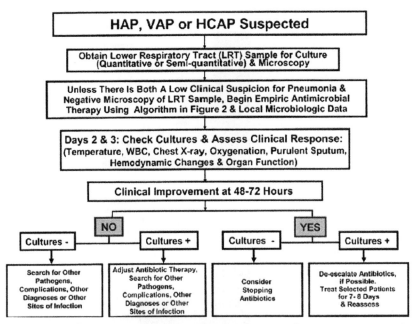

Fig. 6. Algorithm for the diagnosis and treatment of suspected HAP, VAP, or HCAP. (*From* American Thoracic Society. Guidelines for the management of adults with hospital-acquired, ventilator-associated, and healthcare-associated pneumonia. Am J Respir Crit Care Med 2005;171(4):388–416; with permission.)

Antibiotic Treatment

The initiation of early, appropriate, empiric antibiotics to treat HAP, VAP, or HCAP significantly improves patient survival.[3,48] To better understand antibiotic choice, it is important to examine the microbiology of VAP. In the past decade, this has significantly changed (**Fig. 7**). For years (1992–1999), *Staphylococcus aureus* and *Pseudomonas aeruginosa* were the 2 leading causative pathogens for VAP and HAP, each representing approximately 18% of all isolates. *Enterobacter* spp and *Klebsiella pneumoniae* were less common representing 12% and 7% of VAP isolates, respectively.[49,50] The most recent NHSN report of 2006 to 2007 data for VAP from US hospitals confirms a significant change in VAP pathogens.[51] *S aureus* is now the leading VAP pathogen, representing 24.4% of all isolates, and 54.4% of all *S aureus* isolates were identified as methicillin-resistant *S aureus* (MRSA), making MRSA the leading VAP pathogen. *P aeruginosa* decreased from 18% to 16.3% and *Enterobacter* spp decreased from 12% to 8.4%. *Acinetobacter baumannii* is now the third most common VAP pathogen, representing 8.4% of all VAP isolates. This MDR pathogen is very difficult to eradicate, and is a significant issue for infection control.

Because choosing appropriate initial antibiotics has an influence on survival, it is important to discuss the significance of MRSA. The increased prevalence of MRSA in VAP was up to 63% in 2004.[52,53] The mortality associated with MRSA pneumonia can be as high as 56%.[54] In addition, despite appropriate initial therapy, MRSA pneumonia prolongs ICU stay.[55] In a recent phase IV double-blind randomized trial with 1225 patients, intravenous linezolid had a success/cure rate of 57.6% compared with 46.6% for intravenous vancomycin (*P* = .042), but no difference in 60-day

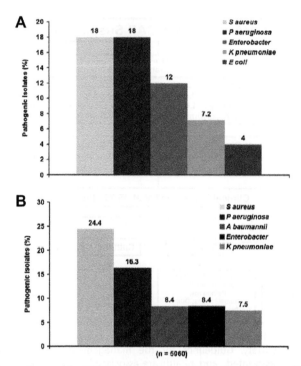

Fig. 7. Causative pathogens for VAP in US hospitals, 1992 to 1999 (*A*) versus 2006 to 2007 (*B*). NHSN report. *Staphylococcus aureus* increased from 18% to 24.4%. Methicillin-resistant *S aureus* is now the leading causative pathogen at 54.4% of all *S aureus* isolates. Note higher rate of *Acinetobacter* in 2006 to 2007. (*Data from* [*A*] Fridkin S, Weibel SF, Weinstein RA. Magnitude and prevention of nosocomial infections in the intensive care unit. Infect Dis Clin North Am 1997;11:479–96; [*B*] Hidron AI, Edwards JR, Patel J, et al. National Healthcare Safety Network Team, Participating National Healthcare Safety Network Facilities. NHSN Annual Update: Antimicrobial-resistant pathogens associated with healthcare-associated infections: Annual summary of data reported to the National Healthcare Safety Network at the Centers for Disease Control and Prevention, 2006-2007. Infect Control Hosp Epidemiol 2008;29:996–1011.)

mortality was identified.[56] This finding is biologically plausible, as the pharmacodynamics of linezolid in the lung are superior to those of vancomycin, and increasing minimum inhibitory concentrations of vancomycin in the MRSA-causative pathogens for pneumonia have been reported worldwide.[54]

Necrotizing pneumonias are an increasing problem and are associated with higher mortality in critically ill patients. Pathogens associated with necrotizing pneumonia include *Pseudomonas* and MRSA. Concurrent with the emergence of community-acquired MRSA (CA-MRSA), there have been increasing reports of community-acquired necrotizing pneumonia in young healthy patients, some after a viral prodrome and influenza infection.[57,58] In the most recent report from the CDC of 51 cases of *S aureus* community-acquired pneumonia, the median age was 16 years and 44% had no underlying comorbidities. Influenza was confirmed in 33% of the cohort and 91% of these patients died. MRSA was confirmed in 37 of the 51 patients and 48% died. Empiric coverage for MRSA pneumonia was provided in only 43% of these patients.[59]

Concomitant use of antibiotics that suppress toxin production has been advocated for the treatment of severe and invasive CA-MRSA infections including pneumonia. The rationale for their use in CA-MRSA pneumonia includes (1) the presumed role of the Panton-Valentine Leucocidin (PVL) toxin, a staphylococcal toxin known to be associated with tissue necrosis,[60] and (2) the high morbidity and mortality observed. Some clinicians therefore advocate treatment with agents that suppress toxin production (clindamycin, linezolid) and urge the avoidance of agents (ie, β-lactams) that can lead to increased production of PVL and other exotoxins in patients with MRSA pneumonia.[61]

The choice of antibiotic treatment in VAP depends on the microorganism isolated. These organisms differ based on the duration of mechanical ventilation. Patients who develop VAP early (<4 days of mechanical ventilation) have different isolates from those who develop VAP later (more than 4 days).[30] The usual pathogens in early VAP are *S aureus* (methicillin-sensitive *S aureus*), *Haemophilus influenzae*, and *Streptococcus pneumoniae*. These pathogens tend to be sensitive to antimicrobial therapy. The pathogens in late VAP tend to be gram negative and MDR. Usual isolates include *P aeruginosa*, *A baumanii*, *S aureus* (MRSA), and *Stenotrophomonas maltophilia*.[62] The antibiotic should be selected based on risk factors for MDR bacteria. Risk factors in addition to duration of mechanical ventilation include recent antibiotic therapy, presence of underlying diseases, sensitivities of hospital or ICU organisms, and the possibility of HCAP.

Rapid initiation of appropriate antibiotic therapy has a significant effect on outcome. Several trials have shown increased mortality in patients who have inappropriate antibiotic therapy. Inadequate antibiotic therapy is a strong predictor of death in patients with VAP, irrespective of underlying disease state and severity of illness.[63,64] One retrospective trial on patients diagnosed with VAP based on positive BAL culture noted mortality in the adequate-therapy group to be 38%, but in the inadequate-therapy group the mortality was as high as 91%.[65] Several other trials have shown similar results but with lower mortality. One prospective cohort study looked at 655 infected patients, and their all-cause and infection-related mortality based on treatment with appropriate antibiotics. All-cause mortality was significantly higher in the group with inadequate antibiotic coverage (52% vs 12%, $P<.001$). Similarly, infection-related mortality was higher in the inadequate antibiotic group (42% vs 17%, $P<.001$).[66] One of the main reasons for inadequate antibiotic selection is poor risk factor assessment, whereby the antibiotics of choice may not cover MDR bacteria. One study found bacterial resistance to be a significant risk factor for inadequate therapy and mortality. Risk factors for inadequate treatment were MDR bacteria, polymicrobial infection, and late-onset VAP.[67]

To avoid inadequate antibiotic therapy, early use of empiric broad-spectrum antibiotics to cover all potential causative pathogens is required. The choice of empiric antibiotics in pneumonia should be based on national guidelines with knowledge of the most common pathogens, and also with consideration of local antibiograms, particularly in surgical ICUs.[3] It is crucial to start antibiotics when a clinical diagnosis is made, immediately after cultures are obtained. To avoid excessive antibiotics, therapy should be modified to a narrower spectrum (de-escalation) as soon as culture results and antimicrobial susceptibilities are available.

The initial choice of empiric antibiotic therapy is based on the patient's risk factors for MDR bacteria (**Box 1**). Initially, the onset time for pneumonia was used to assess the risk for MDR bacteria. However, patients who have previously been on antibiotic therapy or have visited other health care facilities, regardless of time of pneumonia, are considered to have higher risk for MDR bacteria (see **Box 1**).

Box 1
Risk factors for MDR pathogens causing HAP, HCAP, and VAP

- Antimicrobial therapy in preceding 90 days
- Current hospitalization of 5 days or more
- High frequency of antibiotic resistance in the community or in the specific hospital unit
- Presence of risk factors for HCAP:
  - Hospitalization for 2 days or more in the preceding 90 days
  - Residence in a nursing home or extended care facility
  - Home infusion therapy (including antibiotics)
  - Chronic dialysis within 30 days
  - Home wound care
  - Family member with MDR pathogen
- Immunosuppressive disease and/or therapy

Data from American Thoracic Society. Guidelines for the management of adults with hospital-acquired, ventilator-associated, and healthcare-associated pneumonia. Am J Respir Crit Care Med 2005;171(4):388–416.

The 2005 ATS/IDSA consensus gives excellent recommendations for antibiotic choice. Patients with no risk factors for MDR bacteria may be treated with ceftriaxone, quinolones, ampicillin-sulbactam, or ertapenem. Patients with late-onset pneumonia (>5 days) or those with risk factors for MDR bacteria must be treated with a broader spectrum of antibiotics. Particular attention is paid to starting initial combination therapy for possible gram-negative infections (because *Pseudomonas* is most common, 2 agents are recommended so that at least 1 agent may have appropriate susceptibility) with coverage of gram-positive/MRSA infections (**Fig. 8**).

Duration of Antibiotics for Pneumonia

Duration of treatment for pneumonia has been discussed extensively in the literature. Previously it was thought that treatment for 7 to 10 days was adequate for sensitive organisms, with a longer course of 14 to 21 days recommended for resistant organisms.[3,68] A landmark, prospective, randomized, multicenter trial compared 8 days with 15 days of antibiotic treatment in 401 patients in 51 ICUs.[69] No difference in 30-day mortality was identified (18.8% vs 17.2%) and no differences in ventilator-free days, organ failure–free days, length of ICU stay, and 60-day mortality were identified. However, there was a higher recurrence of infection rate for nonfermenting gram-negative bacilli, including *P aeruginosa*. In addition, more MDR pathogens appeared in the 15-day treatment group (42% vs 62%, *P* = .038). Based on the results of this study, optimal duration of therapy for VAP should be 8 days, except in those isolates that are nonfermenting gram-negative bacilli, including *P aeruginosa* and *Acinetobacter* spp, for which longer duration of antimicrobial therapy is recommended.

However, the duration of antimicrobial therapy for HAP or VAP caused by MRSA needs additional evaluation, because the studies that evaluated treatment duration included an insufficient number of patients infected with MRSA. Most clinicians would provide a minimum of 14 days of therapy for MRSA pneumonia, and if there is concomitant bacteremia, more prolonged antibiotic therapy may be required. In

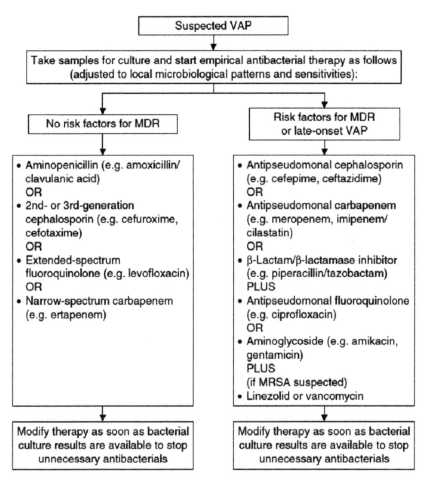

Fig. 8. Initial empiric antibiotic therapy for HAP, VAP, and HCAP with risk for MDR pathogens. (*Data from* American Thoracic Society. Guidelines for the management of adults with hospital-acquired, ventilator-associated, and healthcare-associated pneumonia. Am J Respir Crit Care Med 2005;171(4):388–416.)

addition, duration of therapy probably should also be assessed according to each patient's clinical course.

HAP Prevention

Some institutions have initiated aggressive HAP prevention efforts in surgical patients to reduce postoperative pneumonia.[70] The program consisted of education of physicians and staff and a standardized postoperative electronic order set consisting of incentive spirometer, chlorhexidine oral hygiene, early ambulation, and head-of-bed elevation. This strategy was associated with an 81% decrease in postoperative pneumonia from 2006 to 2008.

VAP Prevention

The foremost strategy for VAP prevention is to avoid intubation or reduce the duration of mechanical ventilation. Noninvasive ventilation may be particularly valuable in this regard because in selected populations it can lead to avoidance of intubation or short-ening of the duration of mechanical ventilation, therefore noninvasive ventilation should be considered if evidence exists to support its use.[71] In addition, basic infection-control principles such as handwashing, adequate ICU staff education, and optimal resource use are necessary.

The development of VAP is related to (1) bacterial colonization of the aerodigestive tract or (2) aspiration of contaminated secretions into the lower airway. The strategies to prevent infection are therefore aimed at (1) reducing bacterial colonization and (2) decreasing the incidence of aspiration. Decreased incidence of aspiration can be achieved through improved positioning, increased head-of-bed elevation, and use of specialty endotracheal tubes that aspirate subglottic secretions. Bacterial coloniza-tion can be reduced by minimizing the days on mechanical ventilation through wean-ing protocols, use of chlorhexidine in the posterior pharynx, and silver-coated endotracheal tubes. Clinical guidelines for VAP prevention review all evidence-based strategies for VAP prevention.[72] Ventilator bundles are used as an effective method to reduce VAP rates in the ICU.[73]

Semirecumbent position

The semirecumbent (45°) position in mechanically ventilated patients has been asso-ciated with a reduced incidence of VAP. A prospective randomized trial with 86 patients found a significant difference in the incidence of VAP. Patients who were supine compared with those with the head of the bed at 45° had a significant differ-ence in VAP rates (34% vs 3%, $P = .003$).[74] Supine position and mechanical ventila-tion longer than 7 days were independent risk factors for VAP. Other studies have not confirmed this finding, but compliance with the target semirecumbent position was not reached in these studies.[75,76]

Endotracheal tubes for continuous aspiration of subglottic secretions

Aspirated secretions may pool above the endotracheal cuff and increase the risk for VAP. Specialty tubes that aspirate these subglottic secretions are commercially avail-able in many different forms. Several prospective randomized trials have shown a decreased rate of VAP in patients with tubes for continuous aspiration of subglottic secretions (CASS). A meta-analysis of 5 studies with 896 patients showed a reduction of VAP by nearly half (relative risk = 0.51), a delay in the onset of VAP by 6.8 days, and reduction in length of stay in the ICU by 3 days. Despite these beneficial outcomes, no improvement in mortality was identified. A study in cardiac surgical patients (n = 714) also confirmed a significant VAP reduction with use of the CASS tube.[77] The CASS tube may be ideal for patients who are expected to require mechanical ventilation for longer than 72 hours, but this may be difficult to predict.[78] Management of CASS tubes requires particular attention to detail for maintenance, frequent moni-toring, and associated increased cost.[79]

Chlorhexidine gluconate

One strategy to reduce bacterial colonization is to use oral chlorhexidine gluconate (0.12%). One trial in cardiac surgical patients documented a significant decrease in the incidence of nosocomial pneumonia and mortality.[80] A prospective, randomized, double-blind, placebo-controlled, multicenter trial also confirmed a significant reduc-tion in VAP with the use of chlorhexidine.[81] A meta-analysis of similar trials concluded that the use of chlorhexidine was associated with a 26% relative risk reduction in VAP.[82] In addition, chlorhexidine in combination with protocol-driven weaning from mechanical ventilation has been shown to reduce the incidence of VAP in surgical ICU patients.[83]

Silver-coated endotracheal tube

Another strategy to reduce bacterial colonization is the use of silver-coated endotracheal tubes. Silver prevents biofilm formation, delays airway colonization, has bactericidal activity, and reduces bacterial burden. The NASCENT randomized, single-blind, multicenter phase III trial enrolled 2003 patients expected to require mechanical ventilation for more than 24 hours. The primary outcome measure was VAP (defined as BAL $>10^4$ CFU/mL). Use of the silver-coated endotracheal tube was associated with a significant reduction in VAP (4.8% vs 7.5%, 36% relative risk reduction), and was associated with a significant delay in time to VAP.

Spontaneous awakening and breathing trials

Prolonged mechanical ventilation is a risk factor for VAP. This risk increases by 1% to 3% with each day of mechanical ventilation.[84] The use of a weaning protocol, a sedation protocol, or both has been shown to reduce the duration of mechanical ventilation.[85] The Awakening and Breathing Controlled (ABC) trial enrolled 336 patients requiring mechanical ventilation at 4 tertiary care hospitals. The group was divided into an intervention group (n = 168) that received daily spontaneous awakening (SAT) and spontaneous breathing trials (SBT), and a control group (n = 168) that received sedation and usual care with spontaneous breathing trials. The study found a significant difference in 1-year mortality between the control and intervention groups (58% vs 44%, $P = .01$). Routine use of SAT and SBT is now standard in all ventilated patients.

Selective decontamination

Selective decontamination of the digestive tract (SDD) and oropharynx (SOD) are strategies aimed at preventing colonization with virulent bacteria. The spectrum of studies includes oral administration of antibiotics via nasogastric tubes, to intravenous administration for up to 4 days.[86] Several studies have shown modest benefit in rates of pneumonia and mortality.[87,88] However, this has not been used widely in the United States because of significant concern regarding the potential emergence of MDR bacteria.[89]

Tracheostomy

Previous studies have suggested that tracheostomy was superior to prolonged intubation for VAP prevention.[90] However, 2 recent, large, prospective, randomized, clinical trials have found no difference in VAP or any other outcomes measures in comparing early (6–8 days) with late (13–15 days) tracheostomy in 419 patients[91] or comparing early (4 days) with late (after 10 days) tracheostomy in 909 patients in the TracMan trial.[92] Thus, early tracheostomy should not be performed for VAP prevention but may be considered for other reasons, such as patient comfort and airway protection, for instance, in patients with severe traumatic brain injury.

ACUTE RESPIRATORY FAILURE

Acute respiratory failure in the postoperative setting can be caused by loss of airway protection, failure to oxygenate (hypoxemic respiratory failure, type 1), or failure to ventilate (hypercapnia respiratory failure, type 2) (**Fig. 9**).

In the postoperative setting, it is crucial to first assess whether the patient's airway is protected. Several risk factors contribute to this, including neurologic impairment, absent cough/gag reflex, or laryngeal edema. For these reasons, close attention must be paid to elderly patients, those with head trauma, and patients who have had a procedure on the upper airway. A single event of aspiration in this setting can be disastrous and often is fatal.

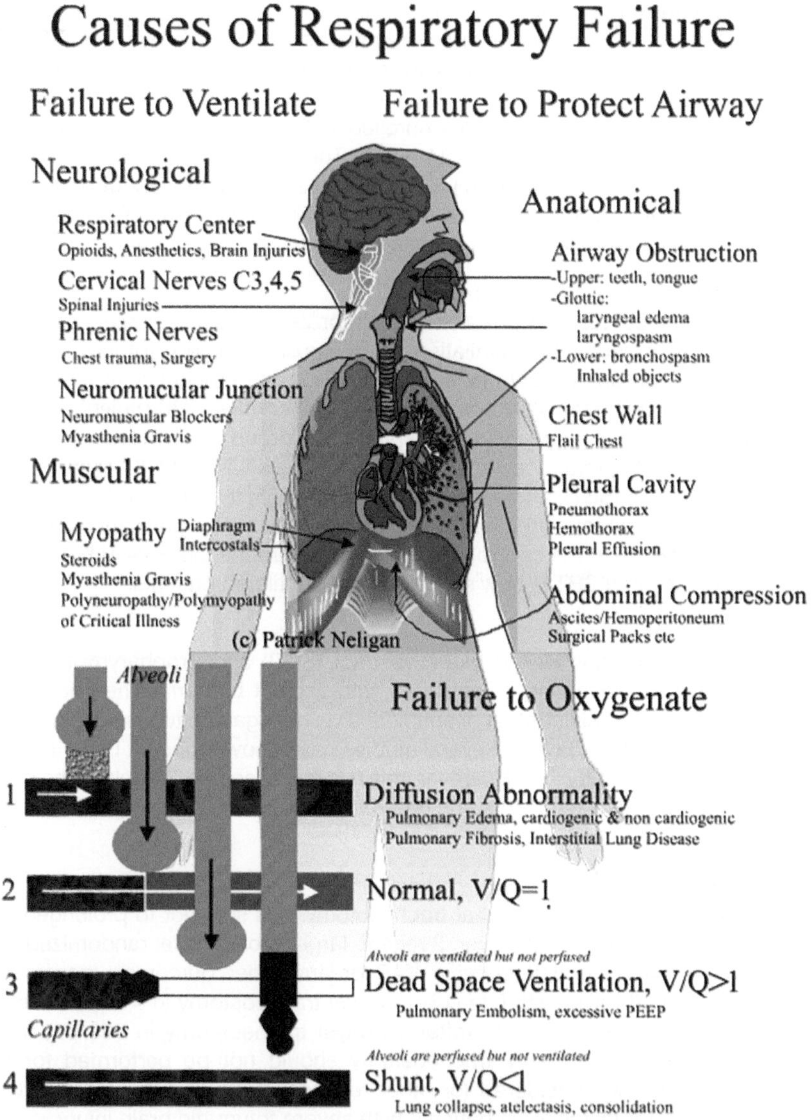

Causes of Respiratory Failure

Failure to Ventilate

Neurological

Respiratory Center
Opioids, Anesthetics, Brain Injuries

Cervical Nerves C3,4,5
Spinal Injuries

Phrenic Nerves
Chest trauma, Surgery

Neuromuscular Junction
Neuromuscular Blockers
Myasthenia Gravis

Muscular

Myopathy   Diaphragm
        Intercostals
Steroids
Myasthenia Gravis
Polyneuropathy/Polymyopathy
of Critical Illness

(c) Patrick Neligan

Failure to Protect Airway

Anatomical

Airway Obstruction
-Upper: teeth, tongue
-Glottic:
    laryngeal edema
    laryngospasm
-Lower: bronchospasm
    Inhaled objects

Chest Wall
Flail Chest

Pleural Cavity
Pneumothorax
Hemothorax
Pleural Effusion

Abdominal Compression
Ascites/Hemoperitoneum
Surgical Packs etc

Alveoli

Failure to Oxygenate

1   **Diffusion Abnormality**
     Pulmonary Edema, cardiogenic & non cardiogenic
     Pulmonary Fibrosis, Interstitial Lung Disease

2   **Normal, V/Q=1**

     Alveoli are ventilated but not perfused

3   **Dead Space Ventilation, V/Q>1**
     Pulmonary Embolism, excessive PEEP

Capillaries

     Alveoli are perfused but not ventilated

4   Shunt, V/Q<1
     Lung collapse, atelectasis, consolidation

Fig. 9. Causes of acute respiratory failure. (*From* http://www.ccmtutorials.com/rs/intubate/in_vent4.htm. Accessed October 11, 2011. © Patrick J. Neligan, MD. Galway, Ireland; with permission.)

Hypoxic respiratory failure (type 1) is defined by a Pao_2 of less than 60 mm Hg (not taking into account chronic illness). Hypocapnia can often accompany hypoxia because of increased ventilatory drive. This type of respiratory failure is more common, and usually the underlying problem is at the pulmonary capillary/alveolar interface. Virtually all processes in type 1 respiratory failure involve either fluid filling or collapse of alveolar units. These injuries are usually categorized into diffusion defects or ventilation-perfusion mismatch. Diffusion defects can be caused by fluid accumulation in the extracellular space leading to pulmonary edema, which leads to impaired oxygenation. There are 2 spectra in ventilation-perfusion mismatch. However, most cases of type 1 respiratory failure have a combination of both. On one side of the spectrum is pure dead space ventilation, where alveoli get ventilation but no perfusion (pulmonary embolism). The other side of the spectrum is shunt, where the alveoli get perfusion but no ventilation.

Hypoxic respiratory failure can be caused by metabolic abnormalities at the cellular level. If the body is unable to extract oxygen at a cellular level, one could still have hypoxia at this level with increasing lactic acid levels, but no evidence of arterial hypoxia. This scenario can be seen in poisoning by carbon monoxide or cyanide, and also in sepsis.

Hypercapneic respiratory failure (type 2) is defined by a $Paco_2$ of greater than 50 mm Hg (not taking into account chronic illness). Hypoxemia can be common in these patients, because increased alveolar CO_2 can displace alveolar O_2. When looking for the underlying cause in type 2 respiratory failure, it is best to proceed in a systematic manner from the brain to the lung. A central loss of ventilation can be due to sedation, narcotic overdose, stroke, or medication. Spinal cord procedures or traumatic injuries can result in loss of diaphragm or accessory muscle use. Trauma causing mechanical injury to the chest can cause broken ribs, flail chest, pneumothorax, hemothorax, or pleural effusions that make ventilation difficult. Attention must also be paid to the obese patient, as obesity can also restrict ventilation. The airway, if already secured via intubation, should be evaluated for distal obstruction (right main stem intubation, foreign object, mucous plug). Attention must be paid at the alveolar level, where problems in gas exchange or V/Q mismatch can cause hyperventilation (atelectasis, pneumonia, contusion, acute lung injury, ARDS).

For most postoperative surgical patients with severe acute respiratory failure, either hypoxemic or hypercapneic, early intubation and initiation of mechanical ventilation should be considered. A brief period of noninvasive ventilation is generally considered if there is a promptly reversible cause of the acute respiratory failure (ie, atelectasis or pulmonary edema). All patients with signs and symptoms of acute respiratory failure must be monitored and treated in an ICU.

SUMMARY

The incidence of postoperative pulmonary complications, particularly postoperative pneumonia and acute respiratory failure, is a significant cause of morbidity and mortality. The clinical diagnosis of pneumonia can be challenging. However, when pneumonia is suspected, it is important first to obtain lower respiratory tract samples for culture. With high clinical suspicion for pneumonia, it is crucial to begin early appropriate empiric antimicrobial therapy to cover all potential causative pathogens. Attention must be paid to the possibility of HCAP and propensity of MDR bacterial pneumonia in high-risk groups. Antibiotics must be tailored to the patient with consideration of both local microbiology and data from national guidelines. National rates of VAP remain highest in surgical, trauma, and burn ICUs. Prevention of VAP can be optimized by reducing the risk of aspiration and bacterial colonization of the airway through evidence-based preventive strategies (chlorhexidine, semirecumbent position, CASS or silver-coated endotracheal tubes, spontaneous awakening and breathing trials, and ventilator-weaning protocols).

REFERENCES

1. Lawrence VA, Hilsenbeck SG, Mulrow CD, et al. Incidence and hospital stay for cardiac and pulmonary complications after abdominal surgery. J Gen Intern Med 1995;10(12):671.

2. Agostini P, Cieslik H, Rathinam S, et al. Postoperative pulmonary complications following thoracic surgery: are there any modifiable risk factors? Thorax 2010; 65(9):815–8.
3. Sheer AJ, Heckman JE, Schneider EB, et al. Congestive heart failure and chronic obstructive pulmonary disease predict poor surgical outcomes in older adults undergoing elective diverticulitis surgery. Dis Colon Rectum 2011;54(11):1430–7.
4. Smetana GW, Lawrence VA, Cornell JE. Preoperative pulmonary risk stratification for noncardiothoracic surgery: systematic review for the American College of Physicians. Ann Intern Med 2006;144:581–95.
5. Hawn MT, Houston TK, Campagna EJ, et al. The attributable risk of smoking on surgical complications. Ann Surg 2011;254(6):914–20.
6. Memtsoudis S, Liu SS, Ma Y, et al. Perioperative pulmonary outcomes in patients with sleep apnea after noncardiac surgery. Anesth Analg 2011;112(1):113–21.
7. Lawrence VA, Cornell JE, Smetana GW. American College of Physicians. Strategies to reduce postoperative pulmonary complications after noncardiothoracic surgery: systematic review for the American College of Physicians. Ann Intern Med 2006;144(8):596–608. Review.
8. Qaseem A, Snow V, Fitterman N, et al. Clinical Efficacy Assessment Subcommittee of the American College of Physicians. Risk assessment for and strategies to reduce perioperative pulmonary complications for patients undergoing noncardiothoracic surgery: a guideline from the American College of Physicians. Ann Intern Med 2006;144(8):575–80.
9. Warner MA, Offord KP, Warner ME, et al. Role of preoperative cessation of smoking and other factors in postoperative pulmonary complications: a blinded prospective study of coronary artery bypass patients. Mayo Clin Proc 1989;64:609.
10. Tarhan S, Moffitt EA, Sessler AD, et al. Risk of anesthesia and surgery in patients with chronic bronchitis and chronic obstructive pulmonary disease. Surgery 1973;74:720.
11. Stein M, Cassara EL. Preoperative pulmonary evaluation and therapy for surgery patients. JAMA 1970;211:787.
12. National Asthma Education and Prevention Program: Expert Panel report III: guidelines for the diagnosis and management of asthma. Bethesda (MD): National Heart, Lung, and Blood Institute; 2007 (NIH publication no. 08-4051). Available at: www.nhlbi.nih.gov/guidelines/asthma/asthgdln.htm. Accessed October 14, 2011.
13. Kabalin CS, Yarnold PR, Grammer LC. Low complication rate of corticosteroid-treated asthmatics undergoing surgical procedures. Arch Intern Med 1995;155:1379.
14. Rodgers A, Walker N, Schug S, et al. Reduction of postoperative mortality and morbidity with epidural or spinal anaesthesia: results from overview of randomised trials. BMJ 2000;321:1493.
15. Pedersen T, Viby-Mogensen J, Ringsted C. Anaesthetic practice and postoperative pulmonary complications. Acta Anaesthesiol Scand 1992;36:812.
16. Berg H, Roed J, Viby-Mogensen J, et al. Residual neuromuscular block is a risk factor for postoperative pulmonary complications. A prospective, randomised, and blinded study of postoperative pulmonary complications after atracurium, vecuronium and pancuronium. Acta Anaesthesiol Scand 1997;41:1095.
17. Hall JC, Tarala RA, Tapper J, et al. Prevention of respiratory complications after abdominal surgery: a randomised clinical trial. BMJ 1996;312:148.
18. Schwieger I, Gamulin Z, Forster A, et al. Absence of benefit of incentive spirometry in low-risk patients undergoing elective cholecystectomy. A controlled randomized study. Chest 1986;89:652.

19. Guimaraes MM, El dib R, Smith AF, et al. Incentive spirometry for prevention of postoperative pulmonary complications in upper abdominal surgery. Cochrane Database Syst Rev 2009;3:CD006058.
20. Zarbock A, Mueller E, Netzer S, et al. Prophylactic nasal continuous positive airway pressure following cardiac surgery protects from postoperative pulmonary complications: a prospective, randomized, controlled trial in 500 patients. Chest 2009;135:1252.
21. Stock MC, Downs JB, Gauer PK, et al. Prevention of postoperative pulmonary complications with CPAP, incentive spirometry, and conservative therapy. Chest 1985;87:151.
22. Tsui SL, Law S, Fok M, et al. Postoperative analgesia reduces mortality and morbidity after esophagectomy. Am J Surg 1997;173:472.
23. Major CP Jr, Greer MS, Russell WL, et al. Postoperative pulmonary complications and morbidity after abdominal aneurysmectomy: a comparison of postoperative epidural versus parenteral opioid analgesia. Am Surg 1996;62:45.
24. Cheatham ML, Chapman WC, Key SP, et al. A meta-analysis of selective versus routine nasogastric decompression after elective laparotomy. Ann Surg 1995; 221:469.
25. Nelson R, Edwards S, Tse B. Prophylactic nasogastric decompression after abdominal surgery. Cochrane Database Syst Rev 2005;1:CD004929.
26. Arozullah AM, Khuri SF, Henderson WG, et al. Development and validation of a multifactorial risk index for predicting postoperative pneumonia after major noncardiac surgery. Ann Intern Med 2001;135(10):847–57.
27. Napolitano LM. Use of severity scoring and stratification factors in clinical trials of hospital-acquired and ventilator-associated pneumonia. Clin Infect Dis 2010; 51(Suppl 1):S67–80.
28. Ozhathil DK, Li Y, Smith JK, et al. Colectomy performance improvement within NSQIP 2005-2008. J Surg Res 2011;171(1):e9–13.
29. Guidelines for the management of adults with hospital-acquired, ventilator-associated, and healthcare-associated pneumonia. Am J Respir Crit Care Med 2005; 171(4):388–416.
30. Hubmayr RD, Burchardi H, Elliot M, et al. Statement of the 4th International Consensus Conference in Critical Care on ICU-Acquired Pneumonia—Chicago, Illinois, 2002. Intensive Care Med 2002;28:1521.
31. Johanson WG, Pierce AK, Sanford JP. Changing pharyngeal bacterial flora of hospitalized patients: emergence of gram-negative bacilli. N Engl J Med 1969; 281:1137.
32. de Jonge E, Schultz MJ, Spanjaard L, et al. Effects of selective decontamination of digestive tract on mortality and acquisition of resistant bacteria in intensive care: a randomized controlled trial. Ann Intern Med 2003;362:1011.
33. Adair CG, Gorman SP, Feron BM, et al. Implications of endotracheal tube biofilm for ventilator-associated pneumonia. Intensive Care Med 1999;25:1072.
34. Napolitano LM. Perspectives in surgical infections: what does the future hold? [review]. Surg Infect (Larchmt) 2010;11(2):111–23.
35. Fàbregas N, Ewig S, Torres A, et al. Clinical diagnosis of ventilator associated pneumonia revisited: comparative validation using immediate post-mortem lung biopsies. Thorax 1999;54:867.
36. Meduri GU. Diagnosis and differential diagnosis of ventilator-associated pneumonia. Clin Chest Med 1995;16:61.
37. Wunderink RG, Woldenberg LS, Zeiss J, et al. The radiologic diagnosis of autopsy-proven ventilator-associated pneumonia. Chest 1992;101:458.

38. Kollef MH, Bock KR, Richards RD, et al. The safety and diagnostic accuracy of minibronchoalveolar lavage in patients with suspected ventilator-associated pneumonia. Ann Intern Med 1995;122:743.
39. Shorr AF, Sherner JH, Jackson WL, et al. Invasive approaches to the diagnosis of ventilator-associated pneumonia: a meta-analysis. Crit Care Med 2005;33:46.
40. Klompas M. Does this patient have ventilator-associated pneumonia? JAMA 2007;297(14):1583–93.
41. Luyt CE, Combes A, Reynaud C, et al. Usefulness of procalcitonin for the diagnosis of ventilator-associated pneumonia. Intensive Care Med 2008;34(8):1434–40.
42. Ramirez P, Garcia MA, Ferrer M, et al. Sequential measurements of procalcitonin levels in diagnosing ventilator-associated pneumonia. Eur Respir J 2008;31(2):356–62.
43. Linssen CF, Bekers O, Drent M, et al. C-reactive protein and procalcitonin concentrations in BAL fluid as a predictor of ventilator-associated pneumonia. Ann Clin Biochem 2008;45:293–8.
44. Gibot S, Cravoisy A, Levy B, et al. Soluble triggering receptor expressed on myeloid cells and the diagnosis of pneumonia. N Engl J Med 2004;350(5):451–8.
45. Determann RM, Millo JL, Gibot S, et al. Serial changes in soluble triggering receptor expressed on myeloid cells in the lung during development of venti-lator-associated-pneumonia. Intensive Care Med 2005;31(11):1495–500.
46. Anand NJ, Zuick S, Klesney-Tait J, et al. Diagnostic implications of soluble trig-gering receptor expressed on myeloid cells-1 in BAL fluid of patients with pulmo-nary infiltrates in the ICU. Chest 2009;135(3):641–7.
47. Oudhuis GJ, Beuving J, Bergmans D, et al. Soluble triggering receptor ex-pressed on myeloid cells-1 in bronchoalveolar lavage fluid is not predictive for ventilator-associated pneumonia. Intensive Care Med 2009;35(7):1265–70.
48. Meduri GU, Johanson WG Jr. International Consensus Conference: clinical inves-tigation of ventilator-associated pneumonia. Chest 1992;102:551S.
49. U.S. Centers for Disease Control and Prevention/National Nosocomial Infections Surveillance—January 1992-May 1999. Am J Infect Control 1999;27:520–32.
50. Fridkin S, Weibel SF, Weinstein RA. Magnitude and prevention of nosocomial infections in the intensive care unit. Infect Dis Clin North Am 1997;11:479–96.
51. Hidron AI, Edwards JR, Patel J, et al. National Healthcare Safety Network Team; Participating National Healthcare Safety Network Facilities. NHSN Annual update: antimicrobial-resistant pathogens associated with healthcare-associated infec-tions: annual summary of data reported to the National Healthcare Safety Network at the Centers for Disease Control and Prevention 2006-2007. Infect Control Hosp Epidemiol 2008;29:996–1011.
52. Lowy FD. Antimicrobial resistance: the example of Staphylococcus aureus. J Clin Invest 2003;111:1265–73.
53. CDC. Available at: http://www.cdc.gov/ncidod/hip/ARESIST/ICU_RESTrend1995-2004.pdf. Accessed August 30, 2005.
54. Rubinstein E, Kollef MH, Nathwani D. Pneumonia caused by methicillin-resistant Staphylococcus aureus. Clin Infect Dis 2008;46(Suppl 5):S378–85. Review.
55. Shorr AF, Combes A, Kollef M, et al. Methicillin-resistant Staphylococcus aureus prolongs intensive care unit stay in ventilator-associated pneumonia, despite initially appropriate antibiotic therapy. Crit Care Med 2006;34:700–6.
56. Wunderink RG, Niederman MS, Kollef MH, et al. Linezolid in methicillin-resistant Staphylococcus aureus nosocomial pneumonia: a randomized, controlled study. Clin Infect Dis 2012. [Epub ahead of print].
57. Napolitano LM, Brunsvold ME, Reddy RC, et al. Community-acquired MRSA pneumonia and ARDS: 1-year followup. Chest 2009;136(5):1407–12.

58. Hidron AI, Low CE, Honig EG, et al. Emergence of community-acquired MRSA strain USA300 as a cause of necrotizing community-onset pneumonia. Lancet Infect Dis 2009;9:384–92.
59. Kallen AJ, Brunkard J, Moore Z, et al. *Staphylococcus aureus* community-acquired pneumonia during the 2006-2007 influenza season. Ann Emerg Med 2009;53(3):358–65.
60. Labandeira-Rey M, Couzon F, Boisset S, et al. *Staphylococcus aureus* Panton-Valentine leukocidin causes necrotizing pneumonia. Science 2007;315:1130–3.
61. Wenzel RP, Bearman G, Edmond MB. Community-acquired methicillin-resistant *Staphylococcus aureus* (MRSA): new issues for infection control. Int J Antimicrob Agents 2007;30:210–2.
62. Rello J, Ollendorf DA, Oster G, et al. Epidemiology and outcomes of ventilator-associated pneumonia in a large US database. Chest 2002;122:2115.
63. Iregui M, Ward S, Sherman G, et al. Clinical importance of delays in the initiation of appropriate antibiotic treatment for ventilator-associated pneumonia. Chest 2002;122:262.
64. Habarth S, Garbino J, Pugin J, et al. Inappropriate initial antimicrobial therapy and its effect on survival in a clinical trial of immunomodulating therapy for severe sepsis. Am J Med 2003;115(7):529–35.
65. Luna CM, Vujacich P, Niederman MS, et al. Impact of BAL data on the therapy and outcome of ventilator-associated pneumonia. Chest 1997;111:676.
66. Kollef MH, Sherman G, Ward S, et al. Inadequate antimicrobial treatment of infections: a risk factor for hospital mortality among critically ill patients. Chest 1999; 115(2):462–74.
67. Teixeira PJ, Seligman R, Hertz FT, et al. Inadequate treatment of ventilator-associated pneumonia: risk factors and impact on outcomes. J Hosp Infect 2007; 65(4):361–7.
68. Rello J, Mariscal D, March F, et al. Recurrent *Pseudomonas aeruginosa* pneumonia in ventilated patients: relapse or reinfection? Am J Respir Crit Care Med 1998;157:912.
69. Chastre J, Wolff M, Fagon JY, et al. Comparison of 8 vs 15 days of antibiotic therapy for ventilator-associated pneumonia in adults: a randomized trial. JAMA 2003;290: 2588.
70. Wren SM, Martin M, Yoon JK, et al. Postoperative pneumonia-prevention program for the inpatient surgical ward. J Am Coll Surg 2010;210:491–5.
71. Demoule A, Girou E, Richard JC, et al. Increased use of noninvasive ventilation in French intensive care units. Intensive Care Med 2006;32(11):1747–55.
72. Muscedere J, Dodek P, Keenan S, et al. Comprehensive evidence-based clinical practice guidelines for ventilator-associated pneumonia: prevention. J Crit Care 2008;23(1):126–37.
73. Wip C, Napolitano L. Bundles to prevent ventilator-associated pneumonia: how valuable are they? Curr Opin Infect Dis 2009;22(2):159–66.
74. Drakulovic MB, Torres A, Bauer TT, et al. Supine body position as a risk factor for nosocomial pneumonia in mechanically ventilated patients: a randomised trial. Ann Intern Med 1999;354:1851.
75. van Nieuwenhoven CA, Vandenbroucke-Grauls C, van Tiel FH, et al. Feasibility and effects of the semirecumbent position to prevent ventilator-associated pneumonia: a randomized study. Crit Care Med 2006;34(2):396–402.
76. Alexiou VG, Ierodiakonou V, Dimopoulos G, et al. Impact of patient position on the incidence of ventilator-associated pneumonia: a meta-analysis of randomized controlled trials. J Crit Care 2009;24(4):515–22.

77. Bouza E, Perez MJ, Munoz P, et al. Continuous aspiration of subglottic secretions in the prevention of ventilator-associated pneumonia in the postoperative period of major heart surgery. Chest 2008;134(5):938–46.

78. Dezfulian C, Shojania K, Collard HR, et al. Subglottic secretion drainage for preventing ventilator-associated pneumonia: a meta-analysis. Am J Med 2005; 118(1):11–8.

79. Diaz E, Rodríguez AH, Rello J, et al. Ventilator-associated pneumonia: issues related to the artificial airway. Respir Care 2005;50(7):900–6 [discussion: 906–9].

80. DeRiso AJ, Ladowski JS, Dillon TA, et al. Chlorhexidine gluconate 0.12% oral rinse reduces the incidence of total nosocomial respiratory infection and nonprophylactic systemic antibiotic use in patients undergoing heart surgery. Chest 1996;109:1556.

81. Koeman M, van der Ven AJ, Hak E, et al. Oral decontamination with chlorhexidine reduces the incidence of ventilator-associated pneumonia. Am J Respir Crit Care Med 2006;173(12):1348–55.

82. Chlebicki MP, Safdar N. Topical chlorhexidine for prevention of ventilator-associated pneumonia: a meta-analysis. Crit Care Med 2007;35(2):595–602.

83. Genuit T, Bochicchio G, Napolitano LM, et al. Prophylactic chlorhexidine oral rinse decreases ventilator-associated pneumonia in surgical ICU patients. Surg Infect (Larchmt) 2001;2(1):5–18.

84. Garrard CS, A'Court CD. The diagnosis of pneumonia in the critically ill. Chest 1995;108(Suppl 2):17S–25S.

85. Girard TD, Kress JP, Fuchs BD, et al. Efficacy and safety of a paired sedation and ventilator weaning protocol for mechanically ventilated patients in intensive care (Awakening and Breathing Controlled trial): a randomised controlled trial. Lancet 2008;371(9607):126–34.

86. de Smet AM, Kluytmans JA, Cooper BS, et al. Decontamination of the digestive tract and oropharynx in ICU patients. N Engl J Med 2009;360:20.

87. D'Amico R, Pifferi S, Leonetti C, et al. Effectiveness of antibiotic prophylaxis in critically ill adult patients: systematic review of randomised controlled trials. BMJ 1998;316:1275.

88. Silvestri L, van Saene HK, Casarin A, et al. Impact of selective decontamination of the digestive tract on carriage and infection due to Gram-negative and Gram-positive bacteria: a systematic review of randomised controlled trials. Anaesth Intensive Care 2008;36:324.

89. Wunderink RG. Welkommen to our world. Emergence of antibiotic resistance with selective decontamination of the digestive tract. Am J Respir Crit Care Med 2010; 181:426.

90. Rumbak MJ, Newton M, Truncale T, et al. A prospective, randomized, study comparing early percutaneous dilational tracheotomy to prolonged translaryngeal intubation (delayed tracheotomy) in critically ill medical patients. Crit Care Med 2004;32(8):1689–94.

91. Terragni PP, Antonelli M, Fumagalli R, et al. Early vs late tracheotomy for prevention of pneumonia in mechanically ventilated adult ICU patients: a randomized controlled trial. JAMA 2010;303(15):1483–9.

92. Cuthbertson BH. The TracMan trial presented at Critical Care Canada Forum on October 28, 2009. Toronto. Available at: http://www.criticalcarecanada.com/pdf/CCCF%202009%20Final%20Programme%20Wednesday.pdf. Accessed October 11, 2011.

Multidrug-Resistant Organisms and Antibiotic Management

Philip S. Barie, MD, MBA[a,b,*]

KEYWORDS

- Antibiotics • Antibiotic resistance
- Multidrug-resistant organisms • Resistant bacteria

Antibiotic resistance describes a set of conditions whereby a microorganism is able to survive exposure to an antibiotic. Whereas a genetic mutation in bacteria, whether spontaneous or induced, may confer resistance to antimicrobial agents, resistance genes can be transferred between bacteria by conjugation, transduction, or transformation. Thus, a gene that has evolved via natural selection or evolutionary stress, such as antibiotic exposure, may be disseminated, often by exchange of genetic material by plasmids or transposons. If a bacterium carries several resistance genes, it is called multidrug-resistant (MDR). Clinically, MDR bacteria are those that are resistant to at least 1 agent from at least 3 classes (eg, β-lactamase inhibitor combination drugs [BLICs], cephalosporins, fluoroquinolones). Extremely drug-resistant (XDR) *Mycobacterium tuberculosis* is recognized as a cause of difficult-to-treat tuberculosis, but XDR terminology has yet to find widespread use with respect to nosocomial infections.

The high and increasing prevalence of MDR infections in clinical practice stems from clinical and veterinary antibiotic use, and animal husbandry (antibiotics are added often to animal feed to promote growth; eg, quinolones in chicken feed). Use of antibiotics can increase selection pressure in a population of bacteria by allowing the resistant bacteria within a clone to survive, and then thrive in the ecological vacuum created by the death of susceptible bacteria.[1] As resistance to antibiotics becomes more common, a vicious circle develops wherein increasingly broad-spectrum agents must be prescribed empirically to ensure that initial antibiotic therapy is adequate to the task, and new, ever more powerful agents are needed for the treatment of MDR bacteria. Unfortunately, in part because of an unfavorable regulatory environment for approval of new drugs in general and antibiotics in particular, a dearth of new agents and drugs is in development.[2] As clinicians we must learn to make do with

[a] Department of Surgery, Weill Cornell Medical College, 525 East 68 Street, P713A, New York, NY 10021, USA
[b] Preston A.(Pep) Wade Acute Care Surgery Service, New York-Presbyterian Hospital-Weill Cornell Medical Center, 525 East 68 Street, New York, NY 10021, USA
* Department of Surgery, Weill Cornell Medical College, 525 East 68 Street, P713A, New York, NY 10021.
E-mail address: pbarie@med.cornell.edu

Surg Clin N Am 92 (2012) 345–391
doi:10.1016/j.suc.2012.01.015
0039-6109/12/$ – see front matter © 2012 Elsevier Inc. All rights reserved.

surgical.theclinics.com

what we have for the foreseeable future, according to the principles of antibiotic stewardship.[3,4]

The situation is abetted by several aspects of contemporary medical practice, and surgical practice in particular (**Box 1**). Risk for hospital-acquired infection is high among several patient populations. The population is aging, with attendant senescent immunity and wound healing; elderly patients require hospitalization and surgery at a higher rate than younger persons. Patients who reside in nursing homes are increasing in number accordingly. The population of patients who receive maintenance renal replacement therapy has increased dramatically. Solid-organ transplantation is commonplace, but requires profound immunosuppression. Trauma, burns, and malignant disease are inherently immunosuppressive.[5] Surgical procedures are inherently risky, as any breach of a natural epithelial barrier (eg, surgical incision, percutaneous catheter placement, catheterization of the aerodigestive or urinary tracts) increases the risk that the host will be invaded by pathogens via the portal thus created.

CAUSES OF ANTIBIOTIC RESISTANCE

The widespread use of antibiotics both within and outside medicine is playing a major role in the emergence of resistant bacteria. Although intrinsic antibiotic resistance is ancient and genetically encoded owing to the presence of compounds with antibacterial activity in the natural environment, evolutionary pressure from clinical antibiotic use, beginning in the late 1930s with the introduction of sulfanilamide and the early 1940s with the introduction of penicillin, has played a crucial role in the development of MDR bacteria and interspecies spread. A major aspect of the problem of emergence of MDR bacteria is the misuse and overuse of antibiotics by doctors (and patients); in some countries, antibiotics are available over the counter without a prescription.[6–8]

Box 1
Risk factors for acquisition of infection caused by MDR pathogens

Chronic indwelling catheter (vascular or urinary)

Chronic renal replacement therapy (dialysis)

Colonization with a MDR pathogen (eg, nasal colonization with MRSA, fecal colonization with VRE)

High total or cumulative antibiotic exposure

High severity of illness/care in an intensive care unit

Prolonged acute-care hospitalization

Prolonged endotracheal intubation/mechanical ventilation

Recent antibiotic therapy (within 3 months)

Recent hospitalization (within 3 months)

Recent surgery

Residence in a skilled-nursing or extended-care facility

Solid-organ or bone marrow transplantation

Abbreviations: MDR, multidrug-resistant; MRSA, methicillin-resistant *Staphylococcus aureus*; VRE, vancomycin-resistant *Enterococcus* spp.

The bacterial species of greatest clinical concern for development of resistance are shown in **Box 2**. For convenience, these bacteria may be recalled as the ESKAPE pathogens (*Enterococcus faecium*, *Staphylococcus aureus*, *Klebsiella pneumoniae*, *Acinetobacter calcoaceticus-baumannii* complex, *Pseudomonas aeruginosa*, and *Enterobacter* spp).[9,10] Certain antibiotic classes are highly associated with emergence of resistance compared with other antibiotic classes (**Table 1**). In the case of methicillin-resistant *S aureus* (MRSA), colonization and infection have been associated with prior exposure to glycopeptides, cephalosporins, and fluoroquinolones. Colonization with *Clostridium difficile* has been associated with cephalosporins, fluoroquinolones, and clindamycin in particular (although any antibiotic, even a single dose of a first-or second-generation cephalosporin used appropriately for surgical prophylaxis and those used for treatment of *C difficile* infection [CDI], may lead to CDI). However, although *C difficile* is increasingly virulent, said virulence is not due to increasing resistance.

The amount of antibiotic prescribed is a major factor in increasing rates of bacterial resistance.[11] Even a single dose of antibiotic leads to a greater risk of infection with an organism resistant to that antibiotic, in that person, for up to a year. Inappropriate overprescribing of antibiotics has been attributed to several factors, including insistence on antibacterial treatment of viral infections by unwitting patients,[7,8] physicians who do not know whether or when to prescribe antibiotics owing to diagnostic uncertainty and who may do so for medical-legal reasons, continuance of broad-spectrum therapy when de-escalation to more narrow-spectrum therapy is possible,[12] or excessive prolongation of a course of therapy or continuance even if objective data refute the presence of infection.

Partial, incomplete, or inappropriate therapy has also been associated with clinical failure, the need to re-treat, and the emergence of resistance.[13–15] These irregularities of therapy could take the form of mistargeted initial therapy, or underdosing for fear of toxicity or because of an underestimate of renal function. For example, many people do not finish a course of outpatient antibiotic therapy because they feel better before therapy is completed as intended. Compliance with once-daily regimens is better than with twice-daily therapy. Suboptimal antibiotic concentrations in critically ill patients

---

Box 2
Bacterial pathogens of greatest clinical concern for the development of resistance

The ESKAPE pathogens:

E: *Enterococcus faecium*

S: *Staphylococcus aureus*

K: *Klebsiella pneumoniae*

A: *Acinetobacter calcoaceticus-baumannii* complex

P: *Pseudomonas aeruginosa*

E: *Enterobacter* spp

Other pathogens of concern:

Coagulase-negative *Staphylococcus* spp

Escherichia coli

Stenotrophomonas maltophilia

Streptococcus pneumoniae

Table 1
Causes and consequences of bacterial resistance as related to antibiotic selection pressure

Initial Therapeutic Agent	Emergent Resistant Bacteria	Treatment of Resistant Bacteria
Fluoroquinolones	MRSA	Vancomycin, others
	MDR gram-negative bacilli	Carbapenem or polymyxin or tigecycline (tigecycline not for *Pseudomonas*)
	Clostridium difficile infection	Vancomycin or metronidazole or fidaxomicin
Vancomycin	VRE	Tigecycline, linezolid, daptomycin
	VISA	Ceftaroline, tigecycline, linezolid, daptomycin
Cephalosporins	VRE	Tigecycline, linezolid, daptomycin
	MDR gram-negative bacilli	Carbapenem or polymyxin or tigecycline (tigecycline not for *Pseudomonas*)
	Clostridium difficile infection	Vancomycin or metronidazole or fidaxomicin
Carbapenems	MDR gram-negative bacilli	Carbapenem or polymyxin or tigecycline (tigecycline not for *Pseudomonas*)
	Stenotrophomonas maltophilia	Trimethoprim/sulfamethoxazole
	Clostridium difficile infection	Vancomycin or metronidazole or fidaxomicin

Abbreviations: MDR, Multidrug-resistant (MDR gram-negative bacilli include producers of extended-spectrum β-lactamases, metallo-β-lactamases, and carbapenemases); MRSA, methicillin-resistant *S aureus*; VISA, vancomycin-intermediate *S aureus*; VRE, vancomycin-resistant *Enterococcus*.

increase the likelihood of the development of resistance. Perhaps paradoxically, shortening the course of antibiotics that have been administered appropriately (ie, in adequate dose, according to established principles of pharmacokinetics [PK] and pharmacodynamics [PD])[16,17] may decrease rates of resistance and the incidence of MDR infections.

Proper infection-control practice is central to decreasing the risk of emergence of MDR organisms.[18] Hand hygiene is the single most effective infection-control tactic yet described, yet poor hand hygiene among hospital staff is a leading cause of nosocomial spread of resistant organisms. Increased hand-washing compliance results in decreased rates of MDR organisms.

MECHANISMS OF BACTERIAL RESISTANCE

There are 4 main mechanisms by which microorganisms develop resistance to antimicrobial agents (**Box 3**)[19–25]: drug modification or destruction, alteration of binding sites, altered metabolism, and interdiction of drug entry into the cell (eg, alteration of membrane permeability by reduced or altered expression of porin channels or efflux pumps).

β-Lactamases

Members of the family Enterobacteriaceae express plasmid-encoded β-lactamase enzymes commonly, which modify or destroy the β-lactam nucleus central to penicillins, cephalosporins, and carbapenems.[20,22] These enzymes are unique to bacteria

---

Box 3
Major mechanisms of bacterial resistance

Drug Inactivation or Modification

Enzymatic deactivation of β-lactam antibiotics in some bacteria through the production of β-lactamases. This mechanism of antibiotic resistance is the most predominant in Enterobacteriaceae, and important in *Pseudomonas* and *Acinetobacter* spp

Enzymatic deactivation of aminoglycosides by transpeptidases.

Alteration of Target Site

Penicillin-binding proteins (PBPs) are carboxypeptidases involved in peptidoglycan cross-linking, and act as the binding site of β-lactam antibiotics. PBPs may become altered, preventing binding of an antibiotic to the cell wall. This process is a major mechanism of resistance among gram-positive cocci

Altered binding of an antibiotic to the bacterial ribosome interferes with protein synthesis, and may be manifest in both gram-positive and gram-negative bacteria

Altered binding to the lipid A moiety of bacterial lipopolysaccharide, which is a mechanism for resistance of gram-negative bacteria to polymyxins

Alteration of Metabolic Pathway

For example, some sulfonamide-resistant bacteria do not require para-aminobenzoic acid (PABA), an important precursor of folic acid and nucleic acid synthesis. Instead, similar to mammalian (eukaryotic) cells, preformed folic acid is used as substrate

Reduced Drug Accumulation

Conformational changes within the cell membrane may decrease drug permeability across the cell surface or increase active efflux (extrusion by active transport) once the drug has gained entry to the cytoplasm. These mechanisms may be manifest in both gram-positive (eg, thickening of the cell wall of vancomycin-resistant enterococci) and gram-negative bacteria (eg, *Pseudomonas aeruginosa*, some Enterobacteriaceae)

---

and are not found elsewhere in nature. The molecular classification of β-lactamases is based on the nucleotide and amino acid sequences of these enzymes. Today 4 classes are recognized in the structural classification of Ambler (A–D) (**Table 2**),[26] correlating with the functional classification. Classes A, C, and D act by a

---

Table 2
Molecular classification of β-lactamases

	β-Lactamases
Class A	TEM, SHV, ESBLs
	CTX-M and ESBLs
	PER, VEB, GES, IBC
	KPC
Class B	IMP, VIM, SPM, GIM, NDM
Class C	Chromosomal Enterobacteriaceae AmpC
	Chromosomal *Pseudomonas* AmpC
	Plasmidic ACC, DHA, FOX, LAT, MIX, MIR, ACT
Class D	Penicillinase types OXA-1, -31, -10, -13
	Carbapenemase types OXA-23, -40, -48, -58

See text for definitions.

serine-based mechanism, whereas class B, or metallo-β-lactamases, need zinc for their action. Bush and colleagues[27] proposed a functional classification system that is arguably less useful outside the arcana of microbiology.

Class A β-lactamases

Class A β-lactamases (encoding genes are denoted with the prefix *bla*) include enzymes of the types TEM, SHV, and CTX. The term TEM is derived from the enzyme isolated from the blood of a Greek patient named Temoniera; more than 140 TEM variants are now described. TEM is plasmid-encoded and transposon-mediated, allowing rapid spread to other gram-negative bacteria. TEM-1 is the most commonly encountered β-lactamase in gram-negative bacteria. Up to 90% of ampicillin resistance in *E coli* is due to the production of TEM-1. Although TEM-type β-lactamases are most often found in *E coli* and *K pneumoniae*, they are also found in other gram-negative bacteria with increasing frequency. The amino acid substitutions responsible for the extended-spectrum β-lactamase (ESBL) phenotype (see later discussion) cluster around the active site of the enzyme and change its configuration, allowing access to oxyimino (a divalent radical of the form R-O-N=)-β-lactam substrates (eg, third- and fourth-generation cephalosporins and the new, unclassified agent ceftaroline). However, this conformational change also typically enhances the susceptibility of the enzyme to β-lactamase inhibitors (eg, sulbactam, tazobactam, clavulanic acid). Single amino acid substitutions can produce the ESBL phenotype, but ESBLs with the broadest spectrum usually have multiple amino acid substitutions.

Although inhibitor-resistant β-lactamases (called IRTs historically) are not ESBLs per se, they are often discussed with ESBLs because they are also derived from classic TEM-type or SHV-type enzymes. All have been renamed with numerical TEM designations. There are at least 19 distinct inhibitor-resistant TEM β-lactamases. Inhibitor-resistant TEM β-lactamases are mainly characteristic of *E coli*, but some strains of *K pneumoniae*, *Klebsiella oxytoca*, *Proteus mirabilis*, and *Citrobacter freundii* may elaborate them. The inhibitor-resistant TEM variants are invariably resistant to inhibition by clavulanic acid and sulbactam. Some strains remain susceptible to inhibition by tazobactam and the combination of piperacillin/tazobactam. To date, these β-lactamases have been detected primarily in Europe.

SHV (sulfhydryl variable) enzymes share substantial sequence homology with TEM and have a similar overall structure; more than 60 variants have been described. The SHV-1 β-lactamase is found in *K pneumoniae* most commonly and is responsible for up to 20% of plasmid-mediated ampicillin resistance in that species, some of which carry the ESBL phenotype. SHV enzymes are the predominant ESBL type in Europe and the United States, and are found worldwide.

Cefotaximases (CTX-M β-lactamases)[28] are a relatively small family of β-lactamases that have relatively low sequence homology with TEM and SHV. These enzymes were named for their greater activity against cefotaxime than other oxyimino-β-lactam substrates. Rather than arising by mutation, CTX-M is acquired only by plasmid transfer. Despite their name, a few are more active against ceftazidime than cefotaxime. CTX-M lactamases have mainly been identified in strains of *Salmonella enterica* serovar Typhimurium and *E coli*, but have also been described in other species of Enterobacteriaceae; they are the predominant ESBL type in parts of South America and are also prevalent in eastern Europe. CTX-M-15 is widespread in *E coli* in the United Kingdom, and is widely prevalent in the community.

In Germany in 1983, a new SHV-2 enzyme was detected from an isolate of *Klebsiella ozaenae* that hydrolyzed cefotaxime and, to a lesser extent, ceftazidime (a mere 2 years after the introduction of these drugs),[29] which was the dawn of the age of the ESBLs.

ESBLs specifically hydrolyze oxyimino–extended-spectrum cephalosporins, as well as the oxyimino-monobactam aztreonam. Thus, ESBLs confer resistance to these antibiotics and related oxyimino-β-lactams. ESBLs are believed initially to have been derived from genes for TEM-1, TEM-2, or SHV-1 by mutations that alter the amino acid configuration around the active site of these β-lactamases, extending the spectrum of β-lactam antibiotics susceptible to hydrolysis by those enzymes, but an increasing number of ESBLs not of TEM or SHV lineage have been described recently. ESBLs are usually plasmid-encoded, by which plasmids also carry genes frequently that encode resistance to other drug classes (eg, aminoglycosides). The combination of a Class A β-lactamase plus another mutation (eg, a porin mutation; see later discussion) may confer resistance to carbapenems. Therefore, antibiotic options in the treatment of ESBL-producing organisms may be limited[30,31] (see later discussion).

K pneumoniae carbapenemase

Carbapenems are stable to most β-lactamases and ESBLs, but carbapenemases are emerging,[32] being a diverse group of β-lactamases that are active not only against the oxyimino-cephalosporins and cephamycins (eg, cefoxitin and cefotetan, called second-generation cephalosporins in a common misnomer). A few class A enzymes, most notably the plasmid-mediated K pneumoniae carbapenemase (KPC) enzymes, are effective carbapenemases. Ten variants are known, KPC-2 through KPC-11, which are distinguished by 1 or 2 amino acid substitutions. The class A KPC is currently the most common carbapenemase, which was first detected in North Carolina in 1996 (reported in 2001),[33] and has since spread worldwide. KPC-producing isolates often coexpress resistance to fluoroquinolones and aminoglycosides,[34] but are usually still susceptible to polymyxins or tigecycline. Alarmingly, panresistant isolates have been reported.[35] Other Enterobacteriaceae that produce KPC are being reported in the United States, but the enzyme remains most prevalent in northeastern states for now.

Other plasmid-mediated ESBLs, such as PER, VEB, GES, and IBC, have been described, but are uncommon and have been found mainly in P aeruginosa and at a limited number of geographic sites. PER-1 has been described in isolates from Turkey, France, and Italy; VEB-1 and VEB-2 in strains from Southeast Asia; and GES-1, GES-2, and IBC-2 in isolates from South Africa, France, and Greece. PER-1 is also common in MDR Acinetobacter spp in Korea and Turkey. Some of these enzymes are found in Enterobacteriaceae as well, whereas other uncommon ESBLs (such as BES-1, IBC-1, SFO-1, and TLA-1) have been found only in Enterobacteriaceae.

Organisms that produce TEM-type and SHV-type ESBLs may appear in vitro to be susceptible to cefepime and piperacillin/tazobactam, but both drugs show an inoculum effect, with diminished susceptibility as the size of the inoculum is increased from 10^5 to 10^7 organisms/mL. Therefore, standard susceptibility tests, which are conducted with standardized low inocula, may be misleading. Hence these agents should not be relied on to treat infections caused by these bacteria. Strains that produce only ESBLs are susceptible to cephamycins and carbapenems in vitro and show little or no inoculum effect.

Class B β-lactamases

Class B β-lactamases differ structurally from class A enzymes, and require the presence of zinc to catalyze their activity, thus all are considered metallo-β-lactamases. These β-lactamases are those of greatest clinical concern at present.

A second family of carbapenemases, the class B Verona integron-encoded metallo-β-lactamase (VIM) family, was discovered in P aeruginosa in Italy in 1996 and now includes 10 members distributed widely in Europe, South America, and Asia, and which have been reported in the United States. The predominant VIM-2 variant is now widespread, as noted.[36] Although VIM enzymes occur mostly in *P aeruginosa*, they have been reported rarely in Enterobacteriaceae.

Plasmid-mediated imipenem (IMP)-type carbapenemases,[37] a form of metallo-β-lactamase of which nearly 20 varieties are known currently, became established in Japan in the 1990s both in enteric gram-negative bacilli and in *Pseudomonas* and *Acinetobacter* spp. IMP enzymes are now distributed widely throughout Asia, Europe, and the Americas. Amino acid sequence homology is about 70% between VIM and IMP. Both are integron-associated, sometimes within plasmids. Both hydrolyze all β-lactams except monobactams, and evade all β-lactam inhibitors currently available.

Originally described in *K pneumoniae* from New Delhi in 2009,[38] the New Delhi metallo-β-lactamase (NDM-1) gene is now widespread in *E coli* and *K pneumoniae* from India and Pakistan.[39] At present, NDM-1-carrying bacteria have been introduced to other countries (including the United States and United Kingdom), owing to the relative ease of global travel. NDM-1 may have originated in the environment, as strains containing the NDM-1 gene have been found in environmental samples from India.

Class C β-lactamases

AmpC type β-lactamases (also called cephalosporinases) are isolated commonly from extended-spectrum cephalosporin-resistant gram-negative bacteria.[40] AmpC β-lactamases are encoded on the chromosome of many gram-negative bacteria, notably *P aeruginosa*, and also *Citrobacter*, *Serratia*, and *Enterobacter* spp, where its expression is usually inducible; it may also occur in *E coli* but is not usually inducible, although it can be hyperexpressed through derepression. AmpC β-lactamases may also be carried on plasmids.

AmpC β-lactamases, in contrast to ESBLs, hydrolyze extended-spectrum cephalosporins (cephamycins and oxyimino-β-lactams) but are never inhibited by β-lactamase inhibitors. AmpC-producing strains are typically resistant to oxyimino-β lactams and cephamycins but are susceptible to carbapenems; however, diminished porin expression or increased efflux pump expression (see later discussion) can make such a strain carbapenem-resistant as well.

AmpC overproduction by *P aeruginosa* can be difficult to parse owing to the multiple resistance mechanisms usually expressed by MDR *Pseudomonas*, but AmpC overproduction is a major factor in persistent bacteremia, and the initial selection of inappropriate therapy. Overproduction can occur by induction of the *ampC* gene after exposure to β-lactam drugs and β-lactamase inhibitors, but the process is reversible after withdrawal of the offending agent. AmpC expression is regulated by 3 genes, *ampG*, *ampD*, and *ampR*, the latter being a global regulator affecting the expression of multiple genes in addition to *ampC*. The process of AmpC induction requires binding of a β-lactam or β-lactamase inhibitor to penicillin-binding proteins (PBPs) (see later discussion).

By contrast, AmpC derepression occurs when proteins in the induction pathway become compromised through chromosomal mutation, resulting in constitutive overproduction even in the absence of a β-lactam agent. Several phenotypes of partial and complete AmpC derepression are prevalent in *Pseudomonas*, more so than in the Enterobacteriaceae. Strains with partial derepression may retain susceptibility to cefepime.

Class D β-lactamases

Oxacillin-hydrolyzing (OXA) β-lactamases are a less common plasmid-mediated β-lactamase family of at least 30 variants that hydrolyze oxacillin and related antistaphylococcal penicillins, and are inhibited poorly by clavulanic acid. These β-lactamases differ structurally from TEM and SHV enzymes. Whereas most ESBLs have been found in *E coli*, *K pneumoniae*, and other Enterobacteriaceae, the OXA-type ESBLs have been found mainly in *P aeruginosa* and confer resistance to cephalosporins primarily, but with some amino acid substitutions may exhibit the ESBL phenotype. At present the OXA β-lactamases occur mainly in *Acinetobacter* spp.[41] OXA carbapenemases hydrolyze carbapenems slowly in vitro, and the high minimum inhibitory concentrations (MICs) (>64 μg/mL) observed for some *Acinetobacter* isolates may reflect secondary resistance mechanisms, such as impermeability or efflux (see later discussion). OXA carbapenemases also tend to have reduced activity against penicillins and cephalosporins, but not to the degree that cephalosporins represent reliable therapy. Strains with IMP-, VIM-, and OXA-type carbapenemases usually remain susceptible to aztreonam, but resistance to non–β-lactam antibiotics is common in strains making any of these enzymes, such that susceptibilities need to be determined directly. Note that resistance to fluoroquinolones and aminoglycosides is especially likely.

Penicillin-Binding Proteins

PBPs are carboxypeptidases characterized by their affinity for binding to penicillin. A normal constituent of many bacteria; the name reflects the way by which the protein was first discovered. All β-lactam antibiotics bind to PBP to block cross-linking and final assembly of peptidoglycans, preventing the bacterium from constructing a cell wall. There are a large number of PBPs, usually several in each organism, and they are found as both membrane-bound and cytoplasmic proteins. Different PBPs occur in different numbers per cell and have varied affinities for penicillin. All PBPs are involved in peptidoglycan synthesis, which is the major component of bacterial cell walls. Bacterial cell wall synthesis is essential to growth, reproduction, and structural maintenance. Inhibition of PBPs leads to structural irregularities such as elongation, loss of selective permeability, and eventual cell death and lysis.

PBPs can be inhibited permanently by penicillin and other β-lactam antibiotics. Bacterial cell wall synthesis and the role of PBPs in synthesis is a good target for antibiotic therapy because the metabolic pathways and enzymes are unique to bacteria. PBPs bind β-lactam antibiotics owing to structural similarity to the modular pieces that form the peptidoglycan. When a PBP binds to a penicillin, the amide bond of the β-lactam ring is ruptured, forming an irreversible covalent bond with the serine residue at the PBP active site, inactivating the carboxypeptidase. Research on PBPs led to the discovery of semisynthetic β-lactams, whereby altering the side chains on the original penicillin molecule increased the affinity of PBPs for penicillin, and thus enhanced its effectiveness.

Resistance to antibiotics has come about through overproduction of PBPs and generation of PBPs that have low binding affinity for penicillins. For example, the *mecA* gene is carried on the *SCCmec* genetic element by MRSA and penicillin-resistant *Streptococcus pneumoniae* (PRSP), conferring resistance to penicillin, methicillin, and other semisynthetic penicillins, most other β-lactams, erythromycin, and tetracyclines (but not tigecycline). *MecA* prevents the action of β-lactam antibiotics to attack transpeptidases active in bacterial cell wall synthesis, hence the bacteria replicate normally. The gene encodes penicillin-binding protein 2A (PBP$_{2A}$). The low affinity of PBP$_{2A}$ for β-lactam antibiotics preserves carboxypeptidase activity, accounting for the antibiotic resistance characteristic of MRSA.

Ribosomal Protection

Antibiotics of the aminoglycoside, macrolide-lincosamide-streptogramin, oxazolidi-none, and tetracycline[25] classes bind in general to bacterial ribosomes and disrupt protein synthesis, most commonly by the prevention of the elongation phase of protein synthesis, although specific binding sites and mechanisms of action may differ slightly. A major resistance determinant for gram-negative and gram-positive bacteria is the generation of ribosomal protection proteins,[24] which dislodge the antibiotic after initial binding to the ribosome and may induce a conformational change in the ribosome that decreases subsequent affinity for tetracyclines while preserving the ability of the ribosome to ligate aminoacyl-tRNA (aa-tRNA) and perpetuate elongation. Ribosomal protection proteins, such as Tet(M) and Tet(O) (the most well characterized of the ribosomal protection proteins, identified in most gram-positive bacteria that are human pathogens; see later discussion), are soluble cytoplasmic proteins that are related to the guanosine triphosphatase translation factor superfamily. However, from an evolutionary perspective they seem to have lost their original function and have adapted to function in tetracycline resistance.

In one proposed model,[24] after the ribosome is bound by tetracycline, the preferred binding site (the A site) for aa-tRNA becomes inaccessible and translation ceases. Tet(O), which cannot bind a ribosome with an occupied A site but which can bind (and may do so with increased avidity) when the A site is blocked, likely induces a conformational change that releases tetracycline from its binding site. It is unknown whether, once released and Tet(O) has disassociated, cytosolic free tetracycline is able to rebind successively in competition with aa-tRNA, or whether ribosomal architecture is altered to favor binding of the aa-tRNA at the expense of the tetracycline.

Porins

Porins are barrel-shaped proteins that extend into the cell membrane and act as a pore through which molecules can diffuse.[42] Porins are sufficiently large to act as molecule-specific (or group of molecules–specific) channels for passive molecular diffusion, typically small moieties such sugars, ions, and amino acids up to 1.5 kDa in size. Porins are present in the cell wall of gram-negative bacteria and some gram-positive bacteria. For an antibiotic to be effective against a bacterium, it must pass through the outer membrane, using a porin to enable diffusion. Bacteria can develop resistance to the antibiotic by mutating the gene that encodes the porin, which changes the conformation of the porin protein and prohibits the antibiotic from passing through the outer membrane.

Certain hydrophilic antibiotics, such as β-lactams, aminoglycosides, tetracyclines, and some fluoroquinolones, traverse the outer membrane through porin channels. Loss of specific porin channels (of which *P aeruginosa* possesses at least 64) can decrease the susceptibility of *P aeruginosa* to specific antibacterial agents. The outer membrane porin OprD transports carbapenems into *P aeruginosa*,[43] and has attracted considerable attention in relation to carbapenem resistance. Loss of OprD has been estimated to reduce the susceptibility of *P aeruginosa* antipseudomonal carbapenems substantially, to a level well above the susceptible breakpoint. The molecular mechanisms of OprD-mediated resistance in *P aeruginosa* are less well understood than regulation of AmpC, but identified mechanisms that affect the expression of *oprD* are linked to the regulation of the multiple efflux pump gene *mexEF-oprN* (see later discussion), highlighting the complexity by which *P aeruginosa* is able to regulate expression of resistance mechanisms, and why it can be difficult to relate phenotypic expression to any single mechanism.

Efflux Pumps

Active efflux is mechanistically responsible for extrusion of toxic substances and antibiotics outside the cell, and is an important mechanism contributing to antibiotic resistance. Efflux systems function via an energy-dependent mechanism (active transport) to extrude unwanted substances (ie, antibiotic) through specific efflux pumps within the cell wall. Some efflux systems are drug specific,[44] whereas others may accommodate multiple drugs, and thus contribute to MDR pathogenesis.

Efflux pumps are ubiquitous in the cytoplasmic membrane of all types of cells. Primary active transporters use adenosine triphosphate as an energy source, whereas secondary active transporters derive energy from the electrochemical potential difference created by transmembrane flux of hydrogen or sodium cations.

Of the 5 major superfamilies of bacterial efflux transporters, which are classified based on their amino acid sequence and the energy source used, the 2 of most relevance to bacterial resistance are the major facilitator superfamily (MFS), which is important in gram-positive bacteria, and the resistance-nodulation-cell division superfamily (RND),[45] which is unique among gram-negative bacteria; both are secondary transporters. Because most antibiotics are amphiphilic molecules, possessing both hydrophilic and hydrophobic characteristics, they are recognized easily by many efflux pumps. Although antibiotics are the most clinically important substrates of efflux systems, it is probable that most efflux pumps have other natural physiologic functions. Ten RND efflux pumps have been identified in *P aeruginosa*,[46] including MexEF-OprN. MexAB-OprM has the broadest substrate profile for the β-lactam class, being able to export carboxypenicillins, aztreonam, extended-spectrum cephalosporins, and meropenem (but not imipenem-cilastatin), and contributes to the intrinsic resistance of *P aeruginosa* to these agents through constitutive expression in wild-type cells. Some efflux pumps appear to be inducible rather than constitutive; for example, the MexXY component of the MexXY-OprM multidrug efflux system of *P aeruginosa* is inducible by antibiotics that act on bacterial ribosomes (eg, tetracyclines, aminoglycosides).

The impact of efflux mechanisms on antimicrobial resistance is substantial owing to several factors. Genes for efflux pumps may be encoded on chromosomes or plasmids, thus contributing to both intrinsic and inducible resistance, respectively. As an intrinsic resistance mechanism, efflux pump genes can survive the presence of antibiotics, which may select mutants that overexpress these genes. Thus, antibiotics can act as inducers and regulators of the expression of some efflux pumps. Expression of several efflux pumps in a given bacterial species may lead to broad-spectrum resistance, whereas one multidrug efflux pump may confer resistance to a wide range of antimicrobials.

FLUOROQUINOLONE RESISTANCE

There are 3 known mechanisms of fluoroquinolone resistance. Efflux pumps can act to decrease the intracellular quinolone concentration (eg, *Acinetobacter* spp).[47] In other gram-negative bacteria, plasmid-mediated resistance genes produce proteins that bind to DNA gyrase, protecting it from the action of quinolones.[48] Finally, mutations at key sites in DNA gyrase or topoisomerase IV (both are type II topoisomerases, not present in human beings, that relax DNA supercoils during unwinding by helicase as part of the process of replication, and remove cross-links thereafter) can decrease their binding affinity to quinolones, decreasing the drug's effectiveness. Research has shown the bacterial protein LexA may play a key role in the acquisition of bacterial mutations giving resistance to quinolones and rifampicin.

TETRACYCLINE AND GLYCYLCYCLINE RESISTANCE

Tetracyclines inhibit bacterial growth by interrupting protein synthesis,[25] but the emergence of bacterial resistance to these antibiotics has limited their use. A wide variety of tetracycline resistance mechanisms exists. These determinants include efflux-based mechanisms found in gram-positive and gram-negative bacteria, enzymatic degradation of tetracyclines found in *Bacteroides* spp, rRNA mutations found in *Helicobacter pylori*, and a host of novel mechanisms as yet uncharacterized. Three of these mechanisms are of particular importance: tetracycline efflux, ribosome protection, and tetracycline modification.

Tetracycline efflux is achieved by an MFS export protein that functions to catalyze the exchange of a tetracycline-divalent metal cation complex for a proton.[25] Ribosome protection is mediated by a soluble protein that shares homology with glutamyl transpeptidases that participate in protein synthesis.[24] The third mechanism involves a cytoplasmic protein that modifies tetracycline chemically in the presence of oxygen and hydrogenated nicotinamide adenine dinucleotide phosphate. The 2 first mechanisms are the most widespread, having been observed in both aerobic and anaerobic gram-negative and gram-positive bacteria; most of the genes are acquired via transferable plasmids or transposons. Tetracycline resistance genes, called *tet*, encode efflux proteins or ribosomal proteins, both of which confer resistance to tetracyclines. To date more than 60 tetracycline resistance genes have been sequenced, organized taxonomically into 6 groups based on sequence homology.

Tigecycline, a novel glycylcycline derived from the conventional tetracycline, minocycline, retains substantial activity against MDR gram-positive cocci and MDR Enterobacteriaceae, and some activity against MDR *Acinetobacter* spp.[49–51] Tigecycline enables high-affinity binding to the 30S ribosomal unit because of a modification at position 9 of its core structure. The 2 tetracycline resistance mechanisms of greatest clinical importance that tigecycline is able to deter are efflux and ribosomal protection. There are 2 possible mechanisms by which tigecycline can overcome efflux resistance mechanisms: either the failure of the efflux pumps to recognize tigecycline, or the inability of efflux transporters to translocate tigecycline across the cytoplasmic membrane. Efflux-mediated resistance of *Acinetobacter* spp to tigecycline has been reported. With respect to ribosomal protection, the exact mechanism has yet to be elucidated, but it has been suggested that ribosomal binding of tigecycline disrupts the tight bond of the ribosomal protection protein with the ribosome.

AMINOGLYCOSIDE RESISTANCE

Aminoglycosides are characterized by the presence of an aminocyclitol ring linked to amino sugars. Bactericidal activity is mediated by irreversible binding to bacterial ribosomes. Three mechanisms of resistance have been recognized: ribosome alteration by methyltransferases, decreased permeability, and inactivation of the drugs by aminoglycoside-modifying enzymes.[52] The latter mechanism is most important clinically because the genes encoding aminoglycoside-modifying enzymes can be disseminated by plasmids or transposons.

High-level resistance to aminoglycosides can result from single-step mutations in chromosomal genes encoding ribosomal proteins, resulting in methylation of the 16S rRNA. Absence of or alteration in the aminoglycoside transport system, inadequate membrane potential, or modification of the lipopolysaccharide (LPS) phenotype can result in cross-resistance to all aminoglycosides. Enzymatic inactivation of aminoglycosides may be mediated by acetyltransferases, nucleotidyltransferases, adenyltransferases, or phosphotransferases.

VANCOMYCIN RESISTANCE

Few gram-positive human pathogens are intrinsically resistant to vancomycin, whereas most gram-negative bacteria are intrinsically resistant because their outer membrane is impermeable to large molecules. Acquired resistance to vancomycin is a growing problem, particularly within health care facilities, owing to its widespread use.[53] Vancomycin-resistant *Enterococcus* (VRE) emerged in 1987. Vancomycin resistance emerged in *S aureus* during the 1990s and 2000s, including vancomycin-intermediate *S aureus* (VISA) (1996, Japan) and vancomycin-resistant *S aureus* (VRSA) (2002, Michigan). There is some suspicion that agricultural use of avoparicin, a similar glycopeptide antibiotic, has contributed to the emergence of VISA organisms, but VRSA possesses the transmissible *vanA* gene that confers resistance among VRE.

Cell wall peptidoglycan is organized into a crystal lattice structure formed from linear chains of 2 alternating amino sugars, namely *N*-acetylglucosamine (GlcNAc or NAG) and *N*-acetylmuramic acid (MurNAc or NAM). The primary mechanism of resistance to vancomycin involves alteration to the terminal amino acid residues of NAM/NAG-peptide subunits (under normal conditions, D-alanyl-D-alanine), to which vancomycin binds. The D-alanyl-D-lactate variation results in the loss of 1 of the 5 hydrogen bonds possible between vancomycin and the peptide, and a 1000-fold decrease in affinity. The D-alanyl-D-serine variation causes a 6-fold loss of affinity between vancomycin and the peptide.

Six different vancomycin resistance genes are expressed by *Enterococcus*: *vanA* to *vanF*, of which only *vanA* to *vanC* have thus far been expressed by clinical isolates.[54] The *vanA* phenotype is most common (~85%), inducible, expressed usually by *Enterococcus faecium*, and confers resistance to both vancomycin and teicoplanin (a glycopeptide that is not marketed in the United States). *vanB* is also inducible and confers resistance to vancomycin but not teicoplanin (unusual, but may be induced in *Enterococcus faecalis*), whereas *vanC* confers constitutive resistance only to vancomycin. In enterococci, these modifications impede the binding of vancomycin to the peptidoglycan subunit. In the United States, linezolid is used commonly to treat VRE because teicoplanin is not available.

LINEZOLID RESISTANCE

Acquired resistance of MDR *E faecium* to linezolid was reported as early as 1999. Linezolid-resistant *S aureus* was first isolated in 2001. Fortunately, resistance to linezolid remains rare, affecting fewer than 0.5% of gram-positive cocci isolates overall, and fewer than 0.1% of *S aureus*. Gram-positive bacteria usually develop resistance to linezolid as the result of a point mutation of the gene (*cfr*) coding for 23S ribosomal RNA, thus causing ribosomal target modification (as has been described for *S aureus*).[55] This mechanism of resistance is the most common in staphylococci, and the only one known to date in isolates of *E. faecium*. Other identified mechanisms include mutations in an RNA methyltransferase that methylates 23S rRNA. The intrinsic resistance of most gram-negative bacteria to linezolid is due to the activity of efflux pumps.

DAPTOMYCIN RESISTANCE

Although genetic mutations have been described, there is still no definitive mechanism described for the development of antimicrobial resistance to daptomycin.[56] Fortunately, resistance among clinical isolates remains rare. Prior vancomycin therapy does not increase the risk of failure of daptomycin therapy.

RESISTANCE TO POLYMYXINS

Although the precise molecular basis of polymyxin resistance remains unknown, it seems clear that LPS modifications and loss of affinity for anionic polymyxins are necessary to the development of resistance to these antibiotics in *Acinetobacter baumannii*. The most important mechanism of polymyxin resistance involves modification of LPS in the bacterial outer membrane,[57,58] mediated by the 2-component response regulator and sensor kinase PmrA/B, which allows bacteria to sense and respond to various environmental conditions (including pH or Fe^{3+} and Mg^{2+} concentrations), affects expression of genes implicated in lipid A modification, and thereby influences susceptibility to polymyxins.[59] Heteroresistance (see later discussion) to polymyxins is associated with exposure to polymyxins, especially in subtherapeutic dosage.[60]

RESISTANCE IN SPECIFIC BACTERIA
Staphylococcus aureus

The rapid evolution of resistance by *S aureus* dates to the introduction of antibiotics into clinical practice, and has been problematic for clinicians. Changes in the PBP on the staphylococcal cell membrane was the mechanism for the emergence of resistance to penicillin and methicillin. Using pulsed-field gel electrophoresis (PGFE), 8 strains of MRSA have been characterized as PGFE USA100 through USA800.[61] The resistance determinant lies in the staphylococcal cassette chromosome within the accessory portion of the genome (*SCCmec*).[62] However, the genetics of resistance varies among these strains. Seven different *SCCmec* gene cassettes have been identified in MRSA; types I, V, VI, and VII typically carry only resistance for β-lactam antibiotics. *SCCmec* type IV has been associated most commonly with the prevalent community-acquired methicillin-resistant staphylococci (CA-MRSA) in the United States (USA300),[63] which has retained susceptibility to non–β-lactam antibiotics such as trimethoprim-sulfamethoxazole (TMP-SMX). By contrast, hospital-acquired (HA)-MRSA has the larger molecular weight *SCCmec* type II and -III gene cassettes, which confer resistance to most non–β-lactam antibiotics as well. Continuing changes within accessory genes, acquisition by plasmid transfer of additional resistance genes, and the increasing presence of CA-MRSA within the hospital environment suggest that the phenotypic differences in susceptibility among all strains of MRSA are likely to become less distinct.[64–66]

A looming threat is VISA and VRSA (referred to also in glycopeptide terms, ie, GISA and GRSA). First reported in 1997,[67] VISA (historically, MICs 4–16 μg/mL) appears to be increasing in frequency. Moreover, although controversial, a "MIC creep" has been observed among susceptible *S aureus* isolates (MIC ≤2 μg/mL), meaning that a greater proportion of isolates have an MIC of 1 μg/mL instead of 0.5 μg/mL historically, and so on. This finding correlates clinically with increased risk of failure of therapy for isolates at the higher end of the range (**Table 3**),[68–70] and has led to revision of the susceptibility breakpoints for *S aureus* to vancomycin by the Clinical and Laboratory Standards Institute (**Table 4**)[71] to decrease the possibility of treatment failure by labeling the formerly borderline vancomycin-susceptible isolates as being either VISA or VRSA, thereby influencing antibiotic choice. Higher reported prevalences of VISA and VRSA will be the inevitable result.

Heteroresistant VISA (hVISA) strains are those for which MICs are conventionally susceptible (≤2 μg/mL) by routine susceptibility testing, except when high-density inocula are used. With such inocula, minority subpopulations emerge for which MICs are in the intermediate range (4–8 μg/mL).[71] The detection of hVISA requires

Table 3
Causes of vancomycin failure in a single-center cohort of 320 patients with documented MRSA bacteremia: logistic regression analysis

Parameter Predicting Failure of Vancomycin Therapy	Adjusted Odds Ratio	95% Confidence Interval
Infective endocarditis	4.55	2.26–9.15
Nosocomial acquisition of infection	2.19	1.21–3.97
Initial vancomycin trough concentration <15 µg/mL	2.00	1.25–3.22
Vancomycin MIC >1 µg/mL	1.52	1.09–2.49

Abbreviation: MIC, minimum inhibitory concentration.
Data from Patel N, Pai MP, Rodvold KA, et al. Vancomycin: we can't get there from here. Clin Infect Dis 2011;52:969–74.

inocula containing greater than 10^6 bacteria, because resistant clones spontaneously occur infrequently ($\sim 1/1,000,000$).[72] The MICs for most heteroresistant clones are usually in the 4- to 8-µg/mL range,[73] but unstable heteroresistance can be detected.[74,75] Clones of S aureus demonstrating unstable heteroresistance grow in the presence of high concentrations of vancomycin (>4 µg/mL), although conventional MICs for such clones are not elevated; that is, nonsusceptible clones revert rapidly to normal phenotypes and therefore cannot be detected by usual laboratory tests. Clinical failure with vancomycin or MICs to vancomycin of 2 µg/mL or more should alert the laboratory to proceed with the more specific methods of population analysis profiling, along with hVISA screening performed by the macro-Etest (MET) to identify hVISA or VISA isolates.[68] Both VISA and hVISA appear to emerge in SCCmec II isolates among vancomycin-exposed patients, and are detected better by MET.[76] Infection with hVISA is associated with high-density inocula, bacteremic infections, prolonged therapy, and clinical failures, although higher mortality has not been substantiated[77,78] and optimal therapy has not been established.

The VISA phenotype is not the consequence of vancomycin-resistance genes transmitted from enterococci. The natural history of VISA phenotypic expression is believed to begin with adaptive thickening of the cell wall of the occasional heteroresistant organism, which leads to its emergence as the dominant phenotype when exposed to environmental pressures, including vancomycin use. The thickened cell wall impedes penetration of the vancomycin molecule, and upregulates expression of peptidoglycan binding sites to create resistance.[71] Unremitting pressure to use vancomycin is likely to continue to exacerbate the situation.

Table 4
Vancomycin MIC interpretive criteria for S aureus

Old Breakpoints (µg/mL)	New Breakpoints (µg/mL)
Susceptible: ≤4	Susceptible: ≤2
Intermediate: 8–16	Intermediate: 4–8
Resistant: ≥32	Resistant: ≥16

Data from Hageman JC, Patel JB, Carey RC, et al. Investigation and control of vancomycin-intermediate and-resistant *Staphylococcus aureus*: a guide for health departments and infection control personnel. Atlanta (GA): Centers for Disease Control and Prevention; 2006.

A total of 11 VRSA infections have now been identified in the United States.[79] By contrast, it appears that the *vanA* gene acquired by plasmid-mediated gene transfer from VRE encodes for VRSA. All VRSA are methicillin resistant. Most are classified as USA100. These clinical infections have been associated with preceding MRSA or enterococcal infections that were treated with vancomycin. Chronic comorbid conditions are present, notably chronic kidney disease and end-stage renal disease. All infections occurred following surgical care, or occurred in patients with complicated soft tissue infections in whose management surgeons are involved.

The pathogen *S aureus* may form small colony variants (SCVs), a naturally occurring, slow-growing subpopulation with distinctive phenotypic characteristics and pathogenic traits.[80] SCVs are defined by mostly nonpigmented and nonhemolytic colonies approximately one-tenth of the size of the parent strain. The tiny size of clinical and experimentally derived SCVs on solid agar is often due to auxotrophy for hemin or menadione, 2 compounds involved in the biosynthesis of electron transport chain components (an auxotroph is a mutant organism, especially a microorganism, that has a nutritional requirement not shared by the parent organism). The morphology and physiology of SCVs present a challenge to microbiologists in terms of recovery, identification, and susceptibility testing of these organisms. Several reports support a pathogenic role for SCVs in patients with persistent or recurrent infections, whether because of difficulties with laboratory diagnosis (and thus treatment), the role of SCVs in biofilm formation, or the propensity of SCVs to persist intracellularly, which may affect the choice of agent for therapy.

Pseudomonas aeruginosa

Pseudomonas aeruginosa is a highly prevalent opportunistic pathogen. One of many concerning characteristics of *P aeruginosa* is its low antibiotic susceptibility, which is attributable to the concerted action of multidrug efflux pumps from chromosomally encoded antibiotic resistance genes (eg, *mexAB-oprM*) (see earlier discussion) and the low permeability of its bacterial cell wall.[23,46,81] Besides intrinsic resistance, *P aeruginosa* has a propensity to develop resistance during therapy, even evolving an MDR phenotype, either by mutation in chromosomally encoded genes or by the horizontal gene transfer of antibiotic resistance determinants, therefore serial culture and susceptibility testing is advisable during therapy, even of ostensibly susceptible isolates. Hypermutation favors the selection of mutation-driven antibiotic resistance in *P aeruginosa* strains, producing chronic infections, whereas the clustering of several different antibiotic resistance genes in integrons favors the acquisition of multiple antibiotic resistance determinants and expression of the MDR phenotype. Phenotypic resistance associated with biofilm formation,[82] or the emergence of SCVs, may be important in the response of *P aeruginosa* populations to treatment.

Acinetobacter calcoaceticus-baumannii Complex

Acinetobacter spp are a key source of infection in debilitated patients in the hospital, in particular the species referred to commonly as *A baumannii*.[83] *Acinetobacter* are strictly aerobic, nonfermenting gram-negative bacilli, which show preponderant coccobacillary morphology on nonselective agar. Bacillary forms predominate in fluid media, especially during early growth. The morphology of *Acinetobacter* spp can be variable in gram-stained human clinical specimens, hindering early identification. Because *A baumannii* can survive on inanimate surfaces for protracted periods, they pose a high risk of spread and contamination in hospitals.

Acinetobacter spp are innately resistant to many classes of antibiotics, including penicillins, chloramphenicol, and often aminoglycosides. Resistance to fluoroquinolones has been reported to develop during therapy, resulting in an MDR phenotype mediated through increased expression of chromosomal genes for efflux systems.[44] RND pump systems are the most prevalent in multiply-resistant *A baumannii*.[84] Overexpression of AdeABC, secondary to mutations in the *adeRS* genes encoding a 2-component regulatory system, constitutes a major mechanism of MDR expression in *A baumannii*. The recently described AdeFGH also confers MDR when overexpressed. Finally, acquired narrow-spectrum efflux pumps, such as the MFS members TetA, TetB, CmlA, and FloR, and the small multidrug resistance (SMR) member QacE, have been detected and are mainly encoded by mobile genetic elements.

A dramatic increase in antibiotic resistance in *Acinetobacter* spp has been reported, making the carbapenems the gold-standard treatment heretofore. However, carbapenem resistance in *A baumannii* is increasing worldwide.[85] Class B metallo-β-lactamases have been reported in *Acinetobacter* spp, but the widespread β-lactamases in *A baumannii* are class D OXA carbapenemases that are specific for the species. These enzymes belong to 3 unrelated groups represented by OXA-23, OXA-24, and OXA-58, which can be either plasmid-encoded or chromosomally encoded. *A baumannii* also possesses an intrinsic carbapenem-hydrolyzing oxacillinase, the expression of which may vary. In addition to mediation by β-lactamases, carbapenem resistance in *A baumannii* may also result from porin or PBP modifications. *Acinetobacter* spp are unusual in that they are susceptible to sulbactam about 50% of the time; this is an example of the intrinsic antibacterial properties of β-lactamase inhibitors.

LABORATORY DETECTION OF ESBL-PRODUCING BACTERIA

Detailed discussion of microbiology laboratory procedures for the characterization of resistant bacterial isolates is beyond the scope of this discussion, but clinicians must be aware that ESBL producers may not be detected by automated systems[21] and thus require laborious, time-consuming, and expensive manual processing that some laboratories may be unable (or unwilling) to perform under budgetary constraints. Thus, clinical suspicion is important to initiate effective treatment as soon as possible, or to alert the laboratory that special handling of a specimen is desired. Underreporting leads to underrecognition, increased treatment failures, higher mortality, greater cost, and ineffectiveness of infection control measures. There is no single, definitive marker for ESBL production, as there is for MRSA or VRE. Ceftazidime resistance was formerly a clue that ESBL production might be present, but as cefepime use has supplanted the former, hospitals are increasingly doing susceptibility testing only for the latter. Not all ESBL-producers are uniformly resistant to β-lactamase inhibitors, or an ESBL-producer may harbor multiple ESBL enzymes or coexpress other enzymes, such as AmpC or a metalloenzyme that may alter the resistance phenotype. The inoculum effect (lower susceptibility at higher bacterial concentrations) may confound the translation of susceptibility tests into clinical effectiveness, because susceptibility testing is conducted on standard, lower inocula.

In general, an isolate is suspected to be an ESBL-producer when it shows in vitro susceptibility to cephamycins but resistance to third-generation cephalosporins and aztreonam. Moreover, one should be suspicious when treatment of a gram-negative infection with these agents fails despite susceptibility reported in vitro. Once an ESBL-producing strain is detected, laboratory standards now require reporting it as resistant to all penicillins, cephalosporins, and aztreonam, even if it appears to be susceptible in vitro. β-Lactamase inhibitors inhibit most ESBLs in vitro, but the clinical effectiveness of BLICs cannot be relied on for therapy. Moreover, the Clinical and Laboratory Standards Institute has lowered the susceptibility breakpoints of Enterobacteriaceae for cephalosporins and carbapenems (**Table 5**),[86] to reduce the burden on microbiology laboratories and ensure that no borderline organisms will be reported as susceptible, although the inevitable result will be reports of increasing prevalences of MDR pathogens.

When performed, the Etest may be used for both screening and phenotypic confirmation of ESBL production. The test device is a two-sided plastic strip on which clavulanic acid is added to one side of a dual oxyimino-β-lactam gradient (cefotaxime or ceftazidime), to look for a reduction of the MIC for the organism in the presence of clavulanate. Sensitivity as a confirmatory test is reported to be 87% to 100%, whereas specificity is reported to be 95% to 100%. Some automated susceptibility test systems (eg, Vitek, MicroScan) have also been introduced, with sensitivity and specificity reported to exceed 90%.

EPIDEMIOLOGY OF MDR INFECTIONS

MDR organisms are prevalent worldwide, but not invariably to the same degree. Prevalence may vary by organism, region, country, hospital, or by unit within a facility. Originally infections caused by MDR organisms were limited to nosocomial infections in hospitals, but now the bacteria may colonize vulnerable patients. Moreover, these pathogens are now prevalent in the community.

Table 6 lists the pathogens isolated most commonly from nosocomial infections in the United States (as reported to the National Healthcare Safety Network [NHSN] of the United States Centers for Disease Control and Prevention [CDC] in 2006–2007),[87,88] and the predominant site of isolation. Overall, central line–associated bloodstream infections (CLABSIs) are most common in intensive care units (ICUs), followed by urinary tract infections (UTIs). However, by comparison with medical ICUs, ventilator-associated pneumonia (VAP) is more prevalent whereas CLABSIs are less so in surgical ICUs (**Tables 7** and **8**).[87,89,90] For VAP, approximately 80% of infections are accounted for by 6 pathogens (in rank order): *S aureus* (a majority are MRSA), *P aeruginosa*, *Klebsiella* spp, *E coli*, *Acinetobacter* spp, and *Enterobacter* spp[87,88] With respect to CLABSI, approximately 70% of infections are accounted for by 4 pathogens (in rank order): coagulase-negative *Staphylococcus* spp, *Enterococcus* spp (a minority are VRE), *Candida* spp (either *albicans* or non-*albicans* spp), and *S aureus* (a majority are MRSA). Regarding UTI, the predominant pathogens (in rank order) are *E coli*, *Enterococcus* spp (a minority are VRE), *Candida* spp (either *albicans* or non-*albicans* spp), and *P aeruginosa*, accounting for about two-thirds of isolates.

Stratified by organism as reported to NHSN for the 2006 to 2007 period, 56% of *S aureus* isolates were MRSA, 33% of enterococcal isolates were VRE, and 25% and 31% of *P aeruginosa* isolates were resistant to fluoroquinolones and carbapenems, respectively. *K pneumoniae* isolates were 21% to 27% resistant to third-generation cephalosporins and 4% to 11% resistant to carbapenems, respectively, depending on the locus of isolation, whereas *K oxytoca* isolates were somewhat less likely to exhibit resistance. *A baumannii* isolates were 26% to 37% carbapenem-resistant, whereas *E coli* exhibited resistance of 23% to 31% to fluoroquinolones, 8% to 11% to third-generation cephalosporins, and 1% to 4% to carbapenems. Resistance is increasing most rapidly for third-generation cephalosporin-resistant (ESBL-producing) *E coli* and *K pneumoniae*, and carbapenem-resistant *P aeruginosa* (usually by a metallo-β-lactamase). However, data as to the specific mechanisms of resistance

Table 5
New susceptibility breakpoints for β-lactam antibiotics against Enterobacteriaceae as defined by the Clinical and Laboratory Standards Institute, 2010

| Drug (Usual Dosage) | MIC (μg/mL) | | | | | |
| | New | | | Old | | |
	Susceptible	Intermediate	Resistant	Susceptible	Intermediate	Resistant
Aztreonam (1 g every 8 h)	≤4	8	≥16	≤8	16	≥32
Cefazolin (2 g every 8 h)	≤2	4	≥8	≤8	16	≥32
Cefotaxime (1 g every 8 h)	≤1	2	≥4	≤8	16–32	≥64
Ceftazidime (1 g every 8 h)	≤4	8	≥16	≤8	16	≥32
Ceftizoxime (1 g every 12 h)	≤1	2	≥4	≤8	16–32	≥64
Ceftriaxone (1 g every 24 h)	≤1	2	≥4	≤8	16–32	≥64
Doripenem (500 mg every 8 h)	≤1	2	≥4	—	—	N/A
Ertapenem (1 g every 24 h)	≤0.25	0.5	≥1	≤2	4	≥8
Imipenem-cilastatin (1 g every 8 h)	≤1	2	≥4	≤4	8	≥16
Meropenem (1 g every 8 h)	≤1	2	≥4	≤4	8	≥16

Data from Lee K, Yong D, Jeong SH, et al. Multidrug-resistant Acinetobacter spp: increasingly problematic nosocomial pathogens. Yonsei Med J 2011;52:879–91.

Table 6
Rank order of pathogens isolated from cases of health care-associated infections, reported to the National Healthcare Safety Network, US Centers for Disease Control and Prevention, 2006–2007

Pathogen	Percentage	Most Common Site
Coagulase-negative *Staphylococcus*	15.3	Bloodstream[1]
S aureus	14.5	Surgical site[1]
Enterococcus spp	12.1	Bloodstream[2]
Candida spp	10.7	Urinary tract[2]
Escherichia coli	9.6	Urinary tract[1]
Pseudomonas aeruginosa	7.9	Respiratory tract[2]
Klebsiella pneumoniae	5.8	Urinary tract[5]
Enterobacter spp	4.8	Respiratory tract[4]
Acinetobacter baumannii	2.7	Respiratory tract[4]
K oxytoca	1.1	Respiratory tract[x]
Other	15.6	

Superscript refers to rank order of prevalence for the site. x, not a top-5 pathogen.

are not available from NHSN. Rates of resistance tend to be much higher in Europe, Asia, Africa, and Latin America than in the United States, with the 2 most notable exceptions being VRE and carbapenem-resistant *K pneumoniae*. The data suggest that fluoroquinolones should be avoided as empiric therapy for the most part, unless detailed knowledge of local susceptibility patterns suggests otherwise.

Recent data from the Study for Monitoring Antimicrobial Resistance Trends (SMART) indicate that bacterial resistance is an increasing global problem for complicated intra-abdominal infections, although not to a large degree, as yet, in North America.[91–93] High rates of ESBL-producing *K pneumoniae* and *E coli* have been reported in China (34% and 59%, respectively), India (47% and 61%), and Thailand (23% and 53%, respectively). These trends are affecting the selection of agents for

Table 7
Rates of and central line–associated bloodstream infection among various ICU types: National Nosocomial Infection Surveillance System and National Healthcare Safety Network, US Centers for Disease Control and Prevention

ICU Type	CVC Use		CLABSI Rate Mean/Median	
	1992–2004	2006–2008	1992–2004	2006–2008
Medical	0.52	0.45	5.0/3.9	1.9/1.0
Pediatric	0.46	0.48	6.6/5.2	3.0/2.5
Surgical	0.61	0.59	4.6/3.4	2.3/1.7
Cardiovascular	0.79	0.71	2.7/1.8	1.4/0.8
Neurosurgical	0.48	0.44	4.6/3.1	2.5/1.9
Trauma	0.61	0.63	7.4/5.2	3.6/3.0

Infection rates are indexed per 1000 patient-days.
Abbreviations: CLABSI, central line-associated bloodstream infection; CVC Use, number of days of catheter placement/1000 patient-days in ICU.
Data from Refs.[87,89,90] Data are available at: www.cdc.gov, and are in the public domain.

Table 8
Rates of health care–associated pneumonia among various ICU types: National Nosocomial Infection Surveillance System and National Healthcare Safety Network, US Centers for Disease Control and Prevention

ICU Type	TT Use		VAP Rate Mean/Median	
	1992–2004	2006–2008	1992–2004	2006–2008
Medical	0.46	0.48	4.9/3.7	2.4/2.2
Pediatric	0.39	0.42	2.9/2.3	1.8/0.7
Surgical	0.44	0.39	9.3/8.3	4.9/3.8
Cardiovascular	0.43	0.39	7.2/6.3	3.9/2.6
Neurosurgical	0.39	0.36	11.2/6.2	5.3/4.0
Trauma	0.56	0.57	15.2/11.4	8.1/5.2

Infection rates are indexed per 1000 patient-days.
Abbreviations: TT Use, Number of days of indwelling endotracheal tube or tracheostomy/1000 patient-days in ICU; VAP, ventilator-associated pneumonia.
Data from Refs.[87,89,90] Data available at: www.cdc.gov, and are in the public domain.

antimicrobial therapy for intra-abdominal infections worldwide,[94–96] noting that resistant pathogens in complicated intra-abdominal infections have been associated with increased mortality.[97]

Although MDR infection has been associated with increased morbidity, mortality, duration of hospitalization, and cost,[98] assignation of attributable mortality for critically ill patients is a slippery slope,[99] and circumspection is advised when interpreting the data. Difficulties arise because, in such complex patients, it can be challenging to parse whether death is due to a particular infection, a coexistent infection acting alone or in concert, delay in effective therapy (particularly of an MDR organism),[100] underlying high severity of illness or serious medical comorbidity, multiple organ dysfunction syndrome caused by active or eradicated infection (the latter because dysfunctional host defenses do not "stand down"), or some serious but undiagnosed ailment or complication (eg, pulmonary embolism). That said, the estimated relative risk of death for patients with VAP is approximately doubled, but evidence of mortality attributable directly to VAP is minimal,[98] and lacking in surgical patients as opposed to medical patients.[99,101] The relative risk of death associated with CLABSI is increased by approximately 80%. Whether excess mortality attributable to MDR bacteria is due to increased virulence or decreased efficacy of initial therapy is unclear, but it does appear to be real, particularly based on studies of inarguably invasive infections (ie, bacteremia).[102–112]

PRINCIPLES OF ANTIBIOTIC THERAPY

Antimicrobial therapy is a mainstay of infection management, but widespread overuse and misuse of antibiotics have led to an alarming increase in MDR pathogens (see **Box 2**). New agents and innovative ways to administer existing antibiotics may allow shorter courses of therapy, desirable for cost savings and control of microbial ecology. Effective, nontoxic therapy requires a careful but expeditious search for the source of infection and an understanding of PK and PD.

Pharmacokinetics and Pharmacodynamics

PK describes principles of drug uptake, distribution, and metabolism.[17] Relationships between dose and response are influenced by dose, dosing interval, and route of administration. Plasma and tissue drug concentrations are also influenced by drug metabolism and excretion. To the extent that serum and tissue concentrations correlate (depending on tissue penetration), relationships between concentration and effect are described by PD.[17]

Pharmacodynamic parameters include bioavailability, half-life, clearance, and volume of distribution (V_D). Bioavailability describes the proportion of drug dose that reaches the systemic circulation after oral administration. Bioavailability is affected by absorption, intestinal transit time, and hepatic metabolism (if any). Half-life ($T_{1/2}$) is the time required for the serum drug concentration to reduce by one-half, reflecting both clearance (see later discussion) and V_D.[17] The V_D is used to estimate the plasma drug concentration achievable from a given dose, and is independent of clearance or $T_{1/2}$, but varies substantially according to pathophysiology (eg, reduced V_D causes a higher concentration for a given dose, whereas fluid overload and hypoalbuminemia [which decreases drug binding] both increase V_D). Consequently, increased doses of hydrophilic drugs (eg, β-lactam antibiotics) may be needed in the early phases of sepsis owing to fluid resuscitation and increased microvascular permeability.[113]

Clearance describes the volume of fluid from which drug is eliminated completely per unit of time, regardless of the mode of elimination; knowledge of drug clearance is important to determine the dose necessary to maintain a steady-state concentration. Most drugs are metabolized hepatically to polar compounds for eventual renal excretion. Renal filtration is determined by molecular size and charge, and by the number of functional nephrons. In general, if 40% or more of active drug (including active metabolites) is eliminated unchanged in the urine, the dose should be decreased if the glomerular filtration rate (GFR) is less than 40 to 50 mL/min.

Drug-patient, drug-microbe, and microbe-patient interactions must be accounted for in planning antimicrobial therapy.[17] Unique in pharmacotherapy, the key drug interaction is with the microbe rather than the host. Microbial physiology, inoculum characteristics (ie, size, quorum sensing, presence of a biofilm on an implant),[114,115] microbial growth phase, mechanisms of resistance, the microenvironment (eg, local pH), and the host's response are also factors to consider. Because of microbial resistance, mere administration of the correct drug may not be microbicidal if suboptimal.

Laboratory-derived PD parameters include MIC, the lowest serum drug concentration that inhibits bacterial growth (MIC_{90} refers to 90% inhibition) (**Fig. 1**). Some antibiotics (eg, aminoglycosides and fluoroquinolones for gram-negative bacteria, and carbapenems against *S aureus*) may suppress bacterial growth appreciably (ie, several hours' duration) at subinhibitory concentrations (the post-antibiotic effect).[113,116] However, MIC testing fails to detect resistant bacterial subpopulations within the inoculum (eg, heteroresistance of *S aureus*), whereby subclones may be selected by therapy, overgrow in the ecological vacuum caused by treatment, and cause clinical failure.

Analytical tools that use both PK and PD include the peak serum concentration (Cmax):MIC ratio, the proportion of time that plasma concentration exceeds MIC (fT>MIC), and the area of the plasma concentration-time curve above the MIC (the area under the curve, or AUC). Aminoglycosides exhibit optimal concentration-dependent killing when Cmax:MIC is greater than 10,[116,117] which can be achieved with single daily-dose administration, whereas β-lactam agents exhibit optimal killing determined when fT > MIC > 40% of the dosing interval,[118] which can be achieved by prolonged intermittent or continuous infusion.[17,119,120] Some agents (eg, fluoroquinolones, vancomycin) exhibit both properties; bacterial killing increases as drug concentration increases up to a saturation point, after which the effect becomes concentration independent, characterized by AUC:MIC greater than 125, which describes the optimal effect and minimized risk of developing resistance.

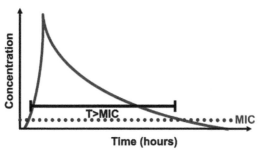

Fig. 1. A stylized elimination curve for a single bolus dose of a parenteral antibiotic. Some drugs (eg, aminoglycosides) exhibit concentration-dependent bactericidal activity; a peak concentration:minimum inhibitory concentration (MIC) ratio of greater than 10 is optimal for bacterial killing. β-Lactam agents exhibit time-dependent bactericidal activity; the proportion (fT) of time above the MIC should be at least 40% for optimal killing. Efficacy of still other drugs (eg, vancomycin, fluoroquinolones) is reflected by the area under the concentration curve (AUC), a method of measurement of the bioavailability of a drug based on a plot of blood concentrations sampled at frequent intervals. The AUC is directly proportional to the total amount of unaltered drug in the patient's blood. An AUC:MIC ratio of greater than 400 is associated with optimal antibacterial effect and minimization of the development of resistance.

Empiric Antibiotic Therapy

Empiric antibiotic therapy must be judicious and expeditious. Injudicious therapy could result in undertreatment of infection, or unnecessary therapy if the patient has only sterile inflammation or bacterial colonization. Inappropriate therapy (eg, delay,[121,122] therapy misdirected against usual pathogens, failure to treat MDR pathogens) leads unequivocally to increased mortality.[13–55] Delay in initiation of empiric antibiotic therapy as brief as 30 to 60 minutes increases mortality[121,122]; current guidelines recommend that empiric antibiotic therapy be instituted with 1 hour of presentation with severe sepsis.[123]

Antibiotic choice is based on several interrelated factors (**Box 4, Tables 9** and **10**). Paramount is activity against identified or likely (for empiric therapy) pathogens. Estimation of likely pathogens depends on the disease process believed responsible; whether the infection is community-acquired, health care–related, or hospital-acquired; and whether MDR organisms are present, or likely. Local knowledge of resistance patterns is essential, even at the unit-specific level. Important patient-related factors include age, debility, immunosuppression, organ function, prior allergy or other adverse reaction, and recent antibiotic therapy (see **Box 4**). Important institutional factors include guidelines that may specify a particular therapy, formulary availability, outbreaks of infections caused by MDR pathogens, and antibiotic stewardship programs.

Antibiotic stewardship programs[3] support optimal antibiotic administration, including physician education and feedback, practitioner prescribing patterns, computerized decision support, administration by protocol, and formulary restriction programs. Owing to the high prevalence of MDR pathogens, it is crucial for initial empiric antibiotic therapy to be targeted appropriately, administered according to PK/PD principles, given in a dose sufficient to ensure bacterial killing, de-escalated[12,124,125] as soon as possible based on microbiology data and clinical response,

Box 4
Factors influencing antibiotic choice

Activity against known/suspected pathogens

Disease believed responsible

Distinguish infection from colonization

Narrow-spectrum coverage most desirable

Antimicrobial resistance patterns

Patient-specific factors

    Location before presentation: home versus health care facility

    Duration of inpatient hospitalization

    Recent prior antibiotic therapy?

    Severity of illness?

    Age?

    Immunosuppression

    Organ dysfunction

    Allergy

Institutional guidelines/restrictions

    Institutional approval required?

    Agent available immediately?

Logistics

    Onset, dose, and dosing interval

    Single or multiple agents?

    Duration of infusion and course of therapy

Table 9
Rank order of key bacterial pathogens in ICU infections (by incidence)

	Bloodstream Infection[a]	Urinary Tract Infection[a]	Pneumonia[b]
Gram-positive	1. Coag-neg staphylococci 2. Enterococcus 3. S aureus	1. Enterococcus 2. Coag-neg staphylococci 3. S aureus	1. S aureus
Gram-negative	1. Enterobacter 2. P aeruginosa 3. K pneumoniae 4. E coli	1. E coli 2. P aeruginosa 3. K pneumoniae 4. Enterobacter	1. P aeruginosa 2. Enterobacter 3. K pneumoniae 4. Acinetobacter 5. E coli

Abbreviation: Coag-neg, coagulase-negative.
  [a] Yeasts are also important pathogens in bloodstream and urinary tract infections.
  [b] Yeasts are seldom pathogens in nosocomial infection, except for solid-organ transplant recipients and patients undergoing antineoplastic chemotherapy.

Table 10
Bacterial resistance: problem infections and pathogens

Infection	Organisms			
	MRSA	VRE	ESBL	Carbapenemases
CAP	+ (CA-MRSA)			
VAP	++++		++	++
UTI		+	++	
Soft tissue	++++ (CA-MRSA)	+	++	+
CLABSI	++++	+	+	+

The number of (+) indicators reflect relative prevalence.

Abbreviations: CA-MRSA, community-acquired methicillin-resistant *S aureus*; CAP, community-acquired pneumonia; CLABSI, central line–associated bloodstream infection; ESBL, extended-spectrum β-lactamase; VAP, ventilator-associated pneumonia; VRE, vancomycin-resistant *Enterococcus*.

and continued only as long as necessary. Appropriate prescribing of antibiotics optimizes patient care, supports infection-control practice, and preserves microbial ecology.[3,124]

Choice of antibiotic

Numerous agents are available for therapy (**Box 5**).[30,126] Agents may be chosen based on spectrum, whether broad or targeted (eg, antipseudomonal, antianaerobic), in addition to the aforementioned factors. If a nosocomial gram-positive pathogen is suspected (eg, skin or soft tissue infection, CLABSI, HAP/VAP) or MRSA is endemic, empiric vancomycin (or linezolid) is appropriate. Some authorities recommend dual-agent therapy for clinically serious (but not necessarily MDR) *Pseudomonas* infections (eg, an antipseudomonal β-lactam drug plus an aminoglycoside), but evidence of efficacy is mixed,[127–130] and may actually worsen outcomes. Meta-analysis of β-lactam monotherapy versus β-lactam/aminoglycoside combination therapy for immunocompetent patients with sepsis (64 trials, 7586 patients) found no difference in either mortality (relative risk 0.90, 95% confidence interval [CI] 0.77–1.06) or the development of resistance.[128] Clinical failure was more common with combination therapy, as was the incidence of acute kidney injury. Regardless, initial empiric therapy for any hospital-acquired infection must include activity against all likely pathogens.[30,94,131,132]

Optimization of therapy

Higher antibiotic doses may be required for MDR isolates.[13,118,133,134] Underdosing of antibiotics is a major factor for the development of resistance during therapy and failure thereof.[118] Dosing of vancomycin and aminoglycosides may be monitored via serum drug concentrations,[117,135,136] and may limit toxicity.[137]

Mathematical modeling such as Monte Carlo simulation has allowed virtual clinical trials to be performed.[138] Such analyses can inform dosing decisions to achieve a higher likelihood of achieving PK/PD targets, and thus better clinical outcomes, for organisms with higher MICs. Modeling of optimal dosing of meropenem and several other antibiotics in critically ill patients[139] found that, at MICs up to 8 μg/mL, the probability of achieving 40% fT > MIC was 96%, 90%, and 61% for 3-hour infusions of meropenem 2 g every 8 hours, 1 g every 8 hours, and 1 g every 12 hours, respectively. By contrast, target attainment was 75%, 65%, and 44% for these same dosing regimens as 0.5-hour infusions. Continuous or prolonged infusion may be the optimal way to administer β-lactam agents (**Figs. 2 and 3**).[140–143] Prolonged

| **Box 5** |
| **Antibacterial agents for potential empiric use** |

Antipseudomonal

Piperacillin-tazobactam

Cefepime, ceftazidime

Imipenem-cilastatin, meropenem, doripenem

? Ciprofloxacin, levofloxacin (depending on local susceptibility patterns)

Aminoglycosides

Polymyxins (polymyxin B, colistin [polymyxin E])

Targeted-spectrum

Gram-positive

    Glycopeptide (eg, vancomycin, telavancin)

    Lipopeptide (eg, daptomycin; not for known/suspected pneumonia)

    Oxazolidinone (eg, linezolid)

Gram-negative

    Third-generation cephalosporin (not ceftriaxone)

    Monobactam

    Polymyxins (polymyxin B, colistin [polymyxin E])

Broad-spectrum

Piperacillin-tazobactam

Carbapenems (not ertapenem for pseudomonas)

Fluoroquinolones (depending on local susceptibility patterns)

Tigecycline (plus an antipseudomonal agent)

Trimethoprim-sulfamethoxazole (used primarily for CA-MRSA, *Stenotrophomonas*)

Antianaerobic

Metronidazole

Carbapenems

β-Lactam/β-lactamase combination agents

Tigecycline

Anti-MRSA

Ceftaroline

Daptomycin (not for use against pneumonia)

Minocycline

Linezolid

Telavancin

Tigecycline (not in pregnancy or for children younger than 8 years)

Vancomycin

fT > MIC is achieved, increasing the likelihood of success, especially against organisms with higher MICs, while minimizing the possibility of resistance developing. Clinical reports support the use of prolonged infusions of β-lactam antibiotics.[119,120,144]

Special Considerations for Therapy for MDR Bacteria

High-dose daptomycin may be effective and safe for treatment of recalcitrant MDR gram-positive infections,[136,145] and there are several options for combination therapy (**Box 6**). Infections caused by MDR gram-negative bacilli pose a major problem, as options for therapy are few. Carbapenems, tigecycline, and polymyxins (see later discussion) retain useful activity against ESBL-producing organisms. At present, carbapenems are preferred for treatment of infections caused by ESBL-producing organisms. Cefepime and piperacillin/tazobactam have been less successful. Several reports have documented failure of cephamycin therapy as a result of resistance caused by porin loss. Some patients have responded to aminoglycoside or quinolone therapy. MDR nonfermenting gram-negative bacilli (eg, *P aeruginosa*, *Acinetobacter* spp, *Stenotrophomonas* spp) and carbapenemase-producing Enterobacteriaceae may require therapy with a polymyxin, high-dose carbapenem by prolonged or continuous infusion, or unusual combinations of agents that have demonstrated synergy in vitro, but remain of uncertain clinical utility.[30,126,146–154]

SPECTRA OF ANTIBIOTIC ACTIVITY USEFUL FOR MDR ORGANISMS

Susceptibility testing of specific organisms is necessary for management of serious infections (including all nosocomial infections). Recommendations focus on agents useful for the treatment of serious/nosocomial infections; not every agent within the class will receive mention. Recommended agents for specific organisms are guidelines only, because in vitro susceptibilities may not correlate with clinical efficacy. Exposure to certain agents has been associated with the emergence of specific MDR bacteria, which require a different empiric antibiotic choice or modification of a regimen if identified or suspected.

Cell Wall–Active Agents: β-Lactam Antibiotics

The β-lactam antibiotic group consists of penicillins, cephalosporins, a monobactam, and carbapenems. Within this group, several agents have been combined with β-lactamase inhibitors to broaden the spectrum of activity, and new extended-spectrum β-

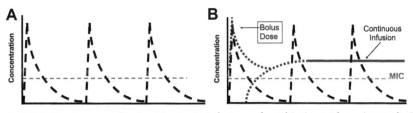

Fig. 2. (*A*) Stylized curves of bolus 30-minute infusions of antibiotic at 6-hour intervals. The proportion of time (fT) above the minimum inhibitory concentration (MIC) must be at least 40% for bactericidal activity in most cases. If the MIC is low, this can be achieved with conventional dosing, but not for organisms with higher MICs. (*B*) Continuous infusion of antibiotic after an initial loading dose (*dotted lines*) is depicted. Not only is fT:MIC higher, but the antibiotic becomes effective against organisms with higher MICs, depending on the rate of continuous infusion. Lower total daily doses of antibiotic may be used against bacteria with low MICs. For drugs that exhibit time-dependent bactericidal activity (eg, β-lactams), this is the ideal mode of administration, provided vascular access is sufficient.

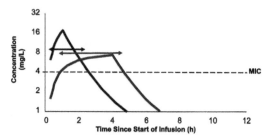

Fig. 3. A conventional bolus dose of antibiotic with a 30-minute infusion and a 6-hour dosing interval is compared with the same drug given as a 4-hour infusion over the same dosing interval. fT:MIC is doubled (compare the lengths of the *short and long double arrows*) while organisms with higher MICs can still be treated. The interruption allows the intravenous line to be used for fluid or other medication during the hiatus, without compromising bactericidal action.

lactamase inhibitors are sought avidly, although none to date has demonstrated the ability to inhibit metalloenzymes.[155] Except for carboxypenicillins and ureidopenicillins, penicillins retain little or no activity against gram-negative bacilli. Carboxypenicillins (eg, ticarcillin) and ureidopenicillins (or acylampicillins, eg, piperacillin) are now used only as a BLIC. Piperacillin-tazobactam has the widest spectrum of activity against gram-negative bacteria, and reasonable potency against *P aeruginosa*. Ampicillin-sulbactam is unreliable against *E coli* and *Klebsiella* spp (resistance rate ~50%), but it has modest effectiveness against *Acinetobacter* spp owing to the activity of the sulbactam moiety. Tazobactam is the most active β-lactamase inhibitor available currently, but the investigational agent avibactam (NXL-104) has enhanced activity (albeit not against metallo-β-lactamases).[155]

The cephalosporin class comprises more than 20 agents, few of which are useful against MDR pathogens. Ceftazidime and cefepime have enhanced activity against gram-negative bacilli and some specific antipseudomonal activity; cefepime is a less potent inducer of ESBLs than is ceftazidime. Activity is reliable only against non–ESBL-producing species of Enterobacteriaceae including *Enterobacter*, *Citrobacter*, *Providencia*, and *Morganella*, but not for empiric monotherapy against nonfermenting gram-negative bacilli. Similar to the carbapenems, cefepime is intrinsically more resistant to hydrolysis by β-lactamases, but not enough to be reliable empirically against ESBL-producing bacteria. Ceftaroline (usual dose, 600 mg intravenously every 12 hours) has not been classified, but has anti-MRSA activity unique among the cephalosporins while retaining modest activity comparable to first-generation agents against gram-negative bacilli.[156]

Imipenem-cilastatin, meropenem, doripenem, and ertapenem are the available carbapenems in the United States. Imipenem-cilastatin, meropenem, and doripenem have the widest (and generally comparable) clinical utility of any antibiotics (subtle differences that are reported in vitro are of uncertain importance). Activity is excellent against aerobic and anaerobic streptococci, methicillin-sensitive staphylococci, and virtually all gram-negative bacilli except *Acinetobacter* spp, *Legionella pneumophila*, *Pseudomonas cepacia*, and *Stenotrophomonas maltophilia*.[157] All carbapenems are superlative antianaerobic agents, thus there is no reason to combine a carbapenem with metronidazole unless CDI and another anaerobic infection coexist.

Meropenem and doripenem have less potential than imipenem-cilastatin for neurotoxicity, which is contraindicated in patients with active central nervous system disease or injury (except the spinal cord), because of the rare (~0.5%) appearance

Box 6
Combination therapy options for the treatment of recalcitrant or highly resistant MDR infections

Management of persistent MRSA bacteremia

Management of vancomycin treatment failures

Search for and eradicate any focus of infection, including debridement or surgical drainage, with:

High-dose daptomycin (10 mg/kg/d)[a] alone or in combination with:

Gentamicin 1 mg/kg/d IV, *or*

Rifampin 600 mg IV/PO daily *or* 300–450 mg IV/PO twice daily, *or*

Linezolid 600 mg IV/PO twice daily, *or*

Televancin 10 mg/kg IV once daily, *or*

Trimethoprim/sulfamethoxazole 5 mg/kg IV twice daily, *or*

A β-lactam antibiotic

If reduced susceptibility to vancomycin or daptomycin are present[b]:

Quinupristin/dalfopristin 7.5 mg/kg IV every 8 hours, *or*

Linezolid 600 mg IV/PO twice daily, *or*

Televancin 10 mg/kg IV once daily, *or*

Trimethoprim/sulfamethoxazole 5 mg/kg IV twice daily

Management of MDR gram-negative bacillary infections when effective conventional monotherapy is not available based on in vitro susceptibility testing, or is contraindicated (eg, hypersensitivity)[c]

High-dose, prolonged-infusion, or continuous-infusion carbapenem with or without a polymyxin or aminoglycoside

Dual carbapenem therapy

Aminoglycoside combined with a β-lactam agent (antipseudomonal cephalosporin or BLIC agent) or antipseudomonal fluoroquinolone, with or without rifampin

Aminoglycoside plus fosfomycin

Intravenous combined with inhalational aminoglycoside (for pneumonia)

Intravenous combined with inhalational polymyxin B plus a carbapenem, aminoglycoside, fluoroquinolone, or aztreonam (for pneumonia)

Antipseudomonal cephalosporin or BLIC agent combined with an antipseudomonal fluoroquinolone

Polymyxin combined with one or more of a carbapenem, aminoglycoside, fluoroquinolone, or β-lactam agent

Polymyxin or aminoglycoside plus tigecycline

Polymyxin combined with rifampin, an antipseudomonal carbapenem (or both), with or without azithromycin or doxycycline

Abbreviations: BLIC, β-lactamase inhibitor combination; IV, intravenous; MDR, multidrug-resistant; MRSA, methicillin-resistant *Staphylococcus aureus*; PO, oral.

[a] Assumes the organism is susceptible in vitro. *Data from* Liu C, Bayer A, Cosgrove SE, et al. Clinical practice guidelines by the Infectious Diseases Society of America for the treatment of methicillin-resistant *Staphylococcus aureus* infections in adults and children. Clin Infect Dis 2011;52:e8–45.

[b] Agents may be given alone or in combination. *Data from* Liu C, Bayer A, Cosgrove SE, et al. Clinical practice guidelines by the Infectious Diseases Society of America for the treatment of methicillin-resistant *Staphylococcus aureus* infections in adults and children. Clin Infect Dis 2011;52:e8–45.

[c] Suggestions are derived from in vitro testing, animal studies, or case reports. No class I data or large class II studies are available.

of myoclonus or generalized seizures in patients who have received high doses (with normal renal function) or inadequate dosage reductions with renal insufficiency. Ertapenem is not useful against *Pseudomonas* spp, *Acinetobacter* spp, *Enterobacter* spp, or MRSA, but its long half-life permits once-daily dosing.[158] Ertapenem is active against ESBL-producing Enterobacteriaceae, and also has less potential for neurotoxicity. With all carbapenems, disruption of host microbial flora may lead to superinfections (eg, fungi, CDI, *S maltophilia*, resistant enterococci).

Cell Wall–Active Agents: Lipoglycopeptides

Vancomycin, a soluble lipoglycopeptide, is bactericidal, but tissue penetration is universally poor, which limits its effectiveness. Most strains of *E faecalis* are inhibited (but not killed) by attainable concentrations, but *E faecium* is increasingly VRE. Both *S aureus* and *Staphylococcus epidermidis* are usually susceptible to vancomycin. Although vancomycin has been a mainstay of therapy for nosocomial infections, MICs for vancomycin against MRSA are increasing, even within the susceptible range. Mortality increases as a function of the vancomycin MIC, even for strains with MIC values within the susceptible range (see **Table 3**).[69,159] As a result, MIC susceptibility breakpoints for resistance of *S aureus* have been revised downward to minimize the chance of ineffective therapy (see **Table 4**),[160] and higher doses of vancomycin are recommended (**Box 7**),[135,136] albeit with greater risk of nephrotoxicity. Vancomycin therapy for MRSA isolates with MICs between 1 and 2 mg/mL should be undertaken cautiously. Adequate therapeutic concentrations probably may not be achievable for

---

Box 7
Summary of vancomycin dosing guidelines

Therapeutic Vancomycin Dose Adjustment and Drug Monitoring

Dosage

- Initial vancomycin dosages should be calculated on the basis of actual body weight, including for obese patients. IV vancomycin 15 to 20 mg/kg (actual body weight) every 8 to 12 h, not to exceed 2 g per dose, is recommended for most patients with normal renal function. For seriously ill patients (eg, those with sepsis, meningitis, pneumonia, or infective endocarditis) with suspected MRSA infection, a loading dose of 25 to 30 mg/kg (actual body weight) may be considered.

- Subsequent dosage adjustments should be based on actual trough serum concentrations, obtained just before the fourth dose, to achieve targeted therapeutic concentrations. Trough vancomycin monitoring is recommended for serious infections and for patients who are morbidly obese, have renal dysfunction (including those receiving renal replacement therapy), or have fluctuating volumes of distribution. For serious infections, such as bacteremia, infective endocarditis, osteomyelitis, meningitis, pneumonia, and severe skin and soft tissue infections (eg, necrotizing fasciitis) caused by MRSA, vancomycin trough concentrations of 15 to 20 μg/mL are recommended.

- Monitoring of peak vancomycin concentrations is not recommended.

- Doses of 1 g should be infused over 1 h. Doses of more than 1 g should be infused over 1.5 to 2 h. Continuous infusion of vancomycin is not recommended.

Adapted from Rybak MJ, Lomaestro BM, Rotschaefer JC, et al. Vancomycin therapeutic guidelines: a summary of consensus recommendations from the Infectious Diseases Society of America, the American Society of Health-System Pharmacists, and the Society of Infectious Diseases Pharmacists. Clin Infect Dis 2009;49:325–7; and Liu C, Bayer A, Cosgrove SE, et al. Clinical practice guidelines by the Infectious Diseases Society of America for the treatment of methicillin-resistant *Staphylococcus aureus* infections in adults and children. Clin Infect Dis 2011;52:e18–55.

S aureus isolates with MICs greater than 2 μg/mL,[69] so alternative therapy should be identified if the patient is slow to respond.

Telavancin, a synthetic derivative of vancomycin, has been approved for treatment of complicated skin and skin structure infections.[161] There appears to be a dual mechanism of action, including cell membrane disruption and inhibition of cell wall synthesis. The drug is active against MRSA, but only vancomycin-susceptible enterococci (MIC <1 μg/mL). The most common side effects are taste disturbance, nausea, vomiting, and headache. There may be a small increased risk of acute kidney injury. The usual dose is 10 mg/kg, infused intravenously over 60 minutes, every 24 hours for 7 to 14 days; dosage reductions are necessary in renal insufficiency. No information is available regarding the prevalence of resistance to telavancin, which remains rare.

Cell Wall–Active Agents: Cyclic Lipopeptides

Daptomycin has potent, rapid bactericidal activity against most gram-positive organisms. The mechanism of action is via rapid membrane depolarization; potassium efflux; arrest of DNA, RNA, and protein synthesis; and cell death. Daptomycin exhibits concentration-dependent killing, and has a long half-life (8 hours). A dose of 4 mg/kg once daily is recommended for nonbacteremic infections, versus 6 mg/kg/d for bacteremia. The dosing interval should be increased to 48 hours when creatinine clearance is less than 30 mL/min. Daptomycin is active against most aerobic and anaerobic gram-positive bacteria, including MDR strains such as MRSA, MR S epidermidis, and VRE. Resistance to daptomycin has been reported for both MRSA and VRE.[146] Myositis is rare and mild, but creatine phosphokinase must be monitored periodically; higher doses seem to be safe for recalcitrant infections (see **Box 6**).[145]

It is important that daptomycin not be used for the treatment of pneumonia or empiric therapy when pneumonia is in the differential diagnosis, even when caused by a susceptible organism, because daptomycin penetrates lung tissue poorly and is also inactivated by pulmonary surfactant.[162]

Cell Wall–Active Agents: Polymyxins

Polymyxins are cyclic, cationic peptide antibiotics that have fatty acid residues[58,163]; 2 (polymyxins B and E, or colistin) have been used clinically. Polymixins bind to the anionic bacterial outer membrane, leading to a detergent effect that disrupts membrane integrity. High-affinity binding to the lipid A moiety of LPS may have an endotoxin-neutralizing effect. Commercial preparations of polymyxin B are standardized, but those of colistimethate (the less toxic prodrug of colistin that is administered clinically) are not, so dosing depends on which preparation is being supplied. Most recent reports describe colistimethate use, but the drugs are therapeutically equivalent.

Dosing of polymyxin B is 1.5 to 2.5 mg/kg (15,000–25,000 U/kg) daily in divided doses, whereas dosing of colistimethate ranges from 2.5 to 6 mg/kg/d, also in divided doses. The diluent is voluminous, adding substantially to daily fluid intake. Scant PK data indicate rapid, concentration-dependent bactericidal activity against most gram-negative bacilli, including MDR E coli, Klebsiella spp, Enterobacter spp, P aeruginosa, S maltophilia, and Acinetobacter spp. Tissue uptake is poor, but both intrathecal and inhalational administration have been described. Clinical response rates for respiratory tract infections appear to be lower than for other sites of infection. Increasing rates of resistance, including heteroresistance, have been observed and are of concern.[163]

Polymyxins fell out of favor because of nephrotoxicity and neurotoxicity, but MDR pathogens have restored their clinical utility. Up to 40% of colistimethate-treated patients (5%–15% for polymyxin B) will develop acute kidney injury, but seldom is renal replacement therapy required. Neurotoxicity (5%–7% for both) usually manifests as muscle weakness or polyneuropathy.

Protein Synthesis Inhibitors

Several classes of antibiotics, although dissimilar structurally and having divergent spectra of activity, exert their effects via binding to bacterial ribosomes and inhibiting protein synthesis. This classification is valuable mechanistically, linking several classes of antibiotics conceptually that have few clinically useful members.

Aminoglycosides

Once disdained owing to toxicity, a resurgence of aminoglycoside use has occurred as resistance to newer antibiotics has developed (especially cephalosporins and fluoroquinolones). Gentamicin, tobramycin, and amikacin are still used frequently. Aminoglycosides bind to the bacterial 30S ribosomal subunit. Gentamicin has modest activity against gram-positive cocci; otherwise the activity and toxicity of the agents is nearly identical, so the choice of aminoglycoside should be based on local resistance patterns. Nevertheless, the potential for toxicity is real, and aminoglycosides are now seldom first-line therapy, except in a synergistic combination to treat a serious *Pseudomonas* infection, enterococcal endocarditis, or an infection caused by a known or suspected MDR gram-negative bacillus. As second-line therapy, these drugs are efficacious against the Enterobacteriaceae, but less active against *Acinetobacter* spp, and limited against *P cepacia*, *Aeromonas* spp, and *S maltophilia*.

Aminoglycosides kill bacteria most effectively with a concentration peak:MIC of greater than 10, therefore a loading dose is necessary and monitoring of serum drug concentration is performed.[117] Marked dosage reductions are necessary in renal insufficiency, but the drugs are dialyzed and a maintenance dose should be given after each hemodialysis treatment.

Single daily-dose aminoglycoside therapy ensures that a peak:MIC ratio greater than 10 will be achieved. A dose of gentamicin or tobramycin (7 mg/kg), or amikacin (20 mg/kg), is administered and a trough concentration is determined at 23 hours postdose (some protocols call for an intermediate determination [~16 hours] so that the elimination curve can be determined with greater precision). A trough concentration of 0.5 to 1 µg/mL is ideal for gentamicin or tobramycin, whereas a trough concentration of 5 to 10 µg/mL is sought for amikacin. Outcomes are comparable or better compared with conventional dosing, with decreased toxicity. Single-daily-dose aminoglycoside therapy has not been validated for children, pregnant women, burns patients, or patients older than 70 years.

Tetracyclines

Tetracyclines bind to the 30S ribosomal subunit, but they are bacteriostatic only. Widespread resistance limits their utility (with the exceptions of doxycycline, minocycline, and tigecycline [intravenous only]). Tetracyclines are active against anaerobes; *Actinomyces* can be treated successfully. Doxycycline is active against *Bacillus fragilis* but is seldom used for this purpose. All tetracyclines are contraindicated in pregnancy and for children younger than 8 years, owing to dental toxicity.

Tigecycline is a novel glycylcycline derived from minocycline (both are now available parenterally).[164] With the major exceptions of *Pseudomonas* spp and *P mirabilis*, the spectrum of activity is broad, including many MDR gram-positive and gram-negative bacteria, including MRSA, VRE, and some isolates of *Acinetobacter* spp. Tigecycline is active against aerobic and anaerobic streptococci, staphylococci, MRSA, MRSE, and enterococci, including VRE. Antianaerobic activity is excellent. Activity against gram-negative bacilli is directed against ESBL-producing Enterobacteriaceae, *Pasteurella multocida*, *Aeromonas hydrophila*, *S maltophilia*, *Enterobacter aerogenes*, and *Acinetobacter* spp. However, clinical evidence of efficacy against MDR pathogens is scant, consisting mostly of retrospective reports[51,150,152,165,166] and a few prospective, observational studies.[165,167–169] In the observational studies, clinical cure rates were reported to be between 67% and 82%, depending on the pathogen and the site of infection.

Concern has been raised recently by a post hoc analysis that the mortality of tigecycline-treated patients is higher in pooled phase 3 and 4 clinical trials, including unpublished registration trials.[170] The adjusted risk difference for all-cause mortality, based on a random effects model stratified by trial weight, was 0.6% (95% CI 0.1–1.2) between tigecycline and comparator agents. However, an independent meta-analysis found no such survival disadvantage in an analysis of 8 published randomized controlled trials (4651 patients).[171] Overall, no difference was identified for the pooled clinically- (odds ratio [OR] 0.92, 95% CI 0.76–1.12) or microbiologically-evaluable populations (OR 0.86, 95% CI 0.69–1.07) from the trials.

Oxazolidinones

Oxazolidinones bind to the ribosomal 50S subunit, preventing complexing with the 30S subunit. Assembly of a functional initiation complex for protein synthesis is blocked, preventing translation of mRNA. This mode of action is novel in that other protein synthesis inhibitors permit mRNA translation but then inhibit peptide elongation. Linezolid is bacteriostatic against most susceptible organisms. The ribosomes of *E coli* are as susceptible to linezolid as those of gram-positive cocci but, with minor exceptions, gram-negative bacteria are oxazolidinone resistant, because oxazolidinones are excreted by efflux pumps.

Linezolid is equally active against methicillin-sensitive *S aureus* and MRSA, vancomycin-susceptible enterococci and VRE, and against susceptible and penicillin-resistant *S pneumoniae*. Most gram-negative bacteria are resistant, but *Bacteroides* spp are susceptible. Linezolid requires no dosage reduction in renal insufficiency and exhibits excellent tissue penetration, but it is uncertain whether this provides clinical benefit in treatment of serious infections.[172] Meta-analysis suggests that linezolid is equivalent to vancomycin for hospital-acquired and ventilator-associated pneumonia.[173]

Drugs That Disrupt Nucleic Acids

Fluoroquinolones

The fluoroquinolones exhibit excellent oral absorption and bioavailability, but the spectrum of activity is diminishing, and there are numerous toxicities (photosensitivity, cartilage [especially in children] and tendon damage, prolongation of the QTc interval) and drug interactions. These agents have a marked propensity to develop and induce resistance (see **Table 1**). Ciprofloxacin, levofloxacin, and moxifloxacin (which has some antianaerobic activity) are available parenterally and orally. Several others have been withdrawn from the market or were never approved owing to toxicity.

Fluoroquinolones are most active against enteric gram-negative bacteria, particularly the Enterobacteriaceae and *Haemophilus* spp. There is some activity against *P aeruginosa*, *S maltophilia*, and gram-negative cocci. Activity against gram-positive cocci is variable, being least for ciprofloxacin and highest for moxifloxacin. Ciprofloxacin is most active against *P aeruginosa*. However, rampant overuse of fluoroquinolones is rapidly causing resistance that may limit severely the future usefulness of these agents.[174] Fluoroquinolone use has been associated with the emergence of resistant *E coli*, *Klebsiella* spp, *P aeruginosa*, and MRSA.[175,176] Fluoroquinolones prolong the QTc interval and may precipitate the ventricular dysrhythmia torsades de pointes, so electrocardiographic measurement of the QTc interval before and during fluoroquinolone therapy is important. Also, fluoroquinolones interact with warfarin to cause a rapid, marked prolongation of the International Normalized Ratio, which must be monitored closely during therapy.

Cytotoxic Antibiotics

Trimethoprim-sulfamethoxazole

Sulfonamides exert bacteriostatic activity by interfering with bacterial folic acid synthesis, a necessary step in DNA synthesis. Resistance is widespread, limiting use. The addition of sulfamethoxazole to trimethoprim (TMP SMX), which prevents the conversion of dihydrofolic acid to tetrahydrofolic acid by the action of dihydrofolate reductase (downstream from the action of sulfonamides), accentuates the bactericidal activity.

The combination TMP-SMX is active against *S aureus*, *Streptococcus pyogenes*, *S pneumoniae*, *E coli*, *P mirabilis*, *Salmonella* and *Shigella* spp, *Yersinia enterocolitica*, *S maltophilia*, *Listeria monocytogenes*, and *Pneumocystis jerovici*. TMP-SMX is a treatment of choice for infections caused by *S maltophilia*, and outpatient (and sometimes inpatient) treatment of infections caused by CA-MRSA.

A fixed-dose combination of TMP-SMX of 1:5 is available for parenteral administration. The standard oral formulation is 80:400 mg, but lesser and greater strength tablets are available. Oral absorption is rapid and bioavailability is nearly 100%. Tissue penetration is excellent. Ten milliliters of the parenteral formulation contains 160:800 mg drug. Full doses (150–300 mg TMP in 3–4 divided doses) may be given if creatinine clearance is greater than 30 mL/min, but the drug is not recommended when the creatinine clearance is less than 15 mL/min.

DURATION OF THERAPY

Class I evidence is scant regarding duration of therapy for serious infections, but there are assuredly no data to indicate that MDR infections require prolonged therapy per se if initial empiric therapy is adequate. There is some evidence to suggest that prompt, effective bacterial killing by timely, appropriate initial empiric therapy may lead to shorter duration of therapy. Moreover, if initial broad-spectrum therapy is adequate, de-escalation of therapy is safe and effective.[177] Consensus recommendations for duration of therapy are shown in **Table 11**.[125] There is evidence emerging that serial measurements of serum procalcitonin concentration may be antibiotic sparing in that it facilitates the earlier termination of antibiotic therapy.[178]

MANAGING THE MICROBIAL ECOLOGY OF THE UNIT

Prescribing the same antibiotic regimen repeatedly is believed to lead to resistance by increasing antibiotic selection pressure on a unit. ICUs are frequently the epicenter of nosocomial infections caused by MDR bacteria. Prevention of bacterial resistance is paramount to achieving good outcomes of critical care, but outbreaks do occur and must be contained. The microbiology laboratory supports the provision of appropriate antibiotic therapy by providing clinicians with antibiograms to aid empiric antibiotic

Table 11
Current recommendations for duration of therapy for selected serious infections

Bacterial meningitis	
Gram-negative bacilli (eg, postoperative)	21 d
CLABSI	
Coagulase-negative *Staphylococcus*	5–7 d
S aureus	14 d[a]
Enterococcus spp	7–14 d
Gram-negative bacilli	7–14 d
Candida spp	14 d after the last positive blood culture
Complicated intra-abdominal infection	4–7 d
Pneumonia	
CAP[b]	≤5 d
VAP[b]	
Bacteria other than NFGNB	7 d
NFGNB	14 d

Abbreviations: CAP, community-acquired pneumonia; CLABSI, central line-associated bloodstream infection; NFGNB, nonfermenting gram-negative bacilli; VAP, ventilator-associated pneumonia.

[a] If the patient is not immunosuppressed or neutropenic, the catheter has been removed, there is no recent placement of a prosthetic intravascular device, and there is no evidence of either endocarditis (by echocardiography) or suppurative thrombophlebitis (by ultrasonography). Fever and bacteremia must resolve within 72 h, and there must be no evidence of metastatic infection by physical examination. If these conditions are not met, 6 weeks of therapy is recommended.

[b] Supported by one or more randomized prospective trials, rather than expert opinion.

Adapted from Hayashi DL, Paterson DL. Strategies for reduction in duration of antibiotic use in hospitalized patients. Clin Infect Dis 2011;52:1232–40.

choice and by providing MICs of key antibiotics so that antibiotic dosing is optimized to PD targets (**Table 12**). Laboratories also play a crucial role in the prevention of antibiotic resistance. Molecular epidemiologic evidence of an oligoclonal outbreak of infections orients prevention measures toward investigation of common environmental sources of infection and prevention of patient-to-patient transmission. The CDC has published several guidelines on management of outbreaks caused by MDR organisms, including hand hygiene, isolation precautions, and environmental controls.[179–182]

By contrast, evidence of polyclonality shifts prevention of antibiotic resistance to antibiotic management strategies; selection strategies for individual patients have been outlined earlier in this article. Restoration of microbial ecology at the unit-specific or institutional level requires a coordinated effort. It has been demonstrated for some time that the selective withdrawal of antibiotics that exert high selection pressure (eg, ceftazidime, vancomycin, fluoroquinolones) is restorative.[183–186] Whether the ecology can be maintained is still hypothetical. The hypothesis states that if homogeneity of prescribing leads to increased antibiotic selection pressure, diversity of prescribing will prevent the development of resistance.[187] Truly random prescribing cannot occur; each clinician will have his or her favored regimens, and bias is inevitable. So-called heterogeneity of prescribing can be enforced through tactics referred to as mixing or cycling. These constructs are not identical, in that in the former one antibiotic at a time is withdrawn from use, whereas cycling uses only a single agent for a defined period. Neither approach is clearly superior,[188] but cycling has been

Table 12
Pharmacokinetics of bacterial killing: implications for antibiotic dosing

Characteristic	Drug	Therapeutic Goal	Tactic
Time-dependent (no or minimal PAE) fT >MIC >70% ideal)	Carbapenems Cephalosporins Linezolid Penicillins	Maintain drug concentration	Maximize duration of exposure with prolonged or continuous infusion[a]
Time-dependent, concentration-enhanced (with PAE) AUC:MIC$_{24h}$ >125; AUC:MIC$_{24h}$ >400 for MDR pathogens?	Clindamycin Glycylcyclines Macrolides Streptogramins Tetracyclines Vancomycin	Maximize effectiveness of bacteriostatic/ weak bactericidal antibiotics with prolonged PAEs. PAE is concentration-dependent	Maximize drug dosage[b] consistent with avoidance of toxicity
Concentration-dependent (with PAE)	Aminoglycosides Daptomycin Fluoroquinolones Ketolides Metronidazole Polymyxins	PAE Is concentration-dependent. Achieve Cmax ([peak]:MIC) >10	Maximize peak concentration[c]

See text for additional explanations.

Abbreviations: AUC, area under the concentration-time curve; Cmax, maximum drug concentration (peak concentration); fT, proportion of time; MDR, multidrug-resistant; MIC, minimum inhibitory concentration; PAE, postantibiotic effect.

[a] Continuous or prolonged infusion of linezolid is not recommended, as efficacy has not been established.

[b] Examples of maximized drug dosages include clindamycin 900 mg every 8 h rather than 600 mg every 6 h, and vancomycin 15 mg/kg/d for patients with normal renal function. Larger doses of tigecycline (a glycylcycline) and streptogramins (eg, quinupristin/dalfopristin) may be limited by increased toxicity.

[c] Examples of dosing to achieve maximized peak drug concentrations include single daily-dose aminoglycoside therapy and metronidazole 1 g every 12 h rather than 500 mg every 8 h. Prolonging the dosing interval is not recommended for polymyxins, owing to a negligible PAE.

tested more extensively and has been found to be an effective tactic for both interdiction and maintenance in surgical ICUs,[121,189–192] but it is not a panacea.[193] Questions to be answered about antibiotic cycling include which agents to cycle and at what interval to cycle them.

REFERENCES

1. Bradley JS, Guidos R, Baragona S, et al. Anti-infective research and development—problems, challenges, and solutions. Lancet Infect Dis 2007;7:68–78.
2. Magee JT. The resistance ratchet: theoretical implications of cyclic selection pressure. J Antimicrob Chemother 2005;56:427–30.
3. Dellit TH, Owens RC, McGowan JE Jr, et al. Infectious Diseases Society of America and Society of Healthcare Epidemiology. Infectious Diseases Society of America and Society of Healthcare Epidemiology of America guidelines for developing an institutional program to enhance antimicrobial stewardship. Clin Infect Dis 2007;44:159–77.
4. Arnold HM, Micek ST, Skrupky LP, et al. Antibiotic stewardship in the intensive care unit. Semin Respir Crit Care Med 2011;32:215–27.

5. Barie PS, Eachempati SR. Infections of trauma patients. In: Peitzman AB, Rhodes M, Schwab CW, et al, editors. The trauma manual. Trauma and acute care surgery. 3rd edition. Philadelphia: Lippincott, Williams & Wilkins; 2008. p. 596–617.

6. Kardas P, Devine S, Golembesky A, et al. A systematic review and meta-analysis of misuse of antibiotic therapies in the community. Int J Antimicrob Agents 2005;26:106–13.

7. Bin Abdulhak AA, Altannir MA, Almansor MA, et al. Non-prescribed sale of antibiotics in Riyadh, Saudi Arabia: a cross sectional study. BMC Public Health 2011;7(11):538.

8. Llor C, Cots JM. The sale of antibiotics without prescription in pharmacies in Catalonia, Spain. Clin Infect Dis 2009;48:1345–9.

9. Rice LB. Federal funding for the study of antimicrobial resistance in nosocomial pathogens: no ESKAPE. J Infect Dis 2009;197:1079–81.

10. Boucher HW, Talbot GH, Bradley JS, et al. Bad bugs, no drugs: no ESKAPE! An update from the Infectious Diseases Society of America. Clin Infect Dis 2009;48:1–12.

11. Filozov A, Visintainer P, Carbonaro C, et al. Epidemiology of an outbreak of antibiotic-resistant *Klebsiella pneumoniae* at a tertiary care medical center. Am J Infect Control 2009;37:723–8.

12. Niederman MS. Use of broad-spectrum antimicrobials for the treatment of pneumonia in seriously ill patients: maximizing clinical outcomes and minimizing selection of resistant organisms. Clin Infect Dis 2006;42:S72–81.

13. Kollef MH, Ward S, Sherman G, et al. Inadequate treatment of nosocomial infections is associated with certain empiric antibiotic choices. Crit Care Med 2000; 28:3456–64.

14. Alvarez-Lerma F. Modification of empiric antibiotic treatment in patients with pneumonia acquired in the intensive care unit: ICU-Acquired Pneumonia Study Group. Intensive Care Med 1996;22:387–94.

15. Garnacho-Montero J, Garcia-Garmendia JL, Barrero-Almodovar A, et al. Impact of adequate empirical antibiotic therapy on the outcome of patients admitted to the intensive care unit with sepsis. Crit Care Med 2003;31:2742–51.

16. Owens RC Jr, Shorr AF. Rational dosing of antimicrobial agents: pharmacokinetic and pharmacodynamic strategies. Am J Health Syst Pharm 2009; 66(12 Suppl 4):S23–30.

17. DiPiro JT, Edmiston CE, Bohnen JMA. Pharmacodynamics of antimicrobial therapy in surgery. Am J Surg 1996;171:615–22.

18. Deege MP, Paterson DL. Reducing the development of antibiotic resistance in critical care units. Curr Pharm Biotechnol 2011. [Epub ahead of print].

19. Harbottle H, Thakur S, Zhao S, et al. Genetics of antimicrobial resistance. Anim Biotechnol 2006;17:111–24.

20. Paterson DL. Resistance in gram-negative bacteria: Enterobacteriaceae. Am J Infect Control 2006;34(5 Suppl 1):S20–8.

21. Champney WS. The other target for ribosomal antibiotics: inhibition of bacterial ribosomal subunit formation. Infect Disord Drug Targets 2006;6:377–90.

22. Al-Jasser AM. Extended-spectrum beta-lactamases (ESBLs): a global problem. Kuwait Med J 2006;38:171–85.

23. Lister PD, Wolter KA, Hanson ND. Antibacterial-resistant *Pseudomonas aeruginosa*: clinical impact and complex regulation of chromosomally encoded resistance mechanisms. Clin Microbiol Rev 2009;22:582–610.

24. Connell SR, Tracz DM, Nierhaus KH, et al. Ribosomal protection proteins and their mechanism of tetracycline resistance. Antimicrob Agents Chemother 2003;47:3675–81.

25. Chopra I, Roberts M. Tetracycline antibiotics: mode of action, applications, molecular biology, and epidemiology of bacterial resistance. Microbiol Mol Biol Rev 2001;65:232–60.

26. Ambler RP. The structure of β-lactamases. Philos Trans R Soc Lond B Biol Sci 1980;289:321–31.

27. Bush K, Jacoby GA, Medeiros AA. A functional classification scheme for β-lactamases and its correlation with molecular structure. Antimicrob Agents Chemother 1995;39:1211–33.

28. Haque SF, Ali SZ, Tp M, et al. Prevalence of plasmid-mediated bla(TEM-1) and bla(CTX-M-15) type extended spectrum beta-lactamases in patients with sepsis. Asian Pac J Trop Med 2012;5:98–102.

29. Knothe H, Shah P, Kremery V, et al. Transferable resistance to cefotaxime cefoxitin, cefamandole, and cefuroxime in clinical isolates of Klebsiella pneumoniae and Serratia marcescens. Infection 1983;11:315–7.

30. Giamarellou H. Multidrug-resistant Gram-negative bacteria: how to treat and for how long. Int J Antimicrob Agents 2010;36(Suppl 2):S50–4.

31. Falagas ME, Karageorgopoulos DE, Nordmann P. Therapeutic options for infections with Enterobacteriaceae producing carbapenem-hydrolyzing enzymes. Expert Opin Drug Metab Toxicol 2011;6:653–66.

32. Patel G, Bonomo RA. Status report on carbepenemases: challenges and prospects. Expert Rev Anti Infect Ther 2011;9:555–70.

33. Yigit H, Queenen AM, Anderson GJ, et al. novel carbepenem-hydrolyzing beta-lactamase, KPC-1, for a carbepenem-resistant strain of Klebsiella pneumoniae. Antimicrob Agents Chemother 2001;45:1151–61.

34. Castanheira M, Sader HS, Jones RN. Antimicrobial susceptibility patterns of KPC-producing or CTX-M-producing Enterobacteriaceae. Microb Drug Resist 2010;16:61–5.

35. Elemam A, Rahimian J, Mandell W. Infection with panresistant Klebsiella pneumoniae: a report of 2 cases and a brief review of the literature. Clin Infect Dis 2009;49:271–4.

36. Lolans K, Queenan AM, Bush K, et al. First nosocomial outbreak of Pseudomonas aeruginosa producing an integron-borne metallo-beta-lactamase (VIM-2) in the United States. Antimicrob Agents Chemother 2005;49:3538–40.

37. Zhao WH, Hu ZQ. IMP-type metallo-β-lactamases in Gram-negative bacilli: distribution, phylogeny, and association with integrons. Crit Rev Microbiol 2011;37:214–26.

38. Yong D, Toleman MA, Giske CG, et al. Characterization of a new metallo-beta-lactamase gene, bla(NDM-1), and a novel erythromycin esterase gene carried on a unique genetic structure in Klebsiella pneumoniae sequence type 14 from India. Antimicrob Agents Chemother 2009;53:5046–54.

39. Deshpande P, Rodrigues C, Shetty A, et al. New Delhi Metallo-beta-lactamase-1 (NDM-1) in Enterobacteriaceae. Treatment options with carbapenems compromised. J Assoc Physicians India 2010;58:147–9.

40. Jacoby GA. AmpC beta-lactamases. Clin Microbiol Rev 2009;22:161–82.

41. Walther-Rasmussen J, Holby N. OXA-type carbepenemases. J Antimicrob Chemother 2006;57:373–83.

42. Fairman JW, Noinaj N, Buchanan SK. The structural biology of β-barrel membrane proteins: a summary of recent reports. Curr Opin Struct Biol 2011;21:523–31.

43. Li H, Luo YF, Williams BJ, et al. Structure and function of OprD protein in Pseudomonas aeruginosa From antibiotic resistance to novel therapies. Int J Med Microbiol 2012. [Epub ahead of print].

44. Peleg AY, Adams J, Paterson DL. Tigecycline efflux as a mechanism for non-susceptibility in *Acinetobacter baumannii*. Antimicrob Agents Chemother 2007;51:2065–9.
45. Blair JM, Piddock LJ. Structure, function, and inhibition of RND efflux pumps in Gram-negative bacteria: an update. Curr Opin Microbiol 2009;12:512–9.
46. Poole K. Multidrug efflux pumps and antimicrobial resistance in *Pseudomonas aeruginosa* and related organisms. J Mol Microbiol Biotechnol 2001;3:255–64.
47. Vila J, Fabrega A, Roca I, et al. Efflux pumps as an important mechanism for quinolone resistance. Adv Enzymol Relat Areas Mol Biol 2011;77:167–235.
48. Rodriguez-Jartinez JM, Cano ME, Velasco C, et al. Plasmid-mediated quinolone resistance: an update. J Infect Chemother 2011;17:149–82.
49. Halstead D, Abid J, Dowzicky MJ. Antimicrobial susceptibility among *Acinetobacter calcoaceticus-baumannii* complex and Enterobacteriaceae collected as part of the Tigecycline Evaluation and Surveillance Trial. J Infect 2007;55:49–57.
50. Namdari H, Tan TY, Dowzickt MJ. Activity of tigecycline and comparators against skin and skin structure pathogens: global results of the Tigecycline Evaluation and Surveillance Trial. Int J Infect Dis 2011. [Epub ahead of print].
51. Garrison MW, Mullers R, Dowzicky MJ. In vitro activity of tigecycline and comparator agents against a global collection of Gram-negative and Gram-positive organisms: Tigecycline Evaluation and Surveillance Trial 2004-2007. Diagn Microbiol Infect Dis 2009;65:288–99.
52. Vaziri F, Peerayeh SN, Nejad QB, et al. The prevalence of aminoglycoside-modifying enzyme genes (aac (6′)-I, aac (6′)-II, ant (2″)-I, and aph (3′)-VI) in *Pseudomonas aeruginosa*. Clinics (Sao Paulo) 2011;66:1519–22.
53. Courvalin P. Vancomycin resistance in gram-positive cocci. Clin Infect Dis 2006; 42(Suppl 1):S25–34.
54. Shlaes DM, Binczewski B. Enterococcal resistance to vancomycin and related cyclic glycopeptide antibiotics. Eur J Clin Microbiol Infect Dis 1990;9:106–10.
55. Rossolini GM, Mantengoli E, Montagnani F, et al. Epidemiology and clinical relevance of microbial resistance determinants versus anti-Gram positive agents. Curr Opin Microbiol 2010;13:582–8.
56. Boucher HW, Sakoulas G. Perspectives on daptomycin resistance, with emphasis on resistance in *Staphylococcus aureus*. Clin Infect Dis 2007;45:601–8.
57. Falagas ME, Rafailidis PI, Matthalou DK. Resistance to polymyxins: mechanisms, frequency, and treatment options. Drug Resist Updat 2010;13:132–8.
58. Landman D, Georgescu C, Martin DA, et al. Polymyxins revisited. Clin Microbiol Rev 2008;21:449–65.
59. Gunn JS. The Salmonella PmrAB regulon: lipopolysaccharide modifications, antimicrobial peptide resistance and more. Trends Microbiol 2008;16:284–90.
60. Hawley JS, Murray CK, Jorgensen JH. Colistin heteroresistance in *Acinetobacter* and its association with previous colistin therapy. Antimicrob Agents Chemother 2008;52:351–2.
61. McDougal LK, Steward CD, Killgore GE, et al. Pulsed-field gel electrophoresis typing of oxacillin-resistant *Staphylococcus aureus* isolates from the United States: establishing a national database. J Clin Microbiol 2003;41:5113–20.
62. Ito T, Okuma K, Ma XX, et al. Insights on antibiotic resistance of *Staphylococcus aureus* from its whole genome: genomic island SCC. Drug Resist Updat 2003;6: 41–52.
63. Daum RS, Ito T, Hiramatsu K, et al. A novel methicillin resistance cassette in community-acquired methicillin-resistant *Staphylococcus aureus* isolates of diverse genetic backgrounds. J Infect Dis 2002;186:1344–7.

64. Rehm SJ. *Staphylococcus aureus*: the new adventures of a legendary pathogen. Cleve Clin J Med 2008;75:177–80.
65. Diep BA, Chambers HF, Graber CJ, et al. Emergence of multidrug-resistant, community-acquired, methicillin-resistant *Staphylococcus aureus* clone USA300 in men who have sex with men. Ann Intern Med 2008;148:249–57.
66. Hawley PM, Jones AM. The changing epidemiology of resistance. J Antimicrob Chemother 2009;64(Suppl):i3–10.
67. Centers for Disease Control. Reduced susceptibility of *Staphylococcus aureus* to vancomycin: Japan, 1996. MMWR Morb Mortal Wkly Rep 1997;46:624–6.
68. Cervera C, Almela M, Martínez-Martínez JA, et al. Risk factors and management of Gram-positive bacteraemia. Int J Antimicrob Agents 2009;34(Suppl 4):S26–30.
69. Patel N, Pai MP, Rodvold KA, et al. Vancomycin: we can't get there from here. Clin Infect Dis 2011;52:969–74.
70. Hageman JC, Patel JB, Carey RC, et al. Investigation and control of vancomycin-intermediate and-resistant *Staphylococcus aureus*: a guide for health departments and infection control personnel. Atlanta (GA): Centers for Disease Control and Prevention; 2006. Available at: www.cdc.gov/ncidod/dhqp/ar_visavrsa_prevention.html. Accessed May 12, 2011.
71. Tenover FC, Biddle JW, Lancaster MV. Increasing resistance to vancomycin and other glycopeptides in *Staphylococcus aureus*. Emerg Infect Dis 2001;7:327–32.
72. Walsh TR, Bolmstöm A, Qwärnström A, et al. Evaluation of current methods for detection of staphylococci with reduced susceptibility to glycopeptides. J Clin Microbiol 2001;39:2439–44.
73. Plipat N, Livni G, Bertram H, et al. Unstable vancomycin heteroresistance is common among clinical isolates of methicillin-resistant *Staphylococcus aureus*. J Clin Microbiol 2005;43:2494–6.
74. Walsh TR, Howe RA. The prevalence and mechanisms of vancomycin resistance in *Staphylococcus aureus*. Annu Rev Microbiol 2002;56:657–75.
75. Khatib R, Jose J, Musta A, et al. Relevance of vancomycin-intermediate susceptibility and heteroresistance in methicillin-resistant *Staphylococcus aureus* bacteraemia. J Antimicrob Chemother 2011;66:1594–9.
76. Cheong JW, Harris P, Oman K, et al. Challenges in the microbiological diagnosis and management of hVISA infections. Pathology 2011;43:357–61.
77. Rong SL. Heterogeneous vancomycin resistance in *Staphylococcus aureus*: a review of epidemiology, diagnosis, and clinical significance. Ann Pharmacother 2010;44:844–50.
78. Van Hal SJ, Paterson DL. Systematic review and meta-analysis of the significance of heterogeneous vancomycin-intermediate *Staphylococcus aureus* isolates. Antimicrob Agents Chemother 2011;55:405–10.
79. Fry DE, Barie PS. The changing face of *Staphylococcus aureus*: a continuing surgical challenge. Surg Infect (Larchmt) 2011;12:191–203.
80. von Eiff C. *Staphylococcus aureus* small colony variants: a challenge to microbiologists and clinicians. Int J Antimicrob Agents 2008;31:507–10.
81. Livermore DM. Multiple mechanisms of antimicrobial resistance in *Pseudomonas aeruginosa*: our worst nightmare. Clin Infect Dis 2002;34:634–40.
82. Mikkelsen H, Sivaneson M, Filloux A. Key two-component regulatory systems that control biofilm formation in *Pseudomonas aeruginosa*. Environ Microbiol 2011;13:1666–81.
83. Lee K, Yong D, Jeong SH, et al. Multidrug-resistant *Acinetobacter* spp.: increasingly problematic nosocomial pathogens. Yonsei Med J 2011;52:879–91.

84. Coyne S, Courvalin P, Périchon B. Efflux-mediated antibiotic resistance in *Acinetobacter* spp. Antimicrob Agents Chemother 2011;55:947–53.
85. Navon-Venezia S, Ben-Ami R, Carmeli Y. Update on *Pseudomonas aeruginosa* and *Acinetobacter baumannii* infections in the healthcare setting. Curr Opin Infect Dis 2005;18:306–13.
86. Available at: http://www.idsociety.org/Content.aspx?id=17429. Accessed January 2, 2012.
87. Edwards JR, Peterson KD, Mu Y, et al. National Healthcare Safety Network (NHSN) report: data summary for 2006 through 2008, issued December 2009. Am J Infect Control 2009;37:783–805.
88. Doyle JS, Buising KL, Thursky KA, et al. Epidemiology of infections acquired in intensive care units. Semin Respir Crit Care Med 2011;32:115–38.
89. National Nosocomial Infections Surveillance System (NNIS) System Report: data summary from January 1992-June 2001, issued August 2001. Am J Infect Control 2001;29:404–21.
90. National Nosocomial Infections Surveillance (NNIS) System Report, data summary from January 1992 to June 2004, issued October 2004. Am J Infect Control 2004;32:470–85.
91. Hsieh PR, Badal RE, Hawser SP, et al, Asia-Pacific SMART Group. Epidemiology and anti-microbial susceptibility profiles of aerobic and facultative gram-negative bacilli isolated from patients with intra-abdominal infections in the Asia-Pacific region: 2008 results from SMART (Study for Monitoring Antimicrobial Resistance Trends). Int J Antimicrob Agents 2010;38:408–14.
92. Baquero F, Hsueh PR, Paterson DL, et al. In vitro susceptibilities of aerobic and facultatively anaerobic gram-negative bacilli isolated from patients with intra-abdominal infections worldwide: 2005 results from Study for Monitoring Antimicrobial Resistance Trends (SMART). Surg Infect (Larchmt) 2009;10:99–104.
93. Brink AJ, Botha RF, Poswa X, et al. Antimicrobial susceptibility of gram-negative pathogens isolated from patients with complicated intra-abdominal infections in South African hospitals (SMART study 2004-2009): impact of the new carbapenem breakpoints. Surg Infect (Larchmt) 2012. [Epub ahead of print].
94. Solomkin JS, Mazuski JE, Bradley JS, et al. Diagnosis and management of complicated intra-abdominal infection in adults and children: guidelines by the Surgical Infection Society and the Infectious Diseases Society of America. Surg Infect (Larchmt) 2010;11:79–109.
95. Eckmann C, Dryden M, Montravers P, et al. Antimicrobial treatment of "complicated" intra-abdominal infections and the new IDSA guidelines-a commentary and an alternative European approach according to clinical definitions. Eur J Med Res 2011;16:115–26.
96. Augustin P, Kermarrec N, Muller-Serieys C, et al. Risk factors for multidrug resistant bacteria and optimization of empirical antibiotic therapy in postoperative peritonitis. Crit Care 2010;14:R20.
97. Montravers P, Gauzit R, Muller C, et al. Emergence of antibiotic-resistant bacteria in cases of peritonitis after intraabdominal surgery affects the efficacy of empirical antimicrobial therapy. Clin Infect Dis 1996;23:486–94.
98. Cosgrove SE. The relationship between antimicrobial resistance and patient outcomes: mortality, length of hospital stay, and health care costs. Clin Infect Dis 2006;42(Suppl 2):S82–9.
99. Muscedere JG, Day A, Heyland DK. Mortality, attributable mortality, and clinical events as end points for clinical trials of ventilator-associated

pneumonia and hospital-acquired pneumonia. Clin Infect Dis 2010;51(Suppl 1):S120–5.

100. Muscedere JG, Shorr AF, Jiang X, et al. The adequacy of timely empiric antibiotic therapy for ventilator-associated pneumonia: an important determinant of outcome. J Crit Care 2011. [Epub ahead of print].

101. Heyland DK, Cook DJ, Griffith L, et al. The attributable morbidity and mortality of ventilator-associated pneumonia in the critically ill patient. The Canadian Critical Trials Group. Am J Respir Crit Care Med 1999;159:1249–56.

102. Cosgrove SE, Sakoulas G, Perencevich EN, et al. Comparison of mortality associated with methicillin-resistant and methicillin-susceptible *Staphylococcus aureus* bacteremia: a meta-analysis. Clin Infect Dis 2003;36:53–9.

103. Bhavnani SM, Rubino CM, Ambrose PG, et al. Impact of the different factors on the probability of clinical response in tigecycline-treated patients with intra-abdominal infections. Antimicrob Agents Chemother 2010;54:1202–7.

104. Holland TL, Fowler VG Jr. Vancomycin minimum inhibitory concentration and outcome in patients with *Staphylococcus aureus* bacteremia: pearl or pellet? J Infect Dis 2011;204:329–31.

105. Holmes NE, Turnidge JD, Munckhof WJ, et al. Antibiotic choice may not explain poorer outcomes in patients with *Staphylococcus aureus* bacteremia and high vancomycin minimum inhibitory concentrations. J Infect Dis 2011;204:340–7.

106. Michalopoulos A, Falagas ME. Treatment of *Acinetobacter* infections. Expert Opin Pharmacother 2010;11:779–88.

107. Zilberberg MD, Chen J, Mody SH, et al. Imipenem resistance of Pseudomonas in pneumonia: a systematic literature review. BMC Pulm Med 2010;10:45.

108. Jean SS, Hsueh PR. Current review of antimicrobial treatment of nosocomial pneumonia caused by multidrug-resistant pathogens. Expert Opin Pharmacother 2011;12:2145–8.

109. Eagye KJ, Kuti JL, Nicolau DP. Risk factors and outcomes associated with isolation of meropenem high-level-resistant *Pseudomonas aeruginosa*. Infect Control Hosp Epidemiol 2009;30:746–52.

110. Aubron C, Chaari A, Bronchard R, et al. High level cephalosporin-resistant Enterobacteriaceae ventilator-associated pneumonia: prognostic factors based on a cohort study. J Hosp Infect 2011;77:64–9.

111. Song JY, Cheong HJ, Choi WS, et al. Clinical and microbiological characterization of carbapenem-resistant *Acinetobacter baumannii* bloodstream infections. J Med Microbiol 2011;60:605–11.

112. Neuner EA, Yeh JY, Hall GS, et al. Treatment and outcomes in carbapenem-resistant *Klebsiella pneumoniae* bloodstream infections. Diagn Microbiol Infect Dis 2011;69:357–62.

113. McKenzie C. Antibiotic dosing in critical illness. J Antimicrob Chemother 2011; 66(Suppl 2):ii25–31.

114. Lazar V, Chifiriuc MC. Architecture and physiology of microbial biofilms. Roum Arch Microbiol Immunol 2010;69:95–107.

115. Wright JS 3rd, Jin R, Novick RP. Transient interference with staphylococcal quorum sensing blocks abscess formation. Proc Natl Acad Sci U S A 2005; 102:169–1696.

116. Mueller EW, Bouchard BA. The use of extended-interval aminoglycoside dosing strategies for the treatment of moderate-to-severe infections encountered in critically ill surgical patients. Surg Infect (Larchmt) 2009;10:563–70.

117. Kashuba AD, Bertino JS Jr, Nafziger AN. Dosing of aminoglycosides to rapidly attain pharmacodynamic goals and hasten therapeutic response by

using individualized pharmacokinetic monitoring of patients with pneumonia caused by gram-negative organisms. Antimicrob Agents Chemother 1998;42: 1842–4.

118. Thomas JK, Forrest A, Bhavnani SM, et al. Pharmacodynamic evaluation of factors associated with the development of bacterial resistance in acutely ill patients during therapy. Antimicrob Agents Chemother 1998;42:521–7.

119. Benko AS, Cappelletty DM, Kruse JA, et al. Continuous infusion versus intermittent administration of ceftazidime in critically ill patients with suspected Gram-negative infections. Antimicrob Agents Chemother 1996;40:691–5.

120. Lau WK, Mercer D, Itani KM, et al. Randomized, open-label, comparative study of piperacillin-tazobactam administered by continuous infusion versus intermittent infusion for treatment of hospitalized patients with complicated intra-abdominal infection. Antimicrob Agents Chemother 2006;50:3556–61.

121. Barie PS, Hydo LJ, Shou J, et al. Influence of antibiotic therapy on mortality of critical surgical illness caused or complicated by infection. Surg Infect (Larchmt) 2005;6:41–54.

122. Kumar A, Roberts D, Wood KE, et al. Duration of hypotension before initiation of effective antimicrobial therapy is the critical determinant of survival in human septic shock. Crit Care Med 2006;34:1589–96.

123. Dellinger RP, Levy MM, Carlet JM, et al. International Surviving Sepsis Campaign Guidelines Committee; American Association of Critical-Care Nurses; American College of Chest Physicians; American College of Emergency Physicians; Canadian Critical Care Society; European Society of Clinical Microbiology and Infectious Diseases; European Society of Intensive Care Medicine; European Respiratory Society; International Sepsis Forum; Japanese Association for Acute Medicine; Japanese Society of Intensive Care Medicine; Society of Critical Care Medicine; Society of Hospital Medicine; Surgical Infection Society; World Federation of Societies of Intensive and Critical Care Medicine. Surviving Sepsis Campaign: international guidelines for management of severe sepsis and septic shock: 2008. Crit Care Med 2008;36:296–327. [Erratum appears in Crit Care Med 2008;36:1394–6].

124. Kollef MH, Micek ST. Strategies to prevent antimicrobial resistance in the intensive care unit. Crit Care Med 2005;33:1845–53.

125. Hayashi DL, Paterson DL. Strategies for reduction in duration of antibiotic use in hospitalized patients. Clin Infect Dis 2011;52:1232–40.

126. Rahal JJ. Novel antibiotic combinations against infections with almost completely resistant Pseudomonas aeruginosa and Acinetobacter species. Clin Infect Dis 2006;43:S95–9.

127. Aarts MA, Hancock JN, Heyland D, et al. Empiric antibiotic therapy for suspected ventilator-associated pneumonia: a systematic review and meta-analysis of randomized trials. Crit Care Med 2008;36:108–17.

128. Paul M, Benuri-Silbiger I, Soares-Weiser K, et al. Beta-lactam monotherapy versus beta-lactam-aminoglycoside combination therapy for sepsis in immunocompetent patients: systematic review and meta-analysis of randomized trials. BMJ 2004;328:668–72.

129. Kumar A, Zarychanski R, Light B, et al. Early combination antibiotic therapy yields improved survival compared with monotherapy in septic shock: a propensity-matched analysis. Crit Care Med 2010;38:1773–85.

130. Ost DE, Hall CS, Joseph G, et al. Decision analysis of antibiotic and diagnostic strategies in ventilator-associated pneumonia. Am J Respir Crit Care Med 2003; 168:1060–7.

131. American Thoracic Society. Guidelines for the management of adults with hospital-acquired, ventilator-associated, and healthcare-associated pneumonia. Am J Respir Crit Care Med 2005;171:388–410.

132. Kollef MH, Kollef KE. Antibiotic utilization and outcomes for patients with clinically suspected VAP and negative quantitative BAL cultures results. Chest 2005;128:2706–13.

133. Hosein S, Udy AA, Lipman J. Physiological changes in the critically ill patient with sepsis. Curr Pharm Biotechnol 2011. [Epub ahead of print].

134. Zelenitsky SA, Ariano RE, Zhanel GG. Pharmacodynamics of empirical antibiotic monotherapies for an intensive care unit (ICU) population based on Canadian surveillance data. J Antimicrob Chemother 2011;66:343–9.

135. Rybak MJ, Lomaestro BM, Rotschaefer JC, et al. Vancomycin therapeutic guidelines: a summary of consensus recommendations from the Infectious Diseases Society of America, the American Society of Health-System Pharmacists, and the Society of Infectious Diseases Pharmacists. Clin Infect Dis 2009;49:325–7.

136. Liu C, Bayer A, Cosgrove SE, et al. Clinical practice guidelines by the Infectious Diseases Society of America for the treatment of methicillin-resistant *Staphylococcus aureus* infections in adults and children. Clin Infect Dis 2011;52: e8–45, e18–55.

137. Lodise TP, Patel N, Lomaestro BM, et al. Relationship between initial vancomycin concentration-time profile and nephrotoxicity among hospitalized patients. Clin Infect Dis 2009;49:507–14.

138. Roberts JA, Kirkpatrick CM, Lipman J. Monte Carlo simulations: maximizing antibiotic pharmacokinetic data to optimize clinical practice for critically ill patients. J Antimicrob Chemother 2011;66:227–31.

139. Crandon JL, Ariano RE, Zelenitsky SA, et al. Optimization of meropenem dosage in the critically ill population based on renal function. Intensive Care Med 2011; 37:632–8.

140. Nicasio AM, Ariano RE, Zelenitsky SA, et al. Population pharmacokinetics of high-dose, prolonged-infusion cefepime in adult critically ill patients with ventilator-associated pneumonia. Antimicrob Agents Chemother 2009;53:1476–81.

141. Kim A, Kuti JL, Nicolau DP. Probability of pharmacodynamic target attainment with standard and prolonged-infusion antibiotic regimens for empiric therapy in adults with hospital-acquired pneumonia. Clin Ther 2009;31:2765–78.

142. Ong CT, Kuti JL, Nicolau DP, OPTAMA Program. Pharmacodynamic modeling of imipenem-cilastatin, meropenem, and piperacillin-tazobactam for empiric therapy of skin and soft tissue infections: a report from the OPTAMA Program. Surg Infect (Larchmt) 2005;6:419–26.

143. Kotapati S, Kuti JL, Nicolau DP. Pharmacodynamic modeling of beta-lactam antibiotics for the empiric treatment of secondary peritonitis: a report from the OPTAMA program. Surg Infect (Larchmt) 2005;6:297–304.

144. Lodise TP Jr, Lomaestro B, Drusano GL. Piperacillin-tazobactam for *Pseudomonas aeruginosa* infection: clinical implications of an extended-infusion dosing strategy. Clin Infect Dis 2007;44:357–63.

145. Kullar R, Davis SL, Levine DP, et al. High-dose daptomycin for treatment of complicated gram-positive infections: a large multicenter, retrospective study. Pharmacotherapy 2011;31:527–36.

146. Kelley PG, Gao W, Ward PB, et al. Daptomycin non-susceptibility in vancomycin-intermediate *Staphylococcus aureus* (VISA) and heterogeneous-VISA (hVISA): implications for therapy after vancomycin treatment failure. J Antimicrob Chemother 2011;66:1057–60.

147. Bulik CC, Nicolau DP. Double-carbapenem therapy for carbapenemase-producing *Klebsiella pneumoniae*. Antimicrob Agents Chemother 2011;55:3002–4.
148. Elemam A, Rahimian J, Doymaz M. In vitro evaluation of antibiotic synergy for polymyxin B-resistant carbapenemase-producing *Klebsiella pneumoniae*. J Clin Microbiol 2010;48:3558–62.
149. Daikos GL, Markogiannakis A. Carbapenemase-producing *Klebsiella pneumoniae*: (when) might we still consider treating with carbapenems? Clin Microbiol Infect 2011;17:1135–41.
150. Peck KR, Kim MJ, Choi JY, et al. In vitro time-kill studies of antimicrobial agents against blood isolates of imipenem-resistant *Acinetobacter baumannii* including colistin-or tigecycline-resistant strains. J Med Microbiol 2011. [Epub ahead of print].
151. Sanchez A, Gattarello S, Rello J. New treatment options for infections caused by multiresistant strains of *Pseudomonas aeruginosa* and other non-fermenting gram-negative bacilli. Semin Respir Crit Care Med 2011;32:151–8.
152. Entenza JM, Moreillon P. Tigecycline in combination with other antimicrobials: a review of in vitro, animal, and case report studies. Int J Antimicrob Agents 2009;34:8. e1–9.
153. Kastoris AC, Rafallidis PI, Voulomanou EK, et al. Synergy of fosfomycin with other antibiotics for Gram-positive and Gram-negative bacteria. Eur J Clin Pharmacol 2010;66:359–68.
154. Grasso C, Bahniuk N, Van Scoy B, et al. The combination of meropenem and levofloxacin is synergistic with respect to both *Pseudomonas aeruginosa* kill rate and resistance suppression. Antimicrob Agents Chemother 2010;54:2646–54.
155. Bebrone C, Lassaux P, Vercheval L, et al. Current challenges in antimicrobial chemotherapy: focus on β-lactamase inhibition. Drugs 2010;70:651–79.
156. Kaushik D, Rathi S, Jain A. Ceftaroline: a comprehensive update. Int J Antimicrob Agents 2011;37:387–95.
157. Rodloff AC, Goldstein EJ, Torres A. Two decades of imipenem therapy. J Antimicrob Chemother 2006;58:916–29.
158. Zhanel GG, Johanson C, Embil JM, et al. Ertapenem: review of a new carbapenem. Expert Rev Anti Infect Ther 2005;31:23–39.
159. Kullar R, Davis SL, Levine DP, et al. Impact of vancomycin exposure on outcomes in patients with methicillin-resistant *Staphylococcus aureus* bacteremia: support for consensus guideline suggested targets. Clin Infect Dis 2011;52:975–81.
160. FDA lowers breakpoints for staph infections. Available at: http://news.idsociety.org/idsa/issues/2008-05-01. Accessed June 20, 2011.
161. Chang MH, Kish TD, Fung HB. Telavancin: a lipoglycopeptide antibiotic for the treatment of complicated skin and skin structure infections caused by gram-positive bacteria in adults. Clin Ther 2010;32:2160–85.
162. Silverman JA, Mortin LI, Vanpraagh AD, et al. Inhibition of daptomycin by pulmonary surfactant: in vitro modeling and clinical impact. J Infect Dis 2005;191:2149–52.
163. Molina J, Cordero E, Pachon J. New information about the polymyxin/colistin class of antibiotics. Expert Opin Pharmacol 2009;10:2811–28.
164. Stein GE, Craig WA. Tigecycline: a critical analysis. Clin Infect Dis 2006;43:518–24.
165. Poulakou G, Kontopidou FV, Paramythiotou E, et al. Tigecycline in the treatment of infections from multi-drug resistant gram-negative pathogens. J Infect 2009;58:273–84.

166. Karageorgopoulos DE, Kelesidis T, Kelesidis I, et al. Tigecycline for the treatment of multidrug-resistant (including carbapenem-resistant) *Acinetobacter* infections: a review of the scientific evidence. J Antimicrob Chemother 2008; 62:45–55.

167. Vasilev K, Reshedko G, Orasan R, et al. A phase 3, open-label, non-comparative study of tigecycline in the treatment of patients with selected serious infections due to resistant Gram-negative organisms including *Enterobacter* species, *Acinetobacter baumannii*, and *Klebsiella pneumoniae*. J Antimicrob Chemother 2008;62(Suppl 1):i29–40.

168. Eckmann C, Heizmann WR, Leitner E, et al. Prospective, non-interventional, multi-centre trial of tigecycline in the treatment of severely ill patients with complicated infections-new insights into clinical results and treatment practice. Chemotherapy 2011;57:275–84.

169. Bassetti M, Nicolini L, Repetto E, et al. Tigecycline use in serious nosocomial infections: a drug use evaluation. BMC Infect Dis 2010;10:287.

170. Available at: www.fda.gov/Drugs/DrugSafety/ucm224370.htm. Accessed June 8, 2011.

171. Cai Y, Wang R, Liang B, et al. Systematic review and meta-analysis of the effectiveness and safety of tigecycline for treatment of infectious disease. Antimicrob Agents Chemother 2011;55:1162–72.

172. Eckmann C, Dryden M. Treatment of complicated skin and soft-tissue infections caused by resistant bacteria: value of linezolid, tigecycline, daptomycin and vancomycin. Eur J Med Res 2010;15:554–63.

173. Walkey AJ, O'Donnell MR, Weiner RS. Linezolid vs. glycopeptide antibiotics for the treatment of suspected methicillin-resistant *Staphylococcus aureus* nosocomial pneumonia. Chest 2011;139:1148–55.

174. Nseir S, Di Pompeo C, Soubrier S, et al. First-generation fluoroquinolone use and subsequent emergence of multiple drug-resistant bacteria in the intensive care unit. Crit Care Med 2005;33:283–9.

175. Livermore DM, Woodford N. The beta-lactamase threat in Enterobacteriaceae, *Pseudomonas* and *Acinetobacter*. Trends Microbiol 2006;14:413–20.

176. Charbonneau P, Parienti JJ, Thibon P, et al. Fluoroquinolone use and methicillin-resistant *Staphylococcus aureus* isolation rates in hospitalized patients: a quasi experimental study. Clin Infect Dis 2006;42:778–84.

177. Joffe AR, Muscadere JG, Marshall JC, et al. The safety of targeted antibiotic therapy for ventilator-associated pneumonia: a multi-center observational study. J Crit Care 2008;23:82–90.

178. Kopterides P, Siempos II, Tsangaris I, et al. Procalcitonin-guided algorithms of antibiotic therapy in the intensive care unit: a systematic review and meta-analysis of randomized controlled trials. Crit Care Med 2010;38:2229–41.

179. Siegel JD, Rhinehart E, Jackson M, et al. The Healthcare Infection Control Practices Advisory Committee. Management of multidrug-resistant organisms in healthcare settings, 2006. Available at: http://www.cdc.gov/hicpac/mdro/mdro_2.html. Accessed June 8, 2011.

180. Siegel JD, Rhinehart E, Jackson M, et al. Healthcare Infection Control Practices Advisory Committee. 2007 Guideline for isolation precautions: preventing transmission of infectious agents in healthcare settings. Available at: http://www.cdc.gov/ncidod/dhqp/pdf/isolation2007.pdf. Accessed June 8, 2011.

181. Sehulster LM, Chinn RY, Arduino MJ, et al. Guidelines for environmental infection control in health-care facilities. Recommendations from CDC and the Healthcare Infection Control Practices Advisory Committee (HICPAC). Chicago: American

Society for Healthcare Engineering/American Hospital Association; 2004. Available at: www.cdc.gov/hicpac/pdf/guidelines/eic_in_HCF_03.pdf. Accessed June 8, 2011.

182. Boyce JM, Pittet D. Guideline for hand hygiene in health-care settings. Recommendations of the Healthcare Infection Control Practices Advisory Committee and the HICPAC/SHEA/APIC/IDSA Hand Hygiene Task Force. Available at: www.cdc.gov/mmwr/preview/mmwrhtml/rr5116a1.htm. Accessed June 8, 2011.

183. Rice LB, Eckstein EC, DeVente J, et al. Ceftazidime-resistant *Klebsiella pneumoniae* isolates recovered at the Cleveland Department of Veterans Affairs Medical Center. Clin Infect Dis 1996;23:118–24.

184. Patterson JE, Hardin TC, Kelly CA, et al. Association of antibiotic utilization measures and control of multiple-drug resistance in *Klebsiella pneumoniae*. Infect Control Hosp Epidemiol 2000;21:455–8.

185. Rahal JJ, Urban C, Segal-Maurer S. Nosocomial gram-negative resistance in multiple gram-negative species: experience at one hospital with squeezing the resistance balloon at multiple sites. Clin Infect Dis 2002;34:499–503.

186. Kollef MH, Vlasnik J, Sharpless L, et al. Scheduled change of antibiotic classes: a strategy to decrease the incidence of ventilator-associated pneumonia. Am J Respir Crit Care Med 1997;156(4 Pt 1):1040–8.

187. Sandiumenge A, Diaz E, Rodriguez A, et al. Impact of diversity of antibiotic use on development of antimicrobial resistance. J Antimicrob Chemother 2006;57: 1197–204.

188. Bal AM, Kumar A, Gould IM. Antibiotic heterogeneity: from concept to practice. Ann N Y Acad Sci 2010;1213:81–91.

189. Raymond DP, Pelletier SJ, Crabtree TD, et al. Impact of a rotating empiric antibiotic schedule on infectious mortality in an intensive care unit. Crit Care Med 2001;29:1101–8.

190. Smith RL, Evans HL, Chong TW, et al. Reduction in rates of methicillin-resistant *Staphylococcus aureus* infection after introduction of quarterly linezolid-vancomycin cycling in a surgical intensive care unit. Surg Infect (Larchmt) 2008;9:423–31.

191. Evans HL, Sawyer RG. Preventing bacterial resistance in surgical patients. Surg Clin North Am 2009;89:501–19.

192. Dortch MJ, Fleming SB, Kauffmann RM, et al. Infection reduction strategies including antibiotic stewardship protocols in surgical and trauma intensive care units are associated with reduced resistant gram-negative healthcare-associated infections. Surg Infect (Larchmt) 2011;12:15–25.

193. Curtis L. Need for both antibiotic cycling and stringent environmental controls to prevent *Pseudomonas* infections. Surg Infect (Larchmt) 2009;10:163–73.

Prevention of Chronic Pain After Surgical Nerve Injury: Amputation and Thoracotomy

Thomas Buchheit, MD*, Srinivas Pyati, MD

KEYWORDS

- Chronic pain • Surgical nerve injury • Amputation
- Thoracotomy • Neuropathic pain

ACUTE POSTSURGICAL PAIN

A surgical incision produces tissue damage, subsequent inflammation, and acute postoperative pain. Although most patients heal without long-term sequelae, procedures, such as amputation, thoracotomy, hernia surgery, coronary artery bypass, and mastectomy, impose a significant burden of persistent postsurgical pain.[1–3] However, amputation and thoracotomy represent two of the higher-risk procedures. These surgeries involve obligatory neurologic injury, often leading to a cascade of postinjury sensitization and chronic neuropathic pain.[1,4]

Although amputation and thoracotomy have different indications and are performed using different techniques, they demonstrate a remarkable similarity both in the severity of acute postoperative pain and in the incidence of persistent postsurgical neuralgic pain.[1] Our ability to control incisional and inflammatory pain in the immediate postoperative period has improved with the combined use of local anesthetics, opioids, and other systemic medications. However, our tools to avoid central sensitization following nerve injury remain limited.

In recent years, an increased emphasis has been placed on the prevention and management of postinjury chronic pain states secondary to the military conflicts in the Middle East and around the globe. Between 2001 and 2010, more than 1600 US military personnel underwent amputation following military trauma.[5] In addition, natural disasters, such as the 2010 Haitian earthquake, have created more than

This work is partly supported by the Congressionally Directed Medical Research Programs (CDMRDP) and the Department of Defense (DM102142).
Department of Anesthesiology, Duke University Medical Center, Box 3094, Durham, NC 27710, USA
* Corresponding author.
E-mail address: Thomas.Buchheit@Duke.edu

6000 amputees.[6] Amputation surgery for medical and vascular disease also remains common, with a national rate of approximately 188 lower extremity amputations per 100,000 people.[7] Given the combination of soft tissue, bone, and neurologic injury that occurs in the course of an amputation, initial management is often problematic; patients experience not only nociceptive pain but also acute neuralgia and occasionally the immediate onset of phantom limb pain.[8]

Similarly, thoracotomy is characterized by a high incidence of both severe acute pain and intractable postoperative pain.[9] Poor analgesia following thoracotomy leads to poor chest wall mechanics, impaired cough, and subsequent respiratory and infectious complications. Given the preexisting tenuous pulmonary function of many thoracotomy patients, further decreases in pulmonary function may lead to significant additional morbidity.[10,11]

An ideal perioperative analgesic regimen for surgeries, such as amputation and thoracotomy, would not only facilitate the immediate relief of suffering but would also reduce the burden of chronic postsurgical pain. Indeed, these goals seem physiologically linked given the correlation between the severity of perioperative pain and the prevalence of chronic pain.[12–14] Despite these observational associations, the prevention of chronic postsurgical pain has been more difficult to accomplish than initially proposed.[15–17] In this review, the authors discuss perioperative pain management techniques and modifiable risk factors to prevent chronic pain following amputation and thoracotomy.

CHRONIC POSTSURGICAL PAIN: AMPUTATION

Patients undergoing amputation experience a high level of both phantom and residual limb pain following surgery. Of these 2 complications, phantom limb pain has been more frequently discussed in the literature, with an estimated prevalence of 51% to 85%.[18–21] Residual limb pain is also reported after amputation, with a frequency of 45% to 74%.[22–24] Although residual limb pain phenomena, such as causalgia[25,26] and neuroma,[22,27] have been reported, they have not been systematically studied as separate entities in the residual limb.[23,27–30] Nonetheless, distinction between the residual limb pain subtypes of neuroma, complex regional pain syndrome, and somatic pain is important for research and clinical care because all postamputation pain subtypes may not equally respond to a given therapy.

The appropriate treatment and prevention of postamputation pain is also of functional significance for patients. In a study of 2694 patients with amputations, 51% had phantom limb pain severe enough to impair lifestyle more than 6 days per month and 27% experienced pain more than 15 hours per day.[20,31] The effects of residual limb pain may have even greater functional implications for the patients with amputations because of its impact on prosthetic use, ambulation, and rehabilitation.[23,32]

In 1984, it was reported that fewer than 10% of patients with phantom limb pain obtained prolonged pain relief from medical treatments,[31] and only limited progress has been made since that time.[22,33] Surgical techniques, including dorsal root entry zone lesions, surgical sympathectomies, and spinal cord stimulation, have also been used.[34–36] Currently, however, there is a lack of evidence to support the efficacy of these techniques.[37] There are promising data regarding improvements in phantom limb pain from body reimaging techniques with mirror box therapy; unfortunately, this intervention does not improve residual limb pain.[38]

CHRONIC POSTSURGICAL PAIN: THORACOTOMY

Persistent post-thoracotomy pain is described as "pain along the incision site that persists or recurs after thoracotomy for at least two months following the surgical procedure."[4] The cause of chronic pain following thoracotomy is undoubtedly similar to that following amputation. Neurologic injury at the time of surgery is likely the source of neuropathic pain, central sensitization, and persistent postsurgical pain in these patients.[4]

Up to 60% of thoracotomy patients report intractable pain a month after surgery and 30% to 50% report pain at 1 to 2 years.[10,39,40] Many of these patients describe significant physical limitations and sleep disturbances months and even years after surgery.[41] Similar to amputation pain, there is a strong correlation between severe perioperative pain and the incidence of chronic post-thoracotomy pain.[42–46]

RISK FACTORS FOR DEVELOPING CHRONIC POSTSURGICAL PAIN

Although all patients who undergo amputation and thoracotomy experience peripheral nerve injury, not all develop persistent neuropathic pain. Therefore, predisposing risk factors must also be present for chronic postsurgical pain to develop. Regarding amputation, identified chronic pain risk factors include severe perioperative pain, psychosocial comorbidity, and genetic predisposition. In particular, the association between severe preoperative pain[12,14,47–49] and postoperative pain[13,46,50] and the development of chronic pain supports the critical importance of acute symptom management. Indeed, both pharmacologic evidence[51] and radiologic demonstration[52–54] suggests central nervous system reorganization and sensitization in patients with amputations. Logically, if the preoperative stimulus is removed, thereby reducing the pain memory, the risk of persistent pain following amputation may decrease. A similar correlation between severe perioperative pain and chronic pain is also well documented in patients undergoing thoracotomy.[42–46] These observed associations between acute symptoms and chronic pain were part of the theoretical foundation behind the preemptive use of regional anesthesia before amputation and thoracotomy.[15,48,55]

Psychosocial factors also have an impact on the risk of chronic postoperative pain. Comorbidities, such as preoperative anxiety[56,57] and depression,[22,47,58,59] correlate strongly with persistent postsurgical pain. A comprehensive preoperative evaluation to identify these risk factors may have an impact on reducing the burden of chronic postsurgical pain.[60]

Gender and genetic risk factors are also increasingly appreciated as important to the development of chronic pain following surgery.[61] Several gene single nucleotide polymorphisms that may contribute to the development of neuropathic pain have been identified. Detailed discussions of these genetic factors may be found in previous publications[62,63] but are outside the scope of this review.

Given our current ability to identify predisposing factors for developing chronic postsurgical pain, we can now risk stratify patients who need more intensive multimodal therapy.[64] In subsequent sections, the authors focus on analgesic interventions that have been studied to reduce the incidence of persistent postsurgical pain.

ACUTE PAIN MANAGEMENT TECHNIQUES

Although there are evidence-based guidelines for acute pain management following thoracotomy,[65] there are no established guidelines for symptom management following amputation because of the inconsistent outcomes and methodological limitations of studies to date.[66] Surgical techniques, such as traction neurectomy and nerve implantation into muscle, may lessen the incidence of symptomatic neuromas.[67] However, these changes in technique have not significantly decreased the prevalence of chronic postamputation pain.[22] Likewise, minimally invasive thoracic surgery has not dramatically improved the incidence of moderate to severe pain following thoracotomy.[68]

Many of the techniques studied in recent years for managing postamputation and post-thoracotomy pain have been initiated preoperatively.[69] This preemptive effect is designed to reduce nociceptive traffic to the spinal cord and central nervous system. In animal models, painful neuropathy can be attenuated with local anesthetic pretreatment[70,71] or by aggressive early treatment of pain.[14] Preemptive and perioperative therapies have been studied in an effort to reduce the burden of both acute and chronic postsurgical pain.

EPIDURAL ANALGESIA: AMPUTATION

Epidural analgesia is a common modality used to control acute pain at the time of amputation. Given the association between severe preoperative pain and chronic pain, investigators have hypothesized that aggressive perioperative pain control with epidural catheter infusion will also lessen the incidence of chronic postamputation pain. In a 1988 unblinded study of preemptive epidural analgesia, 25 patients in the epidural group reported dramatically reduced phantom limb pain at both 6 and 12 months when compared with controls.[15] Similarly, in a 1994 case-controlled study, Jahangiri and colleagues[72] observed only an 8% incidence of phantom limb pain in 24 patients treated with epidural bupivacaine, clonidine, and diamorphine compared with a 73% incidence in the control group treated with systemic opioids.

Unfortunately, these early successes were not repeated in later studies subjected to greater methodological rigor. In a 1997 prospective study, Nikolajsen and colleagues[17] randomized patients to receive preoperative and postoperative epidural blockade or standard postoperative epidural analgesia. At 12 months, both groups had a significant incidence of phantom limb pain: 75% in the preoperative and postoperative block group and 69% in the standard epidural group. Although a nonepidural treatment group was not included in this study, the incidence of phantom limb pain in these 2 study arms was similar to the background prevalence of phantom limb pain noted in other studies.[21,24,73] In a follow-up article, Nikolajsen and colleagues[74] examined the effect of preoperative and intraoperative epidural analgesia on stump sensitization after amputation. Again, they found no significant improvements. These findings are consistent with other clinical studies demonstrating that the timing of an analgesic intervention is not of critical importance.[69]

The current de-emphasis of the preemptive analgesia paradigm, however, has not lessened the significance placed on effective pain relief at the time of surgery. Indeed, the importance of successful analgesia is further supported by the 2011 publication by Karanikolas and colleagues[75] assessing epidural versus systemic analgesia in 65 patients undergoing amputation. Nearly all patients receiving epidural infusion or effective systemic analgesia saw a reduction in the prevalence of phantom limb pain at 6 months when compared with the controls treated with nurse-delivered intramuscular opioids. This article supports the concept that the success of analgesia may be more important than the specific technique used.

EPIDURAL ANALGESIA: THORACOTOMY

Similar to the interventions used for amputation surgery, epidural infusion has also been the gold standard for pain relief following thoracic surgery.[76] Thoracic epidural analgesia provides superior postoperative pain control when compared with parenteral opioids[77,78] and also facilitates early extubation, rehabilitation, and decreased perioperative complications.[79] The Procedure Specific Postoperative

Pain Management working group (www.postoppain.org) recommends thoracic epidural or paravertebral blocks for thoracic surgery as the first-line approach.

Despite the documented efficacy of thoracic epidural analgesia in the perioperative setting, the technique still fails in a significant number of patients.[80] The reason for this is unclear, and multiple hypotheses include catheter malposition, opioid tolerance, or poor drug spread to nerves located on the operative side.[81-84] Currently, there is limited evidence to support the notion that epidural analgesia reduces the incidence of chronic post-thoracotomy pain.

REGIONAL ANALGESIA: AMPUTATION

As an alternative to epidural analgesia, several trials of perineural catheters have been conducted in an effort to improve both acute and chronic pain symptoms following amputation. Initial studies of surgically placed perineural catheters were encouraging. In 1991, Malawer and colleagues[85] reported excellent perioperative analgesia with nerve sheath catheters in patients with amputations, and Fisher and Meller[16] described the complete absence of phantom limb pain in 11 patients treated with this technique.

Additional trials of this technique, however, did not reproduce these initial positive results. In 1994, Elizaga and colleagues[86] observed no significant improvement in acute or chronic pain in patients treated with surgically placed catheters. Other studies have reported either modest[87] or no improvement in the incidence of phantom limb pain.[88] It is also notable that surgically placed perineural catheters seem to provide inferior acute analgesia when compared with other regional anesthesia and epidural techniques.[89] The inadequate perioperative analgesia may be secondary to the distal placement of the catheter with minimal blunting of sensation at the surgical site. It is unknown whether the reduction in acute analgesia from surgical catheters has implications for longer-term postsurgical pain.

Although the previously mentioned studies of surgically placed perineural catheters provided equivocal results for managing postamputation pain, other percutaneous catheter insertion techniques are now commonly used by anesthesiologists and provide some potential advantages.[90] First of all, catheters may be placed preoperatively and used in a preemptive fashion. Secondly, and more importantly, the catheters may be placed in a location proximal to the incision, improving postoperative analgesia.

Previous studies gave sporadic reports of effective management of amputation pain using proximal perineural catheters.[91-93] More recently, Borghi and colleagues[94] evaluated this technique in a more systematic manner and found that prolonged perineural catheter use provided effective acute analgesia and long-term reduction of phantom limb pain. Notable aspects of this study were the lack of preoperative infusion and the prolonged duration of postoperative catheter use (median catheter duration of 30 days). Although not a randomized trial, the investigators did find only a 16% incidence of phantom limb pain at 12 months follow-up. These results have not yet been duplicated but are quite encouraging.

REGIONAL ANALGESIA: THORACOTOMY

Similar to perineural catheter infusions for amputation pain, paravertebral nerve blockade also involves the delivery of local anesthetic to nerves after they exit the spinal canal. Single-injection techniques at multiple dermatomes and continuous paravertebral catheters are generally used to manage pain from thoracotomy surgery. The classic method uses a loss-of-resistance technique; however, nerve stimulator localization[95] and ultrasound techniques are also well described.[96–98] Ultrasound guidance improves accuracy of paravertebral catheter placement and minimizes the risk of pleural puncture.[99,100] Karmarkar and Richardson[101,102] provide additional details about these techniques.

Recent studies suggest that paravertebral nerve block provides comparable analgesia to epidural infusion with greater hemodynamic stability[103] and a better short-term side-effect profile.[104] The side effects associated with thoracic paravertebral blockade are generally low, although local anesthetic toxicity, block failure, bleeding, and pleural puncture may occur.[101,105,106] It is thought that pulmonary function is preserved with paravertebral block, subsequently decreasing pulmonary morbidity.[3,107–109] Thus, paravertebral blockade along with epidural infusion is still recommended.

SYSTEMIC MULTIMODAL ANALGESIA

Despite the recent emphasis placed on the perioperative use of epidural analgesia and peripheral nerve blockade, these techniques alone may not be sufficient for the prevention of chronic postsurgical pain. Circulating humoral inflammatory factors also induce central sensitization and neuropathic pain,[110,111] providing scientific justification for using multimodal systemic analgesia. Multimodal strategies use concurrent therapies in an effort to maximize pain relief and minimize side effects, particularly those related to opioid analgesics.[112] Although opioid analgesics remain an important part of the acute pain protocol for amputation and thoracic surgery, their singular use is often not sufficient to provide effective systemic analgesia. In this review, the authors discuss adjuvant analgesics and novel nonopioid pain control strategies.

Nonsteroidal Antiinflammatory Drugs

Nonsteroidal antiinflammatory drugs (NSAIDs) have been extensively investigated in the perioperative period, and their use improves analgesia, reduces opioid requirements, and reduces opioid-related side effects.[113] Additionally, the question of preemptive analgesia from preoperative NSAID administration has been investigated in more than 20 trials. However, preoperative dosing improved symptom management in only 2 of these trials when compared with intraoperative and postoperative dosing, indicating that there is likely little or no preemptive effect from these drugs.[69]

Cyclooxygenase-2 (COX-2) inhibitors are sometimes preferred in the perioperative period given their decreased effect on platelet function. Similar to other NSAIDs, the COX-2 inhibitor celecoxib demonstrates improvement in acute analgesia with an opioid-sparing effect but no significant preemptive analgesic effect.[114–116] Celecoxib has demonstrated efficacy as part of a multimodal strategy for thoracic surgery.[117] Studies related to NSAID efficacy following amputation are lacking, but these analgesics should be considered given their documented effectiveness for acute pain. However, there is no current evidence that NSAID use prevents either chronic postamputation or post-thoracotomy pain.

Acetaminophen

Oral acetaminophen has enjoyed long-term use for managing acute pain, and intravenous (IV) acetaminophen has recently been approved in the United States. Although both forms have been used in the perioperative period, the IV formulation may have some advantages given its reliable pharmacokinetics and ease of administration.[118,119]

Because acetaminophen improves acute analgesia in patients undergoing thoracotomy, it is increasingly being used in the perioperative period, except in patients with significant liver disease.[120] Although there are concerns about the safety of chronic acetaminophen use, acute administration of up to 4 g/d seems to be safe in most patients.[121] Similar to NSAIDs, however, no studies have demonstrated that acetaminophen reduces chronic postamputation or post-thoracotomy pain. Nonetheless, given its minimal effect on platelet aggregation, perioperative bleeding, and renal function,[122] acetaminophen should be strongly considered in the perioperative setting.

Gabapentinoids: Gabapentin/Pregabalin

There has been significant interest in the use of gabapentinoids for neuropathic pain since their 1993 release in the United States. Because these drugs can inhibit Ca^{2+} currents and reduce neurotransmitter release associated with neural sensitization,[123] they have demonstrated efficacy in multiple neuropathic pain conditions.[124,125]

Gabapentin and pregabalin have been studied as a preemptive measure before surgery with evidence of decreased acute pain, opioid consumption, and improvement in opioid-related side effects.[126–128] Additionally, gabapentin is effective in reducing the severity of chronic phantom limb pain.[33] Despite the demonstrated efficacy of gabapentinoids in acute and chronic neuropathic pain, they have not been shown to prevent chronic phantom limb pain when given in the immediate postoperative period.[129] Although their use following amputation may be appropriate given their beneficial effect on acute postoperative pain, future research is needed to establish optimal timing, dosing, and efficacy of perioperative gabapentenoids.[128,130,131]

Clonidine

Clonidine, an $\alpha2$ adrenergic agonist, plays a potential role in the treatment of neuropathic pain because of the expression of $\alpha2A$ receptors at the site of nerve injury[132] as well as on local infiltrating macrophages and lymphocytes.[133] Clonidine administration decreases the local expression of inflammatory cytokines, such as TNF-α and IL-1β, and improves hypersensitivity following nerve injury.[134] Epidural and perineural clonidine have also been studied as a therapy for neuropathic pain[134] and have been used clinically in the treatment of chronic postamputation pain.[135,136] Because $\alpha2A$-adrenoceptors and inflammatory cytokines play important roles in the production of postamputation chronic pain, clonidine deserves further investigation. It is generally well tolerated, but its clinical use is occasionally limited by dose-dependent side effects, such as hypotension and sedation.[137]

Ketamine

Ketamine is an antagonist of the N-methyl D-aspartate receptor known to be involved in central sensitization and neuropathic pain.[138] It has been used in the treatment and prevention of chronic pain following nerve injury, although randomized controlled efficacy trials are still lacking.[139] Ketamine has been investigated as a systemic drug[51,140] and an epidural drug[141] for amputation surgery and it has been shown to reduce stump sensitivity in the immediate postoperative period.[141] Although ketamine has also been found to reduce acute hyperalgesia and allodynia when given at the time of thoracic surgery,[142] it is not effective for treating chronic postamputation pain[141] or post-thoracotomy pain.[143]

SUMMARY AND FUTURE DIRECTIONS

Growing evidence suggests that multimodal analgesia, using a combination of catheter-based techniques[94,144] and systemic analgesics,[112,145,146] reduces the risk of chronic postsurgical pain. Comprehensive therapy is particularly important for patients undergoing high-risk surgeries, such as amputation and thoracotomy. With the recent demonstration that effective acute pain management, regardless of the method used, decreases the prevalence of phantom limb pain at 6 months,[75] we now have the scientific justification and the ethical obligation to treat these patients with the multiple tools at our disposal. Furthermore, because prolonged perineural catheter infusions may reduce the burden of postamputation pain,[94] we must reevaluate the postoperative treatment period. Therefore, rather than several days of recovery, we may need to consider prolonged therapies during the time of neurologic plasticity. If we can alter this postoperative remodeling process, we will have an additional tool to reduce the incidence of chronic postsurgical pain.

ACKNOWLEDGMENTS

The authors would like to thank Kathy Gage, BS for her editorial assistance in the preparation of this article.

REFERENCES

1. Kehlet H, Jensen TS, Woolf CJ. Persistent postsurgical pain: risk factors and prevention. Lancet 2006;367(9522):1618–25.
2. Ypsilantis E, Tang TY. Pre-emptive analgesia for chronic limb pain after amputation for peripheral vascular disease: a systematic review. Ann Vasc Surg 2010; 24(8):1139–46.
3. Joshi GP, Bonnet F, Shah R, et al. A systematic review of randomized trials evaluating regional techniques for postthoracotomy analgesia. Anesth Analg 2008; 107(3):1026–40.
4. Wildgaard K, Ravn J, Kehlet H. Chronic post-thoracotomy pain: a critical review of pathogenic mechanisms and strategies for prevention. Eur J Cardiothorac Surg 2009;36:170–80.
5. Fisher H. US military casualty statistics: Operation New Dawn, Operation Iraqi Freedom, and Operation Enduring Freedom. In: Department of Defense, editor. Congressional Research Service; 2010. p. 1–11. Available at: http://www.fas. org/sgp/crs/natsec/RS22452.pdf. Accessed October 1, 2011.
6. Iezzoni LI, Ronan LJ. Disability legacy of the Haitian earthquake. Ann Intern Med 2010;152(12):812–4.
7. Goodney PP, Beck AW, Nagle J, et al. National trends in lower extremity bypass surgery, endovascular interventions, and major amputations. J Vasc Surg 2009; 50(1):54–60.
8. Schley MT, Wilms P, Toepfner S, et al. Painful and nonpainful phantom and stump sensations in acute traumatic amputees. J Trauma 2008;65(4):858–64.
9. Hutchison RW. Challenges in acute post-operative pain management. American journal of health-system pharmacy. Am J Health Syst Pharm 2007;64(6 Suppl 4): S2–5.
10. Sabanathan S, Eng J, Mearns AJ. Alterations in respiratory mechanics following thoracotomy. J R Coll Surg Edinb 1990;35(3):144–50.

11. Popping DM, Elia N, Marret E, et al. Protective effects of epidural analgesia on pulmonary complications after abdominal and thoracic surgery: a meta-analysis. Arch Surg 2008;143(10):990–9 [discussion: 1000].
12. Perkins FM, Kehlet H. Chronic pain as an outcome of surgery. A review of predictive factors. Anesthesiology 2000;93(4):1123–33.
13. Callesen T, Bech K, Kehlet H. Prospective study of chronic pain after groin hernia repair. Br J Surg 1999;86(12):1528–31.
14. Coderre TJ, Katz J. Peripheral and central hyperexcitability: differential signs and symptoms in persistent pain. Behav Brain Sci 1997;20(3):404–19 [discussion: 435–513].
15. Bach S, Noreng MF, Tjellden NU. Phantom limb pain in amputees during the first 12 months following limb amputation, after preoperative lumbar epidural blockade. Pain 1988;33(3):297–301.
16. Fisher A, Meller Y. Continuous postoperative regional analgesia by nerve sheath block for amputation surgery–a pilot study. Anesth Analg 1991;72(3):300–3.
17. Nikolajsen L, Ilkjaer S, Christensen JH, et al. Randomised trial of epidural bupivacaine and morphine in prevention of stump and phantom pain in lower-limb amputation. Lancet 1997;350(9088):1353–7.
18. Kooijman CM, Dijkstra PU, Geertzen JH, et al. Phantom pain and phantom sensations in upper limb amputees: an epidemiological study. Pain 2000;87(1):33–41.
19. Sherman RA, Sherman CJ. Prevalence and characteristics of chronic phantom limb pain among American veterans. Results of a trial survey. Am J Phys Med 1983;62(5):227–38.
20. Nikolajsen L, Jensen TS. Phantom limb pain. Br J Anaesth 2001;87(1):107–16.
21. Kern U, Busch V, Rockland M, et al. Prevalence and risk factors of phantom limb pain and phantom limb sensations in Germany. A nationwide field survey. Schmerz 2009;23(5):479–88 [in German].
22. Ephraim PL, Wegener ST, MacKenzie EJ, et al. Phantom pain, residual limb pain, and back pain in amputees: results of a national survey. Arch Phys Med Rehabil 2005;86(10):1910–9.
23. Ehde DM, Czerniecki JM, Smith DG, et al. Chronic phantom sensations, phantom pain, residual limb pain, and other regional pain after lower limb amputation. Arch Phys Med Rehabil 2000;81(8):1039–44.
24. Reiber GE, McFarland LV, Hubbard S, et al. Service members and veterans with major traumatic limb loss from Vietnam war and OIF/OEF conflicts: survey methods, participants, and summary findings. J Rehabil Res Dev 2010;47(4):275–97.
25. Pretty HG. Role of the sympathetic nervous system in traumatic surgery as applied to fractures, causalgias and amputation stumps. Am J Surg 1947;74(5):527–9.
26. Mandl F. Pain after amputation; simple stump pain; phantom sensation; causalgia. Acta Med Orient 1945;4:427–33.
27. Omer GE Jr. Nerve, neuroma, and pain problems related to upper limb amputations. Orthop Clin North Am 1981;12(4):751–62.
28. McIntosh J, Earnshaw JJ. Antibiotic prophylaxis for the prevention of infection after major limb amputation. Eur J Vasc Endovasc Surg 2009;37(6):696–703.
29. Wiffen P, Meynadier J, Dubois M, et al. Diagnostic and treatment issues in post-amputation pain after landmine injury. Pain Med 2006;7:S209–12.
30. Isakov E, Susak Z, Korzets A. Reflex sympathetic dystrophy of the stump in below-knee amputees. Clin J Pain 1992;8(3):270–5.
31. Sherman RA, Sherman CJ, Parker L. Chronic phantom and stump pain among American veterans: results of a survey. Pain 1984;18(1):83–95.

32. Robbins CB, Vreeman DJ, Sothmann MS, et al. A review of the long-term health outcomes associated with war-related amputation. Mil Med 2009;174(6): 588–92.

33. Bone M, Critchley P, Buggy DJ. Gabapentin in postamputation phantom limb pain: a randomized, double-blind, placebo-controlled, cross-over study. Reg Anesth Pain Med 2002;27(5):481–6.

34. Samii M, Moringlane JR. Thermocoagulation of the dorsal root entry zone for the treatment of intractable pain. Neurosurgery 1984;15(6):953–5.

35. Iacono RP, Linford J, Sandyk R. Pain management after lower extremity amputation. Neurosurgery 1987;20(3):496–500.

36. Viswanathan A, Phan PC, Burton AW. Use of spinal cord stimulation in the treatment of phantom limb pain: case series and review of the literature. Pain Pract 2010;10(5):479–84.

37. Wolff A, Vanduynhoven E, van Kleef M, et al. 21. Phantom pain. Pain Pract 2011; 11(4):403–13.

38. Chan BL, Witt R, Charrow AP, et al. Mirror therapy for phantom limb pain. N Engl J Med 2007;357(21):2206–7.

39. Maguire MF, Ravenscroft A, Beggs D, et al. A questionnaire study investigating the prevalence of the neuropathic component of chronic pain after thoracic surgery. Eur J Cardiothorac Surg 2006;29(5):800–5.

40. Steegers MA, Snik DM, Verhagen AF, et al. Only half of the chronic pain after thoracic surgery shows a neuropathic component. J Pain 2008;9(10):955–61.

41. Wildgaard K, Ravn J, Nikolajsen L, et al. Consequences of persistent pain after lung cancer surgery: a nationwide questionnaire study. Acta Anaesthesiol Scand 2011;55(1):60–8.

42. Searle RD, Simpson MP, Simpson KH, et al. Can chronic neuropathic pain following thoracic surgery be predicted during the postoperative period? Interact Cardiovasc Thorac Surg 2009;9(6):999–1002.

43. Pluijms W, Steegers MA, Verhagen AF. Chronic post-thoracotomy pain: a retrospective study. Acta Anaesthesiol Scand 2006;50(7):804–8.

44. d'Amours RH, Riegler FX, Little AG. Pathogenesis and management of persistent postthoracotomy pain. Chest Surg Clin N Am 1998;8(3):703–22.

45. Hazelrigg SR, Cetindag IB, Fullerton J. Acute and chronic pain syndromes after thoracic surgery. Surg Clin North Am 2002;82(4):849–65.

46. Katz J, Jackson M, Kavanagh BP, et al. Acute pain after thoracic surgery predicts long-term post-thoracotomy pain. Clin J Pain 1996;12(1):50–5.

47. Nikolajsen L, Ilkjaer S, Kroner K, et al. The influence of preamputation pain on postamputation stump and phantom pain. Pain 1997;72(3):393–405.

48. Jensen TS, Krebs B, Nielsen J, et al. Phantom limb, phantom pain and stump pain in amputees during the first 6 months following limb amputation. Pain 1983;17(3):243–56.

49. Hanley MA, Jensen MP, Smith DG, et al. Preamputation pain and acute pain predict chronic pain after lower extremity amputation. J Pain 2007;8(2):102–9.

50. Tasmuth T, Estlanderb AM, Kalso E. Effect of present pain and mood on the memory of past postoperative pain in women treated surgically for breast cancer. Pain 1996;68(2–3):343–7.

51. Nikolajsen L, Hansen CL, Nielsen J, et al. The effect of ketamine on phantom pain: a central neuropathic disorder maintained by peripheral input. Pain 1996;67(1):69–77.

52. Reilly KT, Sirigu A. The motor cortex and its role in phantom limb phenomena. Neuroscientist 2008;14(2):195–202.

53. Flor H, Elbert T, Muhlnickel W, et al. Cortical reorganization and phantom phenomena in congenital and traumatic upper-extremity amputees. Exp Brain Res 1998;119(2):205–12.
54. Flor H, Nikolajsen L, Staehelin Jensen T. Phantom limb pain: a case of maladaptive CNS plasticity? Nat Rev Neurosci 2006;7(11):873–81.
55. Amr YM, Yousef AA, Alzeftawy AE, et al. Effect of preincisional epidural fentanyl and bupivacaine on postthoracotomy pain and pulmonary function. Ann Thorac Surg 2010;89(2):381–5.
56. Katz J, Poleshuck EL, Andrus CH, et al. Risk factors for acute pain and its persistence following breast cancer surgery. Pain 2005;119(1–3):16–25.
57. Caumo W, Schmidt AP, Schneider CN, et al. Preoperative predictors of moderate to intense acute postoperative pain in patients undergoing abdominal surgery. Acta Anaesthesiol Scand 2002;46(10):1265–71.
58. Bosmans JC, Geertzen JH, Post WJ, et al. Factors associated with phantom limb pain: a 31/2-year prospective study. Clin Rehabil 2010;24(5):444–53.
59. Dijkstra PU, Geertzen JH, Stewart R, et al. Phantom pain and risk factors: a multivariate analysis. J Pain Symptom Manage 2002;24(6):578–85.
60. Trief PM, Grant W, Fredrickson B. A prospective study of psychological predictors of lumbar surgery outcome. Spine (Phila Pa 1976) 2000;25(20):2616–21.
61. Niederberger E, Geisslinger G. Proteomics in neuropathic pain research. Anesthesiology 2008;108(2):314–23.
62. Hartvigsen J, Christensen K, Frederiksen H, et al. Genetic and environmental contributions to back pain in old age: a study of 2,108 Danish twins aged 70 and older. Spine 2004;29(8):897–901 [discussion: 902].
63. Diatchenko L, Slade GD, Nackley AG, et al. Genetic basis for individual variations in pain perception and the development of a chronic pain condition. Hum Mol Genet 2005;14(1):135–43.
64. Kalkman CJ, Visser K, Moen J, et al. Preoperative prediction of severe postoperative pain. Pain 2003;105(3):415–23.
65. Kehlet H. Prospect Working Group. Procedure specific postoperative pain management 2011; Thoracotomy. Available at: www.postoppain.org. Accessed October 1, 2011.
66. Halbert J, Crotty M, Cameron ID. Evidence for the optimal management of acute and chronic phantom pain: a systematic review. Clin J Pain 2002;18(2):84–92.
67. Mackinnon SE, Dellon AL, Hudson AR, et al. Alteration of neuroma formation by manipulation of its microenvironment. Plast Reconstr Surg 1985;76(3):345–53.
68. Gerner P. Postthoracotomy pain management problems. Anesthesiol Clin 2008; 26(2):355–67, vii.
69. Moiniche S, Kehlet H, Dahl JB. A qualitative and quantitative systematic review of preemptive analgesia for postoperative pain relief: the role of timing of analgesia. Anesthesiology 2002;96(3):725–41.
70. Sotgiu ML, Castagna A, Lacerenza M, et al. Pre-injury lidocaine treatment prevents thermal hyperalgesia and cutaneous thermal abnormalities in a rat model of peripheral neuropathy. Pain 1995;61(1):3–10.
71. Gonzalez-Darder JM, Barbera J, Abellan MJ. Effects of prior anaesthesia on autotomy following sciatic transection in rats. Pain 1986;24(1):87–91.
72. Jahangiri M, Jayatunga AP, Bradley JW, et al. Prevention of phantom pain after major lower limb amputation by epidural infusion of diamorphine, clonidine and bupivacaine. Ann R Coll Surg Engl 1994;76(5):324–6.
73. Wartan SW, Hamann W, Wedley JR, et al. Phantom pain and sensation among British veteran amputees. Br J Anaesth 1997;78(6):652–9.

74. Nikolajsen L, Ilkjaer S, Jensen TS. Effect of preoperative extradural bupivacaine and morphine on stump sensation in lower limb amputees. Br J Anaesth 1998; 81(3):348–54.

75. Karanikolas M, Aretha D, Tsolakis I, et al. Optimized perioperative analgesia reduces chronic phantom limb pain intensity, prevalence, and frequency: a prospective, randomized, clinical trial. Anesthesiology 2011;114(5):1144–54.

76. Powell ES, Cook D, Pearce AC, et al. A prospective, multicentre, observational cohort study of analgesia and outcome after pneumonectomy. Br J Anaesth 2011;106(3):364–70.

77. Block BM, Liu SS, Rowlingson AJ, et al. Efficacy of postoperative epidural analgesia: a meta-analysis. JAMA 2003;290(18):2455–63.

78. Dolin SJ, Cashman JN, Bland JM. Effectiveness of acute postoperative pain management: I. Evidence from published data. Br J Anaesth 2002;89(3):409–23.

79. Watson A, Allen PR. Influence of thoracic epidural analgesia on outcome after resection for esophageal cancer. Surgery 1994;115(4):429–32.

80. Pratt WB, Steinbrook RA, Maithel SK, et al. Epidural analgesia for pancreatoduodenectomy: a critical appraisal. J Gastrointest Surg 2008;12(7):1207–20.

81. Hogan Q. Epidural catheter tip position and distribution of injectate evaluated by computed tomography. Anesthesiology 1999;90(4):964–70.

82. Asato F, Goto F. Radiographic findings of unilateral epidural block. Anesth Analg 1996;83(3):519–22.

83. Taenzer AH, Clark C 5th, Kovarik WD. Experience with 724 epidurograms for epidural catheter placement in pediatric anesthesia. Reg Anesth Pain Med 2010;35(5):432–5.

84. Motamed C, Farhat F, Remerand F, et al. An analysis of postoperative epidural analgesia failure by computed tomography epidurography. Anesth Analg 2006; 103(4):1026–32.

85. Malawer MM, Buch R, Khurana JS, et al. Postoperative infusional continuous regional analgesia. A technique for relief of postoperative pain following major extremity surgery. Clin Orthop Relat Res 1991;(266):227–37.

86. Elizaga AM, Smith DG, Sharar SR, et al. Continuous regional analgesia by intraneural block: effect on postoperative opioid requirements and phantom limb pain following amputation. J Rehabil Res Dev 1994;31(3):179–87.

87. Morey TE, Giannoni J, Duncan E, et al. Nerve sheath catheter analgesia after amputation. Clin Orthop Relat Res 2002;(397):281–9.

88. Pinzur MS, Garla PG, Pluth T, et al. Continuous postoperative infusion of a regional anesthetic after an amputation of the lower extremity. A randomized clinical trial. J Bone Joint Surg Am 1996;78(10):1501–5.

89. Lambert A, Dashfield A, Cosgrove C, et al. Randomized prospective study comparing preoperative epidural and intraoperative perineural analgesia for the prevention of postoperative stump and phantom limb pain following major amputation. Reg Anesth Pain Med 2001;26(4):316–21.

90. Neal JM, Brull R, Chan VW, et al. The ASRA evidence-based medicine assessment of ultrasound-guided regional anesthesia and pain medicine: executive summary. Reg Anesth Pain Med 2010;35(Suppl 2):S1–9.

91. Madabhushi L, Reuben SS, Steinberg RB, et al. The efficacy of postoperative perineural infusion of bupivacaine and clonidine after lower extremity amputation in preventing phantom limb and stump pain. J Clin Anesth 2007;19(3):226–9.

92. Borghi B, Bugamelli S, Stagni G, et al. Perineural infusion of 0.5% ropivacaine for successful treatment of phantom limb syndrome: a case report. Minerva Anestesiol 2009;75(11):661–4.

93. Kiefer RT, Wiech K, Topfner S, et al. Continuous brachial plexus analgesia and NMDA-receptor blockade in early phantom limb pain: a report of two cases. Pain Med 2002;3(2):156–60.

94. Borghi B, D'Addabbo M, White PF, et al. The use of prolonged peripheral neural blockade after lower extremity amputation: the effect on symptoms associated with phantom limb syndrome. Anesth Analg 2010;111(5):1308–15.

95. Lang SA. The use of a nerve stimulator for thoracic paravertebral block. Anesthesiology 2002;97(2):521 [author reply: 521–2].

96. Hara K, Sakura S, Nomura T, et al. Ultrasound guided thoracic paravertebral block in breast surgery. Anaesthesia 2009;64(2):223–5.

97. O Riain SC, Donnell BO, Cuffe T, et al. Thoracic paravertebral block using real-time ultrasound guidance. Anesth Analg 2010;110(1):248–51.

98. Pusch F, Wildling E, Klimscha W, et al. Sonographic measurement of needle insertion depth in paravertebral blocks in women. Br J Anaesth 2000;85(6):841–3.

99. Lonnqvist PA, MacKenzie J, Soni AK, et al. Paravertebral blockade. Failure rate and complications. Anaesthesia 1995;50(9):813–5.

100. Renes SH, Bruhn J, Gielen MJ, et al. In-plane ultrasound-guided thoracic paravertebral block: a preliminary report of 36 cases with radiologic confirmation of catheter position. Reg Anesth Pain Med 2010;35(2):212–6.

101. Richardson J, Lonnqvist PA, Naja Z. Bilateral thoracic paravertebral block: potential and practice. Br J Anaesth 2011;106(2):164–71.

102. Karmakar MK. Thoracic paravertebral block. Anesthesiology 2001;95(3):771–80.

103. Pintaric TS, Potocnik I, Hadzic A, et al. Comparison of continuous thoracic epidural with paravertebral block on perioperative analgesia and hemodynamic stability in patients having open lung surgery. Reg Anesth Pain Med 2011;36(3):256–60.

104. Scarci M, Joshi A, Attia R. In patients undergoing thoracic surgery is paravertebral block as effective as epidural analgesia for pain management? Interact Cardiovasc Thorac Surg 2010;10(1):92–6.

105. Wyatt SS, Price RA. Complications of paravertebral block. Br J Anaesth 2000;84(3):424.

106. Naja Z, Lonnqvist PA. Somatic paravertebral nerve blockade. Incidence of failed block and complications. Anaesthesia 2001;56(12):1184–8.

107. Richardson J, Sabanathan S, Jones J, et al. A prospective, randomized comparison of preoperative and continuous balanced epidural or paravertebral bupivacaine on post-thoracotomy pain, pulmonary function and stress responses. Br J Anaesth 1999;83(3):387–92.

108. Richardson J, Sabanathan S, Shah R. Post-thoracotomy spirometric lung function: the effect of analgesia. A review. J Cardiovasc Surg (Torino) 1999;40(3):445–56.

109. Davies RG, Myles PS, Graham JM. A comparison of the analgesic efficacy and side-effects of paravertebral vs epidural blockade for thoracotomy– a systematic review and meta-analysis of randomized trials. Br J Anaesth 2006;96(4):418–26.

110. Morrison RS, Flanagan S, Fischberg D, et al. A novel interdisciplinary analgesic program reduces pain and improves function in older adults after orthopedic surgery. J Am Geriatr Soc 2009;57(1):1–10.

111. Sinatra R. Causes and consequences of inadequate management of acute pain. Pain Med 2010;11(12):1859–71.

112. Buvanendran A, Kroin JS. Multimodal analgesia for controlling acute postoperative pain. Curr Opin Anaesthesiol 2009;22(5):588–93.
113. Maund E, McDaid C, Rice S, et al. Paracetamol and selective and non-selective non-steroidal anti-inflammatory drugs for the reduction in morphine-related side-effects after major surgery: a systematic review. Br J Anaesth 2011; 106(3):292–7.
114. Fong WP, Yang LC, Wu JI, et al. Does celecoxib have pre-emptive analgesic effect after caesarean section surgery? Br J Anaesth 2008;100(6):861–2.
115. Huang YM, Wang CM, Wang CT, et al. Perioperative celecoxib administration for pain management after total knee arthroplasty - a randomized, controlled study. BMC Musculoskelet Disord 2008;9:77.
116. Sun T, Sacan O, White PF, et al. Perioperative versus postoperative celecoxib on patient outcomes after major plastic surgery procedures. Anesth Analg 2008; 106(3):950–8, table of contents.
117. Senard M, Deflandre EP, Ledoux D, et al. Effect of celecoxib combined with thoracic epidural analgesia on pain after thoracotomy. Br J Anaesth 2010;105(2):196–200.
118. Duggan ST, Scott LJ. Intravenous paracetamol (acetaminophen). Drugs 2009; 69(1):101–13.
119. Jahr JS, Lee VK. Intravenous acetaminophen. Anesthesiol Clin 2010;28(4):619–45.
120. Mac TB, Girard F, Chouinard P, et al. Acetaminophen decreases early post-thoracotomy ipsilateral shoulder pain in patients with thoracic epidural analgesia: a double-blind placebo-controlled study. J Cardiothorac Vasc Anesth 2005;19(4):475–8.
121. Candiotti KA, Bergese SD, Viscusi ER, et al. Safety of multiple-dose intravenous acetaminophen in adult inpatients. Pain Med 2010;11(12):1841–8.
122. Smith HS. Perioperative intravenous acetaminophen and NSAIDs. Pain Med 2011;12(6):961–81.
123. Fink K, Meder W, Dooley DJ, et al. Inhibition of neuronal Ca(2+) influx by gabapentin and subsequent reduction of neurotransmitter release from rat neocortical slices. Br J Pharmacol 2000;130(4):900–6.
124. Bril V, England J, Franklin GM, et al. Evidence-based guideline: treatment of painful diabetic neuropathy: report of the American Academy of Neurology, the American Association of Neuromuscular and Electrodiagnostic Medicine, and the American Academy of Physical Medicine and Rehabilitation. Neurology 2011;76(20):1758–65.
125. Moore RA, Wiffen PJ, Derry S, et al. Gabapentin for chronic neuropathic pain and fibromyalgia in adults. Cochrane Database Syst Rev 2011;3:CD007938.
126. Dauri M, Faria S, Gatti A, et al. Gabapentin and pregabalin for the acute postoperative pain management. A systematic-narrative review of the recent clinical evidences. Curr Drug Targets 2009;10(8):716–33.
127. Tiippana EM, Hamunen K, Kontinen VK, et al. Do surgical patients benefit from perioperative gabapentin/pregabalin? A systematic review of efficacy and safety. Anesth Analg 2007;104(6):1545–56, table of contents.
128. Dahl JB, Mathiesen O, Moiniche S. 'Protective premedication': an option with gabapentin and related drugs? A review of gabapentin and pregabalin in the treatment of post-operative pain. Acta Anaesthesiol Scand 2004;48(9):1130–6.
129. Nikolajsen L, Finnerup NB, Kramp S, et al. A randomized study of the effects of gabapentin on postamputation pain. Anesthesiology 2006;105(5):1008–15.
130. Gilron I. Gabapentin and pregabalin for chronic neuropathic and early postsurgical pain: current evidence and future directions. Curr Opin Anaesthesiol 2007; 20(5):456–72.

131. Clarke H, Pereira S, Kennedy D, et al. Adding gabapentin to a multimodal regimen does not reduce acute pain, opioid consumption or chronic pain after total hip arthroplasty. Acta Anaesthesiol Scand 2009;53(8):1073–83.
132. Gold MS, Dastmalchi S, Levine JD. Alpha 2-adrenergic receptor subtypes in rat dorsal root and superior cervical ganglion neurons. Pain 1997;69(1–2):179–90.
133. Lavand'homme PM, Ma W, De Kock M, et al. Perineural alpha(2A)-adrenoceptor activation inhibits spinal cord neuroplasticity and tactile allodynia after nerve injury. Anesthesiology 2002;97(4):972–80.
134. Lavand'homme PM, Eisenach JC. Perioperative administration of the alpha2-adrenoceptor agonist clonidine at the site of nerve injury reduces the development of mechanical hypersensitivity and modulates local cytokine expression. Pain 2003;105(1–2):247–54.
135. Davis RW. Successful treatment for phantom pain. Orthopedics 1993;16(6):691–5.
136. Danshaw CB. An anesthetic approach to amputation and pain syndromes. Phys Med Rehabil Clin N Am 2000;11(3):553–7.
137. Curatolo M, Schnider TW, Petersen-Felix S, et al. A direct search procedure to optimize combinations of epidural bupivacaine, fentanyl, and clonidine for postoperative analgesia. Anesthesiology 2000;92(2):325–37.
138. Woolf CJ, Thompson SW. The induction and maintenance of central sensitization is dependent on N-methyl-D-aspartic acid receptor activation; implications for the treatment of post-injury pain hypersensitivity states. Pain 1991;44(3):293–9.
139. Collins S, Sigtermans MJ, Dahan A, et al. NMDA receptor antagonists for the treatment of neuropathic pain. Pain Med 2010;11(11):1726–42.
140. Hayes C, Armstrong-Brown A, Burstal R. Perioperative intravenous ketamine infusion for the prevention of persistent post-amputation pain: a randomized, controlled trial. Anaesth Intensive Care 2004;32(3):330–8.
141. Wilson JA, Nimmo AF, Fleetwood-Walker SM, et al. A randomised double blind trial of the effect of pre-emptive epidural ketamine on persistent pain after lower limb amputation. Pain 2008;135(1–2):108–18.
142. Ozyalcin NS, Yucel A, Camlica H, et al. Effect of pre-emptive ketamine on sensory changes and postoperative pain after thoracotomy: comparison of epidural and intramuscular routes. Br J Anaesth 2004;93(3):356–61.
143. Ryu HG, Lee CJ, Kim YT, et al. Preemptive low-dose epidural ketamine for preventing chronic postthoracotomy pain: a prospective, double-blinded, randomized, clinical trial. Clin J Pain 2011;27(4):304–8.
144. Senturk M, Ozcan PE. The effects of three different analgesia techniques on long-term postthoracotomy pain. Anesth Analg 2002;94(1):11–5.
145. Loftus RW, Yeager MP, Clark JA, et al. Intraoperative ketamine reduces perioperative opiate consumption in opiate-dependent patients with chronic back pain undergoing back surgery. Anesthesiology 2010;113(3):639–46.
146. Lavand'homme P, De Kock M, Waterloos H. Intraoperative epidural analgesia combined with ketamine provides effective preventive analgesia in patients undergoing major digestive surgery. Anesthesiology 2005;103(4):813–20.

Postoperative Complications: Delirium

Steven R. Allen, MD[a],*, Heidi L. Frankel, MD[b,c]

KEYWORDS

- Delirium • Postoperative complications
- Cholinergic transmission • Serum anticholinergic activity

Delirium is defined as an acute alteration of attention and cognition with waxing and waning disturbance of consciousness. A person is less able to focus and maintain attention. It is a common complication after surgery. *The Diagnostic and Statistical Manual of Mental Disorders, 4th Edition Text Revision*[1] (*DSM-IV-TR*) defines the standards necessary for a diagnosis of delirium. These include disturbance in consciousness; change in cognition, such as memory deficit or disorientation; acute development of the disturbance (hours to days) and tendency to fluctuate; and (from history, physical examination, or laboratory results) that the disturbance comes from direct physiologic consequences of a general medical condition (**Boxes 1**and **2**).

The incidence of postoperative delirium (POD) is between 10% and 55% in postoperative patients depending on the type of procedure the patient underwent, with a higher percentage in orthopedics compared with general surgery patients.[2] Additionally, the incidence of POD is significantly higher in elderly patients. It is estimated that up to 50% of elderly patients suffer from delirium after surgery.[3] Additionally, over 40% of hospitalized patients with delirium suffer from psychotic features, including visual hallucinations. It typically manifests itself within 24 to 48 hours postoperatively, with exacerbation of symptoms at night due to circadian disturbances. The implications of POD are significant. It is associated with increased morbidity and a 1 year mortality that approaches 40%.[4] The estimated health care–associated costs related to delirium are astronomic. They made up nearly $7 billion dollars of Medicare expenditures in 2004.[4] Despite the relative frequency and profound cost of delirium, POD often goes unrecognized and underappreciated.

[a] Division of Traumatology, Surgical Critical Care and Emergency Surgery, University of Pennsylvania, 3400 Spruce Street, 5 Maloney, Philadelphia, PA 19104, USA
[b] Division of Trauma, Acute Care and Critical Care Surgery, Penn State Hershey Medical Center, 500 University Drive, Hershey, PA 17033, USA
[c] Division of Surgical Critical Care, University of Maryland R Adams Cowley Shock Trauma Center, 22 South Greene Street, Baltimore, MD 21201, USA
* Corresponding author.
E-mail address: steve.allen@uphs.upenn.edu

Surg Clin N Am 92 (2012) 409–431
doi:10.1016/j.suc.2012.01.012
0039-6109/12/$ – see front matter © 2012 Published by Elsevier Inc.

Box 1
DSM-IV-TR **diagnostic criteria for delirium**

1. Disturbance in consciousness manifested by a reduced clarity of awareness of the environment

2. Accompanying change in cognition, which may include memory impairment, disorientation, or language disturbance

3. Development of a perceptual disturbance, which may include misinterpretations, illusions, or hallucinations

4. The disturbance develops over a short period of time (usually hours to days) and tends to fluctuate during the course of the day. There is evidence from the history, physical examination, or laboratory tests that the delirium is a direct physiologic consequence of a general medical condition, substance intoxication or withdrawal, use of a medication, toxin exposure, or a combination of these factors

Data from APA, Diagnostic and statistical manual of mental disorders. 4th edition. Washington, DC: American Psychiatric Association; 1994. Electronic resource.

Delirium is distinct from dementia despite many overlapping features. It has been estimated that as many as two-thirds of hospitalized patients with dementia have superimposed delirium that often worsens functional and mental decline. Delirium may present as a state of agitation, restlessness, hypervigilance, and combativeness known as hyperactive delirium. However, there is also a hypoactive form of delirium in which lethargy and inattentiveness are the notable presenting factors. Elderly patients most commonly suffer from hypoactive delirium. A mixed picture of delirium with hyperactive and hypoactive characteristics is very common. Hyperactive delirium is often recognized during routine care of the patient and has been associated with lower mortality when compared with the hypoactive motor type. Robinson and colleagues[5] classified the motor subtypes of delirium using the Richmond Agitation-Sedation Scale (RASS). Patients with positive daily RASS scores are defined as hyperactive, whereas those with neutral or negative RASS scores are classified as hypoactive delirium. The mixed subtype of delirium was classified as those with both positive and neutral or negative RASS scores.[5] Although the hyperactive form is easily recognized because patients tend to be agitated or combative, the hypoactive delirium often goes unrecognized and is misdiagnosed as depression or sedation. It is crucial that hypoactive delirium is identified in a timely manner because it has been correlated with worse outcomes, including prolonged hospital stay and higher incidence of decubitus ulcers.[5,6] The surgeon must work to prevent the development of delirium. However, should delirium occur, early identification and treatment are paramount to reduce the associated complications and long-term morbidity and mortality.[7]

CAUSES OF DELIRIUM

Post-operative delirium is typically multifactorial[4,8] and includes cognitive decline, preexisting medical comorbidities, and interactions with psychoactive medications. It has been suggested that patients considered vulnerable to delirium due to dementia or multiple chronic medical problems may require only a minor precipitating factor, such as administration of a medication for sleep, for delirium to develop. In contrast, those patients who are not seen to be vulnerable may require a series of precipitating factors such as major surgery, psychoactive medications, and infectious insult[4,9] (to name only a few) to elicit signs and symptoms of delirium.

Box 2
The Confusion Assessment Method for the Intensive Care Unit (CAM-ICU)

Delirium is diagnosed when both Features 1 and 2 are positive, along with either Feature 3 or Feature 4.

Feature 1. Acute onset of mental status changes or fluctuating course

- Is there evidence of an acute change in mental status from the baseline?
- Did the (abnormal) behavior fluctuate during the past 24 hours; come and go or increase or decrease in severity?

    Sources of information: Serial Glasgow Coma Scale or sedation score ratings over 24 hours and available input from bedside critical care nurse or family.

Feature 2. Inattention

- Did the patient have difficulty focusing attention?
- Is there a reduced ability to maintain and shift attention?

    Sources of information: Attention screening examinations by using either picture recognition or Vigilance A random letter test. Neither of these tests requires verbal response and are ideally suited for mechanically ventilated patients.

Feature 3. Disorganized thinking

- Was the patient's thinking disorganized or incoherent, such as rambling or irrelevant conversation, unclear or illogical flow of ideas, or unpredictable-switching from subject to subject?
- Was the patient able to follow questions and commands throughout the assessment?

    1. "Are you having any unclear thinking?"

    2. "Hold up this many fingers."

    3. "Now, do the same thing in the other hand." (Not repeating the number of fingers)

Feature 4. Altered level of consciousness

- Any level of consciousness other than "alert."
- Alert—normal, spontaneously fully aware of environment and interacts appropriately
- Vigilant—hyperalert
- Lethargic—Drowsy but easily aroused, unaware of some elements in the environment, or not spontaneously interacting appropriately with the interviewer; becomes fully aware and appropriately interactive when prodded minimally
- Stupor—Difficult to arouse, unaware of some or all elements in the environment, or not spontaneously interacting with the interviewer; becomes incompletely aware and inappropriately interactive when prodded strongly
- Coma— Unable to arouse, unaware of all elements in the environment, with no spontaneous interaction or awareness of the interviewer, so that the interview is difficult or impossible even with maximal prodding.

Adapted from Ely EW, Margolin R, Francis J, et al. Evaluation of delirium in critically ill patients: validation of the Confusion Assessment Method for the Intensive Care Unit (CAM-ICU). Crit Care Med 2001;29:1370; Copyright 2002, E. Wesley Ely, MD, MPH and Vanderbilt University, all rights reserved.

PATHOPHYSIOLOGY OF DELIRIUM

Delirium is a multifactorial phenomenon with environmental and pathophysiologic components. Several biochemical causes have been proposed, but the exact pathogenesis remains poorly understood. Evaluation with neuropsychological methods and imaging have revealed a defect in higher cortical function with abnormalities in multiple areas of the brain, including the prefrontal cortex, frontal and temporoparietal cortex and thalamus, among others.[4,10]

Abnormal levels of acetylcholine and dopamine (DA), abnormal melatonin metabolism, and inflammatory changes in the brain have been implicated in this process.[3,4] It has been identified that the cholinergic system is involved in arousal, attention, and memory. Low levels of acetylcholine (ACh) in plasma and cerebrospinal fluid have been found in patients with delirium. This allows the hypothesis that delirium is a result of impaired central cholinergic transmission.[11–19] It is well established that anticholinergic medications induce delirium, especially in older patients. The association with age and delirium may be due to the decreased volume of ACh-producing cells as well as decreased cerebral oxidative metabolism, which leads to an expected decline in ACh production. These normal declines may be magnified by mild hypoxia. This hypoxic state results in decreased oxygen supply to the brain and, subsequently, decreased ACh production.[15,20–23]

Studies performed in medical and surgical populations have demonstrated a high correlation between serum anticholinergic activity (SAA) and delirium, with a positive predictive value for delirium as high as 100%.[12,14,15,24–27] One study by Flacker and colleagues[12] demonstrated a dose response relationship between delirium and SAA. Additionally, although studies have shown that SAA is higher in delirious patients compared with those who are not delirious others have supported these findings by demonstrating decreased SAA in those with resolving delirium. Initial hypotheses suggested that the increased SAA is the result of exogenous substances administered to the patient; however, several studies have demonstrated elevated SAA in patients who have not received medications with anticholinergic effects. This suggests the presence of endogenous anticholinergic substances that may be elevated during acute illness.[13,28,29]

Animal models have supported the influence of anticholinergic activity in the development of delirium. In one such study, rats were injected with atropine into their brains. This model of delirium was supported by electroencephalogram (EEG) tracings, maze performance, and observation of behavior that mimicked delirium in humans. The EEG tracings demonstrated higher amplitudes and slower frequencies, significantly longer mean maze time. The rats suffered with inattention and memory problems, sleep-wake problems, and abnormal behavior.[15,30] Other animal models have been used to study the results of impaired cholinergic neurotransmission in the face of encephalopathy, hypoxia, thiamine deficiency, hepatic failure, and hypoglycemia. Additionally, these animal studies have demonstrated that immobility may cause significantly decreased ACh activity and may mimic the effects of the bedridden, critically ill patient.[11,15,30–33]

Inflammatory mediators such as interleukin (IL)-1, IL-2, IL-6, tumor necrosis factor α (TNF-α), and interferon have been implicated in delirium.[34,35] It is hypothesized that these mediators of inflammation affect the permeability of the blood-brain-barrier and alter neurotransmission. Less well-studied causes include, but are not limited to, chronic hypercortisolism and activation of the hypothalamic-pituitary-adrenocortical axis. Multiple causes of delirium have been demonstrated. Likely based on the multifactorial nature of delirium, each of these particular pathways influences the clinical course of delirium.

Medications that Elicit Delirium

Multiple factors related to medications lead to the development of delirium. The presence of polypharmacy (usually the administration of three or more different medications), the use of psychoactive medications, and a specific agent's anticholinergic effects all lead to increased risk of developing delirium.

Polypharmacy may be the combination of pharmacokinetic and pharmacodynamic effects of multiple medications. Medications with psychoactive effects, such as opiates, benzodiazepines, even including corticosteroids, nonsteroidal anti-inflammatory agents (NSAIDs), and chemotherapeutic agents have been implicated in as many as 75% of patients who develop delirium. Evidence has demonstrated that more than 80% of ventilated patients develop delirium, as the vast majority receive some combination of benzodiazepines and opiates to manage pain and anxiety associated with intubation.

Medications with anticholinergic properties may lead to physical and mental impairment. It is suspected that low ACh levels result in the disorientation, sleepiness, and cognitive deficits identified in delirious patients. As described above, studies have demonstrated a dose response relationship between a drug's anticholinergic activity, as measured by SAA, and delirium.[8,12,14,15,27,36-42] Other studies have demonstrated the cumulative effects of medications with subtle anticholinergic potential and their ability to cause delirium.[15,27,36,39,42,43] A study by Blazer and colleagues[44] demonstrated the likelihood of anticholinergic toxicity among geriatric (>65 years) long-term care residents. Within this study, drug administration and drug quantity was determined. It was determined that 60% of residents received medications with significant anticholinergic properties. Polypharmacy was also an issue because 10% of these patients received three or more medications with these properties.[45]

The opioid class of medications is associated with the development of delirium and has been implicated in over 50% of cases of delirium, specifically in patients with advanced malignancy.[15,46-49] Their mechanism of action is thought to be increased activity of DA and glutamate, in addition to decreased ACh activity.[15] One such opiate strongly associated with the development of delirium is meperidine, which is metabolized to normeperidine. The metabolite normeperidine is a potent neurotoxic agent with significant anticholinergic activity. The combination of direct neurotoxic effect and strong anticholinergic activity may contribute to delirium.[15,50]

Additionally, other agents used for postoperative sedation may contribute to delirium by interfering with normal sleep patterns which may lead to a centrally mediated acetylcholine deficient state. It is postulated that at the level of the basal forebrain and hippocampus there is an interruption of cholinergic muscarinic transmission leading to central ACh deficiency.[45,51-53] Still another pathway that may lead to delirium is the abolition of melatonin release in the normal circadian rhythm as is seen in deeply sedated patients in the intensive care unit (ICU).[54-56]

Gamma amino-butyric acid (GABA)-ergic medications have also been associated with the formation of delirium.[45,51-53,57,58] GABA is the primary inhibitory neurotransmitter within the central nervous system. A complex of five proteins form each GABA receptor and combine to form a channel that allows the passage of chloride ions into cells and leads to neuronal inhibition. This inhibition is thought to be responsible for the sedative and anxiolytic effects of drugs such as alcohol, benzodiazepines, and propofol.[59,60]

Dopaminergic medications such as levodopa and bupropion also cause delirium due to dopaminergic excess. This is likely due to dopamine's effect on acetylcholine release. Antipsychotics, which are dopamine antagonists, effectively treat delirium based on this mechanism. Less well characterized biochemical causes of delirium include derangements of norepinephrine, serotonin, and γ-aminobutyric acid with pathways effecting cholinergic and dopaminergic pathways.[61]

EVALUATION OF THE PATIENT

To effectively identify and treat delirium, the surgeon must perform a complete evaluation of the patient and determine the acuity of the change in mental status. Often a history is unobtainable. In the acute setting, the surgeon must assume that the patient is suffering from delirium. A brief assessment of a patient's cognition must be performed with a formal instrument such as the Mini-Mental State Examination (MMSE), Confusion Assessment Method for the Intensive Care Unit (CAM-ICU), RASS, and the Memorial Delirium Assessment Scale (MDAS). Formal evaluation with validated, reliable instruments is necessary because less formal evaluations may miss the diagnosis of delirium. To adequately assess patients, they must be awoken on rounds and critically evaluated for the presence of delirium, with a heightened concern for the hypoactive form.[4]

MMSE

The MMSE is an 11-question bedside screening tool that measures cognitive function. First described by Meyer in 1918, the MMSE assesses attention, calculation, recall, orientation, and language.[62] A score of 0 represents profound cognitive impairment and a score of 30 suggests intact cognition. A score of less than 24 indicates cognitive impairment. Its original use was for the evaluation of psychiatric patients, but it has been validated for use in several other diagnoses that may affect cognition. Multiple studies have demonstrated high reliability among stable patients. Validity was also found to be quite good as proven by several separate studies.[63–66]

The CAM-ICU, RASS, and MDAS are instruments used to assess patients for the development and presence of delirium and have been developed and validated for the identification of delirium in the ICU.

CAM-ICU

The CAM was developed by Inouye and colleagues[67] to assist with the identification of delirium by those who were not trained in psychiatry. This tool was built based on definitions set forth by the DSM-3rd revised edition and the opinion of experts within psychiatry. It has been used over the past decade to assess the incidence, risk factors, and outcomes of delirium. The CAM has since been modified for use in the ICU, described as the CAM-ICU. This modified tool allows for assessment of mechanically ventilated and non-verbal patients.

The CAM-ICU consists of a four-item diagnostic algorithm to identify delirium and is a validated tool to monitor delirium. The presence of two primary symptoms includes acute onset and fluctuating course, as well as inattention. One secondary feature is also required, such as disorganized thinking or an altered level of consciousness. The CAM-ICU is easy and quick to conduct and has good reliability and validity. The original CAM was designed to detect delirium in patients who were able to communicate verbally. It has recently been adapted by Ely and colleagues[68] to the CAM-ICU (see **Box 1**) for use in nonverbal, mechanically ventilated patients in the ICU. This was augmented by the use of the Attention Screening Examination, which includes a visual recognition component and has been validated by Hart and colleagues[69,70] in other tools such as the Cognitive Test for Delirium. The initial study by Ely and colleagues[71] to assess validity and reliability of the CAM-ICU was performed in adult medical coronary ICUs. Within this study, 471 daily paired evaluations were completed. Demonstrated sensitivities of 100% and 93%, specificities of 98% and 100%, and high inter-rater reliability. Additionally, the mean time to administer the tool was 2 minutes. It was concluded that the CAM-ICU is a quick and user friendly, tool to assess delirium in the ICU. From these results, Guenther and colleagues[6] devised a CAM-ICU flow sheet as an easy algorithm to assess the four criteria in mechanically ventilated patients. Using a psychiatrist as the reference rater and two physician investigators, it was determined that the CAM-ICU was highly sensitive (88% and 92%) and specific (100%) with high inter-rater reliability. In addition, it took an average of only 50 seconds to complete in those with delirium.

One drawback of the CAM-ICU is that those who cannot respond to verbal stimuli are not able to be assessed and are considered comatose.

RASS

The RASS is used to assess the level of sedation in patients and is a 10-point scale centered at 0. Zero indicates alert and calm. A positive RASS score ranges from restlessness (+1) to combative (+4). A negative RASS score ranges from lethargy (-1) to responsive only to physical stimulus (-4). A RASS score of -5 indicates a patient is unresponsive. The RASS is very time efficient and may be assessed in a matter of seconds in most cases. Studies have demonstrated high inter-rater reliability and close correlation with the Glasgow Coma Scale (GCS).[7,72,73]

MDAS

The MDAS is used to quantify delirium based on 10 features. Each feature is scored from 0 to 3 for a possible high score of 30, which represents the worst score. Each item assessed in the MDAS (reduced level of consciousness, disorientation, short-term memory impairment, impaired digit span, reduced ability to maintain and shift attention, disorganized thinking, perceptual disturbance, delusions, altered psychomotor activity, and disrupted sleep-wake cycle) represents the diagnostic criteria set forth by the *DSM-IV-TR*. The MDAS may also be completed quickly—requiring less than 5 minutes in many instances. It also includes objective cognitive assessment with behavior observations. The MDAS was validated and found to be a useful adjunct to other assessment tools such as CAM-ICU.[74]

RISK FACTORS

Due to the clinical implications of perioperative delirium there has been intense focus on prevention as a main strategy to reduce the incidence and severity of POD. The identification of specific risk factors— such as age (older patients have been found to be at higher risk of developing POD), gender, mental illness (depression), medical comorbidities, polypharmacy, and alcohol consumption—have allowed some physicians, in a multidisciplinary forum, to minimize POD (**Box 3**).[75,76] Scoring systems help risk-stratify patients have been attempted with relatively unsuccessful results largely due to the multifactorial nature of POD. The goal is to intervene in the care of these patients to reduce the incidence of delirium in those considered high risk.

PREOPERATIVE
Aging

Elderly patients are predisposed to develop POD. Biologic changes that occur with aging are proposed causes of the increased incidence of delirium in elderly patients, including cerebral atrophy, decreased cerebral blood flow, and altered levels of neurotransmitters. A patient's chronologic age may not be consistent with their biologic age, which is affected by existing medical comorbidities. Leading one to be significantly more frail thus more susceptible to delirium for the reasons described above.

Box 3
Risk factors for delirium

1. Advanced age
2. Cardiopulmonary complications (coronary artery disease with infarction, hypotension, hypoxia)
3. Preexisting dementia or other CNS disease
4. Electrolyte disturbances
5. Malnutrition with hypoalbuminemia
6. Infection and sepsis (urinary tract, pneumonia)
7. Multiple medical comorbidities
8. Polypharmacy ($\geq$3 different medications, opioids, or psychotropic medications)
9. Environmental disturbances (lighting, constant sounds, unfamiliar environment)

Preexisting Psychiatric and Cognitive Conditions

Patients with known depression are at increased risk of developing POD. These patients are known to have deficiencies of the serotonergic and noradrenergic transmitter systems that may predispose them to delirium. An increase in cortisol levels in patients with depression may also be a factor that predisposes patients to delirium in the postoperative period.

Those with dementia are more vulnerable to POD. It is estimated that two-thirds of cases of delirium occur in patients with dementia. This is likely due to deficiencies in the cholinergic system, effects of altered cerebral blood flow, and inflammation, which negatively affect normal cognitive function and sleep-wake cycles and lead to signs and symptoms of delirium. Hypoxia and administration of anticholinergic medications and other insults superimposed on dementia exacerbate signs of delirium in these patients. Due to this relationship of delirium and dementia, and the overlapping signs and symptoms of each condition, it has recently been proposed that delirium and dementia represent a spectrum of cognitive disorders, as opposed to two different conditions.[4]

Whether delirium may lead to dementia remains controversial. However, delirium has been shown to worsen dementia. Delirium in the face of underlying dementia may lead to rapid decline in cognition and functional losses with worse long-term outcomes. To this end, patients with delirium superimposed on dementia have worse outcomes and a larger number of these patients require institutionalization and have significantly higher mortality.[4,77–80]

Endocrine and Metabolic Derangements

Dehydration, especially in the elderly, may exacerbate POD. The overzealous use of diuretics may result in intravascular depletion and electrolyte abnormalities such as hyponatremia, hypokalemia, hypomagnesemia, and metabolic alkalosis. Other endocrine abnormalities, including diabetic ketoacidosis, hyperglycemia, hyperthyroid or hypothyroid dysfunction, as well as renal or hepatic insufficiency have been demonstrated to predispose a patient to POD.[15]

OPERATIVE

It has been hypothesized that intraoperative events, such as the type of anesthetic agent used, episodes of hypotension, blood loss, and the amount of fluid and blood products transfused, affect the incidence of delirium in the postoperative period. An early study by Marcantonio and colleagues[81] evaluated how these factors influence the development of delirium. The investigators studied a population of adult patients older than 50 years who were to undergo major, noncardiac surgery. Their results demonstrated a significant association between intraoperative blood loss and units of blood transfused with an increased risk of delirium.[81] In this cohort, those who developed delirium lost more than twice as much blood as the non-delirium group (1150 mL + 1860 mL vs 510 mL + 710 mL, $P<.001$) and received nearly three times the amount of transfused blood (3.3 + 5.6 units vs 1.2 + 1.5 units). Lowest postoperative hematocrit (<30%) was also a multivariable predictor of delirium.

Several studies have shown that other intraoperative factors, including the type of anesthetic agent used during the procedure, have no bearing on the development of delirium.[82–85] Marcantonio and colleagues[81] compared general anesthetic to several other modalities, including spinal and epidural analgesia, and found no significant difference in the incidence of delirium (range 7%–12%, P = ns). In a randomized, controlled clinical trial of 262 patients, Williams-Russo and colleagues[85] compared epidural to general anesthesia and concluded that the type of anesthesia did not affect the magnitude or pattern of delirium. More recently, a meta-analysis by Mason and colleagues[86] confirmed these results. They concluded that the route of anesthesia seemed to have little bearing on the development of POD. There was also an insignificant difference between general anesthesia and non-general anesthesia in the incidence of postoperative cognitive dysfunction (POCD), although a standardized definition of POCD remains to be determined.[86] These results were echoed by Slor and colleagues[87] who compared general anesthesia to regional anesthesia and measured the incidence of POD using the DSM-IV-TR and CAM-ICU criteria. Compared with regional anesthesia, general anesthesia had no effect on POD, even when controlled for preoperative cognitive impairment in patients who were otherwise at risk of developing POD.

POSTOPERATIVE
Polypharmacy

Postoperatively, patients, especially elderly patients, are often on multiple medications, predisposing the patient to adverse drug reactions. Drugs that are associated with the highest incidence of adverse reactions include opioids, benzodiazepines, anti-parkinsonism drugs, anti-hypertensives, psychotropics, and cardiac medications. Additionally, long-term use of benzodiazepines has been associated with the development of POD, especially in the case of withdrawal of benzodiazepines and other sedative-hypnotic medications.[45]

Opioids are drugs which mimic the effects of endogenous opioid peptides on the various opioid receptors (μ-, δ-, κ-opioid receptors) and activate potassium channels postsynaptically or suppress calcium channels presynaptically and postsynaptically. These actions reduce excitability and impulses to the central and peripheral nervous system and provide analgesic effects. These effects may lead to sedation and signs of hypoactive delirium in postoperative patients. Additionally, patients may experience cognitive impairment and hallucinations if they receive an excessive amount of the specific opioid.[88]

Benzodiazepines are a class of drugs with a high affinity for the GABA receptor within the central nervous system. A strong correlation with the development of POD was demonstrated by Marcantonio and colleagues.[45,58] These findings have been confirmed by others including Pandharipande and colleagues.[45,58,89] The investigators performed a cohort study and evaluated 198 mechanically ventilated patients to determine the likelihood of transition to delirium due to sedative and analgesic administration during the previous 24 hours. Within this study, lorazepam was found to be an independent risk factor for delirium with an odds ratio of 1.2 (95% CI, 1.1–1.4; P = .003).[89]

Propofol is an intravenous anesthetic agent that has gained popularity in anesthesia. This enthusiasm has led to increased use in the ICU because of the rapid onset and short half-life. These features allow the anesthesiologist to quickly sedate a patient who may be mechanically ventilated and allow a patient to quickly wake up when the propofol is discontinued for serial examinations as may be necessary in head-injured patients. Propofol affects the GABA pathway in several different capacities, both presynaptic and postsynaptic. It increases the GABA binding, as well as GABA uptake and release, and exerts its effects on the $GABA_A$ receptor. As described above, these effects on the GABA pathway results in inhibitory effects on the central nervous system that lead to sedative and anxiolytic consequences.[90]

Alcohol Withdrawal

Alcohol is the most commonly abused drug in the world and has a significant impact on perioperative outcomes. Patients classified as alcohol abusers (defined in the *DSM-IV-TR* as those who drink more than five drinks [60 g ethanol] daily for a protracted period of time) have significantly increased morbidity compared with those who drink less.[1] Withdrawal from alcohol abuse encompasses a wide range of symptoms ranging from anxiety to delirium tremens (DTs), also known as alcohol withdrawal syndrome (AWS). Up to 25% of alcohol abusers develop AWS. Morbidity relates to 50% longer hospital stay and poorer 3-month postoperative results.[91] With appropriate preventive measures and effective treatment, morbidity and mortality may be significantly reduced.

Prevention of AWS begins in the preoperative period with screening for high-risk patients. Questionnaires such as the CAGE, a mnemonic for attempts to cut back on alcohol intake, feeling annoyed by criticism about drinking, guilt about drinking and the use of alcohol as an eye opener, is commonly used to identify those patients at high-risk for AWS. Those patients identified to be at risk for AWS may be advised to stop drinking preoperatively.[91] A randomized, controlled trial by Tonnesen and colleagues[92] demonstrated that those who abstained from alcohol for 1 month before elective colorectal surgery had fewer postoperative complications (74% in drinkers vs 31% in those who abstained). Despite recommendations of abstinence, patients may continue to drink and have a significant risk of developing POD.

Patients who develop AWS usually develop symptoms within the first several hours to days postoperatively. The timing of symptoms is related to many factors, including the amount consumed, previous withdrawal events, and associated medical conditions. First symptoms may be seen as early as 5 after the alcoholic beverage consumed, peak in 48 to 72 hours, and subside by day 7. Symptoms include tachycardia, hypertension, diaphoresis, tremors, insomnia, hallucinations (10%–25% of hospitalized patients with a history of chronic alcohol use), nausea and vomiting, psychomotor agitation, anxiety, and seizures.[91]

Successful treatment of DTs is multifactorial requiring behavioral, nutritional, and pharmacologic support. Benzodiazepines are the mainstay of pharmacologic treatment to control symptoms and prevent seizures. Benzodiazepines act on the GABA receptors and control hyperactivity of the autonomic system. Beta-blockers and clonidine are used to reduce the autonomic signs of alcohol withdrawal. Other pharmacologic strategies include propofol (intubated patients), valproic acid, barbiturates, phenytoin, and intravenous or enteric ethanol.[91]

Benzodiazepines remain the drug class of choice for the treatment of DTs. Within this class of medications are several suitable options based on the clinical situation. The physician may prefer to use a shorter acting drug in the elderly population or in postoperative patients to reduce the likelihood of oversedation. Diazepam, a longer acting option, may be beneficial in the prevention of seizures. Additionally, because of the longer duration of action there may be fewer breakthrough symptoms and a smoother withdrawal period.[93] Benzodiazepines must be given at doses high enough to overcome the autonomic hyperactivity that patients experience. Those going through alcohol withdrawal must be observed closely and the dosages adjusted accordingly. Traditionally, fixed dosing schedules were used to control the symptoms of alcohol withdrawal. However, a "symptom triggered" strategy proposed by Saitz and colleagues[94] has proven effective and has become the preferred method by which to control symptoms of alcohol withdrawal. This protocol requires frequent assessment of the patient using a validated and reliable tool such as the revised clinical institute withdrawal assessment for alcohol scale (CIWA-Ar) scale (**Fig. 1**). The patient receives a dose of a benzodiazepine when the CIWA-Ar score is eight or greater. Patients who were dosed on an as-needed basis based on symptoms received a smaller amount of benzodiazepine (100 mg of a benzodiazepine, specifically chlordiazepine, for "symptom triggered" vs 425 mg for the "scheduled" group, $P<.001$) for a shorter period (9 hours) compared with those on a fixed dosing schedule (68 hours); $P<.001$.

Sleep Deprivation

Sleep deprivation and delirium share many of the same symptoms and they considered related, especially in the ICU. The effects of sleep deprivation are magnified in elderly patients. Sleep in the ICU is often fragmented along with disruption of the sleep-wake cycle because of environmental factors such as the persistent lighting and noise in the ICU that affect the sleep-wake cycle. Sleep is described in distinct stages. Light sleep is characterized as stages I and II. Rapid eye movement sleep and deep sleep or delta sleep (stages III and IV) follow. The sleep-wake cycle is affected by the circadian rhythm that is controlled by the suprachiasmatic nucleus within the hypothalamus. The sleep-wake cycle may be abolished in the ICU setting owing to the environmental factors as well as neurochemical alterations, such as melatonin from the pineal gland, which maintains the circadian rhythm and sleep-wake cycles. The effects of sleep deprivation include inattention, fluctuating mental status, and cognitive dysfunction. Sleep deprivation is most similar to hypoactive delirium in the most common symptoms of drowsiness and impaired cognition.[95,96]

Sleep deprivation and delirium have been shown to affect the same areas of the brain, including the prefrontal cortex, and basal ganglia. The compromise of these areas of the brain results in disturbances of the associated neurotransmitters such as the cholinergic pathway and dopaminergic stimulation, which leads to signs of delirium. The temporal effects of these disturbances may be devastating as they have been found to last, months or years after recovery from critical illness.[96–98]

The relationship between sleep deprivation and delirium remains controversial. One must consider whether sleep deprivation causes delirium or vice versa. Sleep deprivation may be a risk factor for the development of delirium. Many studies have set out to answer this question, some with contradictory results. Harrell and colleagues[99] and Johns and colleagues[100] each studied populations of patients after cardiac surgery and concluded that patients were sleep deprived due because they were delirious.[54]

Patient: _____ Date: _____ Time: _____:_____

Pulse or heart rate, taken for one minute: _____ Blood pressure: _____/_____

Nausea and vomiting. Ask "Do you feel sick to your stomach? Have you vomited?"
Observation:
0—No nausea and no vomiting
1—Mild nausea with no vomiting
2—
3—
4—Intermittent nausea with dry heaves
5—
6—
7—Constant nausea, frequent dry heaves, and vomiting

Tremor. Ask patient to extend arms and spread fingers apart.
Observation:
0—No tremor
1—Tremor not visible but can be felt, fingertip to fingertip
2—
3—
4—Moderate tremor with arms extended
5—
6—
7—Severe tremor, even with arms not extended

Paroxysmal sweats
Observation:
0—No sweat visible
1—Barely perceptible sweating; palms moist
2—
3—
4—Beads of sweat obvious on forehead
5—
6—
7—Drenching sweats

Anxiety. Ask "Do you feel nervous?"
Observation:
0—No anxiety (at ease)
1—Mildly anxious
2—
3—
4—Moderately anxious or guarded, so anxiety is inferred
5—
6—
7—Equivalent to acute panic states as occur in severe delirium or acute schizophrenic reactions

Agitation
Observation:
0—Normal activity
1—Somewhat more than normal activity
2—
3—
4—Moderately fidgety and restless
5—
6—
7—Paces back and forth during most of the interview or constantly thrashes about

Tactile disturbances. Ask "Do you have you any itching, pins-and-needles sensations, burning, or numbness, or do you feel like bugs are crawling on or under your skin?"
Observation:
0—None
1—Very mild itching, pins-and-needles sensation, burning, or numbness
2—Mild itching, pins-and-needles sensation, burning, or numbness
3—Moderate itching, pins-and-needles sensation, burning, or numbness
4—Moderately severe hallucinations
5—Severe hallucinations
6—Extremely severe hallucinations
7—Continuous hallucinations

Auditory disturbances. Ask "Are you more aware of sounds around you? Are they harsh? Do they frighten you? Are you hearing anything that is disturbing to you? Are you hearing things you know are not there?"
Observation:
0—Not present
1—Very mild harshness or ability to frighten
2—Mild harshness or ability to frighten
3—Moderate harshness or ability to frighten
4—Moderately severe hallucinations
5—Severe hallucinations
6—Extremely severe hallucinations
7—Continuous hallucinations

Visual disturbances. Ask "Does the light appear to be too bright? Is its color different? Does it hurt your eyes? Are you seeing anything that is disturbing to you? Are you seeing things you know are not there?"
Observation:
0—Not present
1—Very mild sensitivity
2—Mild sensitivity
3—Moderate sensitivity
4—Moderately severe hallucinations
5—Severe hallucinations
6—Extremely severe hallucinations
7—Continuous hallucinations

Headache, fullness in head. Ask "Does your head feel different? Does it feel like there is a band around your head?"
Do not rate for dizziness or lightheadedness; otherwise, rate severity
0—Not present
1—Very mild
2—Mild
3—Moderate
4—Moderately severe
5—Severe
6—Very severe
7—Extremely severe

Orientation and clouding of sensorium. Ask "What day is this? Where are you? Who am I?"
Observation:
0—Orientated and can do serial additions
1—Cannot do serial additions or is uncertain about date
2—Date disorientation by no more than two calendar days
3—Date disorientation by more than two calendar days
4—Disorientated for place and/or person

Total score: _____ (maximum = 67)   Rater's initials _____

Fig. 1. CIWA-Ar (*From* Sullivan JT, Sykora K, Schneiderman J, et al. Assessment of alcohol withdrawal: the revised clinical institute withdrawal assessment for alcohol scale (CIWA-Ar). Br J Addict 1989;84(11):1353–7. This scale is not copyrighted and may be used freely).

Yet, multiple other studies have demonstrated that sleep deprivation was not a risk factor leading to delirium.[54,75] However, other investigators suggest that sleep-deprived patients are more likely to develop delirium. Helton and colleagues[101] studied 62 patients from medical and surgical ICUs and correlated the patients' sleep deprivation with development of mental status changes. It was concluded that mental status changes were more frequent in the sleep-deprived patients. To optimize patient care, further studies are required to better understand the dynamics between sleep and delirium.

PREVENTION AND TREATMENT

The prevention of delirium should be one major focus of patient care to reduce the frequency and inherent complications of delirium. Due to the multifactorial nature of delirium, approaches which include strategies from multiple disciplines have been shown to be most effective in its prevention. This was best demonstrated in the Yale Delirium Prevention Trial[102] that targeted prevention strategies toward six risk factors (see later discussion). Another group of investigators demonstrated the effectiveness of multifactorial strategy in patients suffering from hip fractures. This randomized, controlled, clinical trial showed that intervention of 10 specific domains was effective in reducing delirium in this population (**Box 4**).[4,103]

Once POD has been identified, the underlying cause must be determined and addressed. Complications such as infection (pneumonia, urinary tract infection), sepsis, hypoxia, and myocardial infarction may cause POD and must be identified and properly treated. To identify and treat the underlying cause, a comprehensive work up, including history of present illness, medical and medication history, physical examination, and laboratory tests (chemistry panels, blood, and urine cultures) must be completed. Computed tomography and other appropriate imaging should be undertaken if an adequate history is not obtainable or a complete neurologic examination cannot be completed to evaluate for organic causes of the change in mental status. The medication history must be comprehensive because medications are the most common iatrogenic cause of POD. Sedative-hypnotics, narcotics, and any medication with anticholinergic effects must be identified and discontinued from the patient's formulary.

Multidisciplinary Intervention

In most cases, the development of delirium is multifactorial with a number of risk factors coming into play. It has been demonstrated that, as the number of risk factors increases, so does the risk of delirium.[8,104] Inouye and colleagues[102] conducted a controlled clinical trial to prevent delirium by reducing risk factors for delirium. Within the study, standardized protocols for six of the major risk factors were established. The six risk factors included cognitive impairment, hearing impairment, visual impairment, sleep deprivation, immobility, and dehydration. This study demonstrated that with management of these risk factors the incidence of delirium in the intervention

---

Box 4
Ten targeted domains to reduce delirium

1. Oxygen delivery to the brain
2. Fluid and electrolyte balance
3. Appropriate pain management
4. Decreased use of psychoactive medications
5. Optimization of bowel and bladder function
6. Nutritional support
7. Early mobilization
8. Prevention of postoperative complications
9. Appropriate environmental stimuli
10. Treatment of delirium symptoms

group was only 9.9% compared with 15% of the control group. Additionally, the total number of days of delirium and the number of episodes were significantly less in the intervention group. Therefore, a multifaceted approach to address the many risk factors associated with delirium has been shown to be beneficial. It also demonstrated that these interventions had no effect on the severity of delirium once it developed, pointing towards the fact that prevention of delirium is the preferred treatment strategy.[102]

Once delirium occurs, supportive care, including airway protection, fluid resuscitation, and optimizing nutritional status, are integral in the care of the delirious patient. Additionally, the prevention of complications associated with delirium should be paramount. Patients should be positioned and mobilized to prevent pressure ulceration and deep venous thrombosis. The use of physical restraints should be minimized.[45]

Nonpharmacologic management of patients with delirium should be the first line of treatment. One must ensure a calm, quiet environment. Clocks, calendars, and frequent reorientation by care providers should be used to help keep the patient oriented. Other nonpharmacologic methods to help manage delirium include the use of familiar family members, limiting room and staff changes, and minimizing nighttime disruptions to allow for uninterrupted sleep. The maintenance of normal sleep-wake cycles is critical. This may be accomplished by opening blinds and promoting wakefulness during the daylight hours and supplying a quiet, calm, and low-light environment during the evening. Additionally, patients should have access to personal eyeglasses and hearing aids to assist with communication and efforts at reorientation.[4]

Pharmacologic management of delirium may be prophylactic (to prevent the development of delirium) or therapeutic (after delirium has developed). Pharmacologic management should be reserved for those who are a danger to themselves or others, especially those who managed with mechanical ventilation or other life-supportive measures. Before psychotropic medications are administered to a patient suffering with delirium, the physician must rule out reversible causes of delirium such as hypoxia, infection or sepsis, hypoglycemia, metabolic derangements, and shock. The treatment of delirium with psychotropic medications must be individualized to minimize complications associated with these medications.[4]

Antipsychotics

When delirium requires pharmacologic support, haloperidol is typically the medication of choice. Haloperidol is an antipsychotic and its effectiveness has been demonstrated in multiple randomized controlled trials.[105] The downfall of intravenous haloperidol is the short half-life. Adverse effects of haloperidol include extrapyramidal symptoms and prolonged QT interval on electrocardiogram, and it should be avoided in patients with hepatic insufficiency and a history of neuroleptic malignant syndrome (**Table 1**).[4]

Atypical Antipsychotics

Atypical antipsychotic medications include risperidone, and olanzapine, which may be used to treat delirium. Only small, uncontrolled trials have evaluated the efficacy of these medications on delirium and have been associated with increased mortality in elderly patients with dementia. Atypical antipsychotics have similar adverse effects to those of haloperidol including extrapyramidal effects and prolongation of the QT interval (see **Table 1**).[4]

Table 1
Medications for the pharmacologic treatment of delirium

Drug Class	Representative Medications	Dosages	Mechanism of Action	Pitfalls
Benzodiazepines	Lorazepam Midazolam	0.5–1 mg as needed Lowest dose possible for effect	Bind Cl channel of GABA receptor, increase Cl channel opening, hyperpolarizes the cell, prevents nerve firing	May exacerbate delirium Paradoxic reaction Use sparingly Respiratory depression
Antipsychotics	Haloperidol	1–5 mg/h as needed Not to exceed 20 mg/24 h Note: elderly patients, low dose preferred	Antagonizes dopamine-mediated neurotransmission	Extra-pyramidal signs Prolongation of QTc (>25% of baseline or >500ms) Increased risk of arrhythmia in patients with cardiac disease Decreases seizure threshold Neuroleptic malignant syndrome
Atypical antipsychotics	Risperidone	0.5mg twice daily	Antagonist of 5-HT receptor and D2, D3, and D4 receptors	Extrapyramidal side effects, dizziness, hyperactivity or sedation
α2-Adrenoreceptor agonists	Dexmedetomidine	Parenteral formulation Loading bolus over 10–20 min Infusion and titrated to effect 0.2–0.6 μg/kg/h	Selective for alpha receptor, similar to clonidine but much higher affinity to alpha receptor	Hypotension in volume depleted patients Lacks amnestic effect, may require use with benzodiazepine with synergistic respiratory depression

Data from Inouye SK. Delirium in older persons. N Engl J Med 2006;354:1157.

Benzodiazepines

Benzodiazepines such as lorazepam should be reserved as alternative agents. These agents should be reserved for those with sedative and alcohol withdrawal. Especially in the elderly, these agents are associated with worsening and prolongation of delirium symptoms. Adverse events such as paradoxical excitement, over-sedation or respiratory depression may be associated with benzodiazepines (see **Table 1**).[4]

Alpha-2 Adrenoreceptor Agonists

In light of the effects of benzodiazepines and propofol on GABA receptors, new sedatives that are GABA receptor–sparing have shown promise in providing sedation and reducing the incidence of delirium and cognitive dysfunction. Dexmedetomidine, an α2-receptor agonist, has been shown to significantly reduce POD and duration of mechanical ventilation compared with midazolam.[106]

Dexmedetomidine, an α2-adrenoreceptor agonist provides sedation and anxiolysis without respiratory depression. The mechanism of action is focused on receptors of the locus ceruleus for the anxlolytic affects, whereas pain control is via spinal cord receptors. In a prospective, multi-institutional (multinational), double-blind, randomized study by Riker and colleagues[107] in 2009, it was demonstrated that there was no difference in time at goal sedation level based on the study protocol compared to midazolam. Patients who received dexmedetomidine experienced less delirium and spent less time on the ventilator versus those who received midazolam. Dexmedetomidine may provide a beneficial treatment strategy for patients on mechanical ventilation compared with benzodiazepines such as midazolam for the reasons described above (see **Table 1**).

Other Medications

Cholinesterase inhibitors may be administered with benefit in patients with delirium, even in cases of delirium not induced with drugs.[4,108,109] Other medication classes such as antidepressants may also be useful in the treatment of delirium; however, medications such as trazodone have been tested only in small, uncontrolled studies. Oversedation is the major downfall of these drugs (see **Table 1**).

Long-term Consequences of Delirium

Delirium is a significant problem in the postoperative period with an incidence as high as 81% and carries significant morbidity and mortality. Multiple studies have demonstrated worse outcomes for those with delirium compared with patients without delirium in both morbidity and mortality. Those who suffer from delirium experience significantly longer hospital lengths of stay with an average of 5 to 10 days longer than patients who were not delirious.[45,57,110,111]

Delirium offers significant long term morbidity as well, with the sequelae of delirium lasting beyond 6 months in some cases. One study demonstrated that only 14% of those with delirium are discharged at their baseline cognitive function. Other studies have confirmed these findings such as Levkoff and colleagues,[112] with only 4% reaching baseline cognitive function by discharge. Three-month resolution was 20% and 6-month resolution was nearly 18% in this same population.[45,113] Patients who suffer from delirium are more likely to require discharge to a skilled nursing facility or rehabilitation center rather than to their home. One study demonstrated that 16% of those with delirium are discharged to a facility rather than home compared with 3% of those who did not suffer from delirium.[45,114] A study by Robinson and colleagues[76] reinforces the findings of other investigators that these patients experience longer hospital stays, higher hospital costs, higher 30-day (9% vs 1%, $P = .045$) and 6-month mortality (20% vs 3%, $P = .001$), and many patients require institutionalization after hospital discharge.[110,115,116]

The economic implications of delirium are also significant with longer hospital and ICU stays. The cost of medical care in those who develop delirium is astronomic with figures similar to those from falls and diabetes. Specifically, it has been estimated that delirium accounts for 48% of all hospital days of care in patients over the age of 65 years. Additionally, delirium accounts for more than 17.5 million inpatient days and results in multibillion dollars worth of health care expenditures when the increased need for institutionalization and rehabilitation is taken into account.[102]

Mortality is also significantly increased in patients who suffer from delirium. Six-month mortality has been shown to be as high as 34% in delirious patients compared with 15% in non-delirious patients.[45,110] Ouimet and colleagues[117] demonstrated that delirium increased the risk of death when acute physiology and chronic health evaluation scores and patient age were considered. Those with delirium were more likely to die in the ICU (20% vs 10%, $P<.005$) compared to those who did not delirium. In-hospital mortality was also significantly higher at 31% in the delirious patients compared with 24% in patients without delirium, $P<.005$.

SUMMARY

Delirium is an acute alteration in attention and cognitive impairment and is a common feature of the postoperative period, especially in elderly patients. Delirium leads to increased morbidity and mortality and significant health care costs. Multiple factors such as age, medications, and specific biochemical changes have been proposed to predispose a patient to the development of delirium, which may manifest as hypoactive, hyperactive, or mixed forms. The physician must rule out and treat reversible medical causes of delirium such as infection, sepsis, hypoxia, and myocardial infarction. Various tools have been validated for the quick and accurate identification of delirium to ensure timely and effective multidisciplinary intervention and treatment. Delirium is a devastating complication in the hospitalized patient. The effects may be noticeable for weeks, months, or even longer after hospital discharge. A significant percentage of patients may require placement in skilled nursing facilities or similar care environments because of the long-lasting effects of delirium. For these reasons, the physician must be vigilant in the search for and identification of all forms of delirium and effectively treat the underlying medical condition and symptoms of delirium.

REFERENCES

1. Diagnostic and statistical manual of mental disorders. 4th edition. Arlington (VA): Association AP; 2004.
2. Michota FA, Frost SD. Perioperative management of the hospitalized patient. Med Clin North Am 2002;86:731.
3. Ansaloni L, Catena F, Chattat R, et al. Risk factors and incidence of postoperative delirium in elderly patients after elective and emergency surgery. Br J Surg 2010;97:273.
4. Inouye SK. Delirium in older persons. N Engl J Med 2006;354:1157.
5. Robinson TN, Raeburn CD, Tran ZV, et al. Motor subtypes of postoperative delirium in older adults. Arch Surg 2011;146:295.
6. Guenther U, Popp J, Koecher L, et al. Validity and reliability of the CAM-ICU flowsheet to diagnose delirium in surgical ICU patients. J Crit Care 2010; 25:144.

7. Peterson JF, Pun BT, Dittus RS, et al. Delirium and its motoric subtypes: a study of 614 critically ill patients. J Am Geriatr Soc 2006;54:479.

8. Inouye SK, Charpentier PA. Precipitating factors for delirium in hospitalized elderly persons. Predictive model and interrelationship with baseline vulnerability. JAMA 1996;275:852.

9. Gleason OC. Delirium. Am Fam Physician 2003;67:1027.

10. Burns A, Gallagley A, Byrne J. Delirium. J Neurol Neurosurg Psychiatry 2004;75:362.

11. Beresin EV. Delirium in the elderly. J Geriatr Psychiatry Neurol 1988;1:127.

12. Flacker JM, Cummings V, Mach JR Jr, et al. The association of serum anticholinergic activity with delirium in elderly medical patients. Am J Geriatr Psychiatry 1998;6:31.

13. Flacker JM, Wei JY. Endogenous anticholinergic substances may exist during acute illness in elderly medical patients. J Gerontol A Biol Sci Med Sci 2001;56:M353.

14. Golinger RC, Peet T, Tune LE. Association of elevated plasma anticholinergic activity with delirium in surgical patients. Am J Psychiatry 1987;144:1218.

15. Maldonado JR. Pathoetiological model of delirium: a comprehensive understanding of the neurobiology of delirium and an evidence-based approach to prevention and treatment. Crit Care Clin 2008;24:789.

16. Plaschke K, Thomas C, Engelhardt R, et al. Significant correlation between plasma and CSF anticholinergic activity in presurgical patients. Neurosci Lett 2007;417:16.

17. Trzepacz PT. Anticholinergic model for delirium. Semin Clin Neuropsychiatry 1996;1:294.

18. Trzepacz PT. Is there a final common neural pathway in delirium? Focus on acetylcholine and dopamine. Semin Clin Neuropsychiatry 2000;5:132.

19. Tune LE, Bylsma FW, Hilt DC. Anticholinergic delirium caused by topical homatropine ophthalmologic solution: confirmation by anticholinergic radioreceptor assay in two cases. J Neuropsychiatry Clin Neurosci 1992;4:195.

20. Gibson GE, Blass JP. Impaired synthesis of acetylcholine in brain accompanying mild hypoxia and hypoglycemia. J Neurochem 1976;27:37.

21. Gibson GE, Peterson C. Aging decreases oxidative metabolism and the release and synthesis of acetylcholine. J Neurochem 1981;37:978.

22. Gibson GE, Peterson C. Decreases in the release of acetylcholine in vitro with low oxygen. Biochem Pharmacol 1982;31:111.

23. Gibson GE, Peterson C, Sansone J. Decreases in amino acids and acetylcholine metabolism during hypoxia. J Neurochem 1981;37:192.

24. Mussi C, Ferrari R, Ascari S, et al. Importance of serum anticholinergic activity in the assessment of elderly patients with delirium. J Geriatr Psychiatry Neurol 1999;12:82.

25. Thomas RI, Cameron DJ, Fahs MC. A prospective study of delirium and prolonged hospital stay. Exploratory study. Arch Gen Psychiatry 1988;45:937.

26. Tune L, Coyle JT. Serum levels of anticholinergic drugs in treatment of acute extrapyramidal side effects. Arch Gen Psychiatry 1980;37:293.

27. Tune LE, Damlouji NF, Holland A, et al. Association of postoperative delirium with raised serum levels of anticholinergic drugs. Lancet 1981;2:651.

28. Mach JR Jr, Dysken MW, Kuskowski M, et al. Serum anticholinergic activity in hospitalized older persons with delirium: a preliminary study. J Am Geriatr Soc 1995;43:491.

29. Mulsant BH, Pollock BG, Kirshner M, et al. Serum anticholinergic activity in a community-based sample of older adults: relationship with cognitive performance. Arch Gen Psychiatry 2003;60:198.

30. Trzepacz PT, Leavitt M, Ciongoli K. An animal model for delirium. Psychosomatics 1992;33:404.
31. Fatranska M, Budai D, Oprsalova Z, et al. Acetylcholine and its enzymes in some brain areas of the rat under stress. Brain Res 1987;424:109.
32. Lipowski ZJ. Delirium (acute confusional states). JAMA 1987;258:1789.
33. Takayama H, Mizukawa K, Ota Z, et al. Regional responses of rat brain muscarinic cholinergic receptors to immobilization stress. Brain Res 1987;436:291.
34. Broadhurst C, Wilson K. Immunology of delirium: new opportunities for treatment and research. Br J Psychiatry 2001;179:288.
35. Cole MG. Delirium in elderly patients. Am J Geriatr Psychiatry 2004;12:7.
36. Bruera E, Pereira J. Acute neuropsychiatric findings in a patient receiving fentanyl for cancer pain. Pain 1997;69:199.
37. Kobayashi K, Higashima M, Mutou K, et al. Severe delirium due to basal forebrain vascular lesion and efficacy of donepezil. Prog Neuropsychopharmacol Biol Psychiatry 2004;28:1189.
38. Milusheva E, Sperlagh B, Kiss B, et al. Inhibitory effect of hypoxic condition on acetylcholine release is partly due to the effect of adenosine released from the tissue. Brain Res Bull 1990;24:369.
39. Tune L, Carr S, Cooper T, et al. Association of anticholinergic activity of prescribed medications with postoperative delirium. J Neuropsychiatry Clin Neurosci 1993;5:208.
40. Tune L, Carr S, Hoag E, et al. Anticholinergic effects of drugs commonly prescribed for the elderly: potential means for assessing risk of delirium. Am J Psychiatry 1992;149:1393.
41. Tune LE. Anticholinergic effects of medication in elderly patients. J Clin Psychiatry 2001;62(Suppl 21):11.
42. Tune LE. Serum anticholinergic activity levels and delirium in the elderly. Semin Clin Neuropsychiatry 2000;5:149.
43. Tune L, Folstein MF. Post-operative delirium. Adv Psychosom Med 1986;15:51.
44. Blazer DG 2nd, Federspiel CF, Ray WA, et al. The risk of anticholinergic toxicity in the elderly: a study of prescribing practices in two populations. J Gerontol 1983;38:31.
45. Maldonado JR. Delirium in the acute care setting: characteristics, diagnosis and treatment. Crit Care Clin 2008;24:657.
46. Centeno C, Sanz A, Bruera E. Delirium in advanced cancer patients. Palliat Med 2004;18:184.
47. Dubois MJ, Bergeron N, Dumont M, et al. Delirium in an intensive care unit: a study of risk factors. Intensive Care Med 2001;27:1297.
48. Inouye SK. Predisposing and precipitating factors for delirium in hospitalized older patients. Dement Geriatr Cogn Disord 1999;10:393.
49. Inouye SK, Schlesinger MJ, Lydon TJ. Delirium: a symptom of how hospital care is failing older persons and a window to improve quality of hospital care. Am J Med 1999;106:565.
50. Eisendrath SJ, Goldman B, Douglas J, et al. Meperidine-induced delirium. Am J Psychiatry 1987;144:1062.
51. Meuret P, Backman SB, Bonhomme V, et al. Physostigmine reverses propofol-induced unconsciousness and attenuation of the auditory steady state response and bispectral index in human volunteers. Anesthesiology 2000; 93:708.
52. Pain L, Jeltsch H, Lehmann O, et al. Central cholinergic depletion induced by 192 IgG-saporin alleviates the sedative effects of propofol in rats. Br J Anaesth 2000;85:869.

53. Wang Y, Kikuchi T, Sakai M, et al. Age-related modifications of effects of ketamine and propofol on rat hippocampal acetylcholine release studied by in vivo brain microdialysis. Acta Anaesthesiol Scand 2000;44:112.

54. Figueroa-Ramos MI, Arroyo-Novoa CM, Lee KA, et al. Sleep and delirium in ICU patients: a review of mechanisms and manifestations. Intensive Care Med 2009; 35:781.

55. Olofsson K, Alling C, Lundberg D, et al. Abolished circadian rhythm of melatonin secretion in sedated and artificially ventilated intensive care patients. Acta Anaesthesiol Scand 2004;48:679.

56. Shilo L, Dagan Y, Smorjik Y, et al. Patients in the intensive care unit suffer from severe lack of sleep associated with loss of normal melatonin secretion pattern. Am J Med Sci 1999;317:278.

57. Ely EW, Gautam S, Margolin R, et al. The impact of delirium in the intensive care unit on hospital length of stay. Intensive Care Med 2001;27:1892.

58. Marcantonio ER, Juarez G, Goldman L, et al. The relationship of postoperative delirium with psychoactive medications. JAMA 1994;272:1518.

59. Mlhic SJ, Harris RA. GABA and the GABAA receptor. Alcohol Health Res World 1997;21:127.

60. Tabakoff B, Hoffman PL. Alcohol addiction: an enigma among us. Neuron 1996; 16:909.

61. Shigeta H, Yasui A, Nimura Y, et al. Postoperative delirium and melatonin levels in elderly patients. Am J Surg 2001;182:449.

62. Meyer A. Outlines of examinations. New York: Bloomingdale Hospital Press; 1918.

63. Anthony JC, LeResche L, Niaz U, et al. Limits of the 'Mini-Mental State' as a screening test for dementia and delirium among hospital patients. Psychol Med 1982;12:397.

64. Dick JP, Guiloff RJ, Stewart A, et al. Mini-mental state examination in neurological patients. J Neurol Neurosurg Psychiatry 1984;47:496.

65. Fillenbaum GG, Heyman A, Wilkinson WE, et al. Comparison of two screening tests in Alzheimer's disease. The correlation and reliability of the Mini-Mental State Examination and the modified Blessed test. Arch Neurol 1987;44:924.

66. Mitrushina M, Satz P. Reliability and validity of the Mini-Mental State Exam in neurologically intact elderly. J Clin Psychol 1991;47:537.

67. Inouye SK, van Dyck CH, Alessi CA, et al. Clarifying confusion: the confusion assessment method. Ann Intern Med 1990;113:941–8.

68. Ely EW, Margolin R, Francis J, et al. Evaluation of delirium in critically ill patients: Validation of the Confusion Assessment Method for the Intensive Care Unit (CAM-ICU). Crit Care Med 2001;29(7):1370–9.

69. Hart RP, Levenson JL, Sessler CN, et al. Validation of a cognitive test for delirium in medical ICU patients. Psychosomatics 1996;37:533.

70. Hart RP, Best AM, Sessler CN, et al. Abbreviated cognitive test for delirium. J Psychosom Res 1997;43:417.

71. Ely EW, Inouye SK, Bernard GR, et al. Delirium in mechanically ventilated patients: validity and reliability of the confusion assessment method for the intensive care unit (CAM-ICU). JAMA 2001;286:2703.

72. Ely EW, Truman B, Shintani A, et al. Monitoring sedation status over time in ICU patients: reliability and validity of the Richmond Agitation-Sedation Scale (RASS). JAMA 2003;289:2983.

73. Teasdale G, Jennett B. Assessment of coma and impaired consciousness. A practical scale. Lancet 1974;2:81.

74. Marcantonio E, Ta T, Duthie E, et al. Delirium severity and psychomotor types: their relationship with outcomes after hip fracture repair. J Am Geriatr Soc 2002;50:850.
75. Dyer CB, Ashton CM, Teasdale TA. Postoperative delirium. A review of 80 primary data-collection studies. Arch Intern Med 1995;155:461.
76. Robinson TN, Raeburn CD, Tran ZV, et al. Postoperative delirium in the elderly: risk factors and outcomes. Ann Surg 2009;249:173.
77. Baker FM, Wiley C, Kokmen E, et al. Delirium episodes during the course of clinically diagnosed Alzheimer's disease. J Natl Med Assoc 1999;91:625.
78. Fick D, Foreman M. Consequences of not recognizing delirium superimposed on dementia in hospitalized elderly individuals. J Gerontol Nurs 2000;26:30.
79. McCusker J, Cole M, Dendukuri N, et al. Delirium in older medical inpatients and subsequent cognitive and functional status: a prospective study. CMAJ 2001; 165:575.
80. Rockwood K, Cosway S, Carver D, et al. The risk of dementia and death after delirium. Age Ageing 1999;28:551.
81. Marcantonio ER, Goldman L, Orav EJ, et al. The association of intraoperative factors with the development of postoperative delirium. Am J Med 1998;105:380.
82. Haan J, van Kleef JW, Bloem BR, et al. Cognitive function after spinal or general anesthesia for transurethral prostatectomy in elderly men. J Am Geriatr Soc 1991;39:596.
83. Jones MJ, Piggott SE, Vaughan RS, et al. Cognitive and functional competence after anaesthesia in patients aged over 60: controlled trial of general and regional anaesthesia for elective hip or knee replacement. BMJ 1990;300:1683.
84. Nielson WR, Gelb AW, Casey JE, et al. Long-term cognitive and social sequelae of general versus regional anesthesia during arthroplasty in the elderly. Anesthesiology 1990;73:1103.
85. Williams-Russo P, Sharrock NE, Mattis S, et al. Cognitive effects after epidural vs general anesthesia in older adults. A randomized trial. JAMA 1995;274:44.
86. Mason SE, Noel-Storr A, Ritchie CW. The impact of general and regional anesthesia on the incidence of post-operative cognitive dysfunction and post-operative delirium: a systematic review with meta-analysis. J Alzheimers Dis 2010;22(Suppl 3):67.
87. Slor CJ, de Jonghe JF, Vreeswijk R, et al. Anesthesia and postoperative delirium in older adults undergoing hip surgery. J Am Geriatr Soc 2011;59:1313.
88. Yennurajalingam S, Braiteh F, Bruera E. Pain and terminal delirium research in the elderly. Clin Geriatr Med 2005;21:93.
89. Pandharipande P, Shintani A, Peterson J, et al. Lorazepam is an independent risk factor for transitioning to delirium in intensive care unit patients. Anesthesiology 2006;104:21.
90. Trapani G, Altomare C, Liso G, et al. Propofol in anesthesia. Mechanism of action, structure-activity relationships, and drug delivery. Curr Med Chem 2000;7:249.
91. Chang PH, Steinberg MB. Alcohol withdrawal. Med Clin North Am 2001;85:1191.
92. Tonnesen H, Rosenberg J, Nielsen HJ, et al. Effect of preoperative abstinence on poor postoperative outcome in alcohol misusers: randomised controlled trial. BMJ 1999;318:1311.
93. Lohr RH. Treatment of alcohol withdrawal in hospitalized patients. Mayo Clin Proc 1995;70:777.
94. Saitz R, Mayo-Smith MF, Roberts MS, et al. Individualized treatment for alcohol withdrawal. A randomized double-blind controlled trial. JAMA 1994;272:519.

95. Durmer JS, Dinges DF. Neurocognitive consequences of sleep deprivation. Semin Neurol 2005;25:117.

96. Weinhouse GL, Schwab RJ, Watson PL, et al. Bench-to-bedside review: delirium in ICU patients - importance of sleep deprivation. Crit Care 2009;13:234.

97. Hopkins RO, Weaver LK, Pope D, et al. Neuropsychological sequelae and impaired health status in survivors of severe acute respiratory distress syndrome. Am J Respir Crit Care Med 1999;160:50.

98. Jackson JC, Hart RP, Gordon SM, et al. Six-month neuropsychological outcome of medical intensive care unit patients. Crit Care Med 2003;31:1226.

99. Harrell RG, Othmer E. Postcardiotomy confusion and sleep loss. J Clin Psychiatry 1987;48:445.

100. Johns MW, Large AA, Masterton JP, et al. Sleep and delirium after open heart surgery. Br J Surg 1974;61:377.

101. Helton MC, Gordon SH, Nunnery SL. The correlation between sleep deprivation and the intensive care unit syndrome. Heart Lung 1980;9:464.

102. Inouye SK, Bogardus ST Jr, Charpentier PA, et al. A multicomponent intervention to prevent delirium in hospitalized older patients. N Engl J Med 1999;340:669.

103. Marcantonio ER, Flacker JM, Wright RJ, et al. Reducing delirium after hip fracture: a randomized trial. J Am Geriatr Soc 2001;49:516.

104. Inouye SK, Viscoli CM, Horwitz RI, et al. A predictive model for delirium in hospitalized elderly medical patients based on admission characteristics. Ann Intern Med 1993;119:474.

105. Breitbart W, Marotta R, Platt MM, et al. A double-blind trial of haloperidol, chlorpromazine, and lorazepam in the treatment of delirium in hospitalized AIDS patients. Am J Psychiatry 1996;153:231.

106. Shehabi Y, Riker RR, Bokesch PM, et al. Delirium duration and mortality in lightly sedated, mechanically ventilated intensive care patients. Crit Care Med 2010; 38:2311.

107. Riker RR, Shehabi Y, Bokesch PM, et al. Dexmedetomidine vs midazolam for sedation of critically ill patients: a randomized trial. JAMA 2009;301:489.

108. Han L, McCusker J, Cole M, et al. Use of medications with anticholinergic effect predicts clinical severity of delirium symptoms in older medical inpatients. Arch Intern Med 2001;161:1099.

109. Roche V. Southwestern internal medicine conference. Etiology and management of delirium. Am J Med Sci 2003;325:20.

110. Ely EW, Shintani A, Truman B, et al. Delirium as a predictor of mortality in mechanically ventilated patients in the intensive care unit. JAMA 2004; 291:1753.

111. Francis J, Martin D, Kapoor WN. A prospective study of delirium in hospitalized elderly. JAMA 1990;263:1097.

112. Levkoff SE, Evans DA, Liptzin B, et al. Delirium: The occurence and persistence of symptoms among elderly hospitalized patients. Arch Intern Med 1992;152(2): 334–40.

113. Newman MF, Grocott HP, Mathew JP, et al. Report of the substudy assessing the impact of neurocognitive function on quality of life 5 years after cardiac surgery. Stroke 2001;32:2874.

114. O'Keeffe S, Lavan J. The prognostic significance of delirium in older hospital patients. J Am Geriatr Soc 1997;45:174.

115. Edelstein DM, Aharonoff GB, Karp A, et al. Effect of postoperative delirium on outcome after hip fracture. Clin Orthop Relat Res 2004;(422):195.

116. Marcantonio ER, Flacker JM, Michaels M, et al. Delirium is independently associated with poor functional recovery after hip fracture. J Am Geriatr Soc 2000;48:618.
117. Ouimet S, Kavanagh BP, Gottfried SB, et al. Incidence, risk factors and consequences of ICU delirium. Intensive Care Med 2007;33:66.

Rescue Therapies in the Surgical Patient

Samuel A. Tisherman, MD[a,b],*

KEYWORDS

- Acute respiratory failure • Extracorporeal life support
- Cardiac arrest • Therapeutic hypothermia • Stroke

Because of the significant physiologic changes that occur as a result of major operations, general anesthesia, and comorbid conditions, surgical patients are at high risk of developing acute complications. Patients can suddenly experience hypoxemia, shortness of breath, dysrhythmia, or hypotension. They may suddenly develop neurologic changes, including seizures. Clinicians need to be aware of the potential critical events that can occur in the perioperative period and be prepared to intervene in an expeditious and a potentially lifesaving manner.

MEDICAL EMERGENCY TEAMS

To rapidly respond to critical events in the hospital, medical emergency teams (METs) or rapid response teams (RRTs) have been developed.[1] The terminology is sometimes interchangeable, although some recommend using the latter term for teams that do not provide complete intensive care unit (ICU) level of care. Although the initial evaluation of a serious adverse event may suggest that it was acute in nature, frequently there are warning signs to suggest pending physiologic instability. Patient safety initiatives have focused on establishing a hospital culture in which all health care providers feel empowered to call for an MET or RRT any time they suspect significant changes in patient physiology. It has been difficult to consistently demonstrate improved outcomes from the use of METs, but there seems to be some benefit in preventing more serious events such as death after myocardial infarction.[2]

When organizing a rapid response system, a medical emergency needs to be defined first. One definition is when a patient's needs cannot be met by the resources available in the patient's current location. The specific needs vary but may include

Disclosure: Dr Tisherman is the coauthor of a patent entitled, "Emergency Preservation and Resuscitation Methods."
[a] Department of Critical Care Medicine, University of Pittsburgh, 638 Scaife Hall, 3550 Terrace Street, Pittsburgh, PA 15261, USA
[b] Department of Surgery, University of Pittsburgh, Pittsburgh, PA, USA
* Department of Critical Care Medicine, University of Pittsburgh, 638 Scaife Hall, 3550 Terrace Street, Pittsburgh, PA 15261.
E-mail address: tishermansa@upmc.edu

specific personnel or equipment as well as a specific frequency of observation. It is critical to define criteria that would trigger initiation of the rapid response. These criteria need to be well publicized within the system. The use of additional technological monitoring with appropriate alarms can certainly help in reducing the time lag between warning signs of an event and activation of the rescue team. In a surgical patient, the most common changes that should trigger a response include respiratory distress, hypoxemia, and hypotension.

The exact conduct and personnel involved in METs vary between institutions. The team should include the personnel and resources to provide airway management, vascular access, medication administration, and cardiac arrest resuscitation. Ideally, METs should be led by physicians with critical care training, although this optimum membership may be difficult to meet in all settings. The team should be able to provide a level of care similar to that in the ICU in any location within the hospital, at least for a brief period. Rapid triage of the patient to an appropriate location within the hospital should allow ongoing, optimal, and timely care. It is not infrequent, however, that METs require the expertise of specific physicians or services not part of the original response team. In some institutions, this need has been met by developing additional subspecialty teams that can be rapidly deployed to provide a specific service. One such example is a difficult or threatened airway team.

A difficult airway team might include an anesthesiologist, as presumably, the most able airway manager in the hospital; a surgeon skilled in emergency surgical airway techniques (eg, cricothyrotomy); and advanced airway management devices (eg, video laryngoscopy). A chest pain team might include high-level cardiology personnel who could rapidly assess the need for, and then facilitate, percutaneous coronary intervention. Similarly, a stroke team might include high-level neurology personnel who could rapidly evaluate an individual with a presumed stroke for potential lytic therapy or intravascular therapies, within the recommended time windows. These are all examples of serious adverse events that can occur in the perioperative period for which timely intervention by skilled specialists is critical.

RESPIRATORY EVENTS

Respiratory complications are common in surgical patients. Examples include pneumonia, aspiration pneumonia or pneumonitis, atelectasis from mucous plugging, and pulmonary embolism. Patients who underwent major surgical procedures and have significant comorbid conditions may have little physiologic reserve, allowing minor physiologic perturbations to cause life-threatening events very quickly. Because hypoxemia or inadequate ventilation (hypercarbia) can rapidly lead to metabolic acidosis and deterioration in the patient's physiology and, possibly, cardiac arrest, these are frequent indications for an MET response.

Airway management is the first priority. Most of the time, rapid institution of standard ICU management strategies suffice if tracheal intubation is needed. Relatively simple changes in technique, such as optimizing patient positioning, bimanual manipulation of the larynx with pressure on the tracheal cartilage (backward, upward, right, and posterior pressure), and choice of laryngoscope blade or appropriately sized endotracheal tube, can make a significant difference in successfully intubating the airway. Sometimes, specific rescue therapies are indicated.

For patients with a difficult airway,[3] the ability to apply rescue therapies within minutes is essential, which is why difficult airway teams are sometimes deployed. Recognition of the potential for, or existence of, a difficult airway is critical. Once recognized, the first step in management is to have the most experienced airway manager available, typically an anesthesiologist or a senior nurse anesthesiologist. The second step is to provide the airway manager with all the tools that might be necessary to secure the airway. A variety of laryngoscope blades and endotracheal tube sizes can be very helpful. For a patient who needs ventilatory assistance but for whom bag-valve-mask ventilation is ineffective, rescue devices might include the laryngeal mask airway or esophageal-tracheal devices such as the Combitube (Covidien, Boulder, CO, USA) or King Airway (King Systems, Noblesville, IN, USA). Rescue devices that assist in placing an endotracheal tube include a gum elastic bougie and video laryngoscope or bronchoscope. The third step is to have an expert available during placement of a surgical airway, typically a cricothyrotomy. The expert may be a senior surgical resident or an attending surgeon. The availability of such a person is critical for the management of a dislodged tracheostomy tube in a patient with a difficult airway. Deployment of a difficult airway team can decrease the need for an emergency surgical airway.[4]

Once the airway has been secured, patients may still have difficulty with oxygenation or ventilation despite administration of high levels of oxygen and increasing levels of airway pressure. Of utmost concern in this situation is the development of acute respiratory distress syndrome or preceding acute lung injury. Although there are no rescue therapies that have been proved to improve outcomes in these circumstances, several approaches have been used.[5]

Ventilation with pressure-controlled modes can sometimes improve pulmonary recruitment, while deleteriously limiting high peak, mean, and plateau airway pressures. Increasing the inspiratory to expiratory (I:E) ratio can further recruit alveoli. This approach has been taken to the extreme with airway pressure release ventilation, a modified form of continuous positive airway pressure that does not use traditional cyclic ventilation and, therefore, does not have a typical I:E ratio. More extraordinary is the use of high-frequency ventilation, which has taken many forms, including high-frequency positive pressure ventilation, high-frequency jet ventilation, and high-frequency oscillatory ventilation. These modes provide relatively constant mean airway pressure with very rapid shallow breaths, which may minimize ventilator-induced lung injury. This mode may be most useful during operative interventions on the airway or in patients with bronchopulmonary fistulas because it is generally accompanied by carbon dioxide (CO_2) retention, respiratory acidosis, and deep sedation of neuromuscular blockade to enable patient tolerance of the mode.

A separate approach to improving oxygenation is using inhaled nitric oxide (iNO). The desired physiologic effect of iNO is to cause local vasodilatation in lung zones that have the best ventilation, thus improving ventilation/perfusion matching, particularly in patients with pulmonary hypertension. Because of the extremely short half-life of iNO once in contact with hemoglobin, there are minimal systemic effects. To date, although improvements in oxygenation may be realized, no durable improvements in patient survival, ventilator-free days, or ICU length of stay have been achieved.

Ventilation/perfusion matching can also be improved with prone positioning, taking advantage of gravitational forces. When the patient is initially placed prone, blood flow increases to the well-recruited lung segments while the previously atelectatic/dependent lung segments are recruited. Routine shifting from supine to prone and back is then instituted. Care must be taken when placing a patient in this position to avoid the development of pressure injuries and tube dislodgement. Not all patients respond to prone positioning, and there is no consensus regarding the duration of prone positioning, the number of times per day a patient should be in the prone position, or the number of days for which prone positioning should be continued. Moreover, no improvement in outcome has been ascribed to prone positioning, relegating it to an adjunctive role in rescuing a patient from hypoxemic respiratory failure.

For patients with severe pulmonary disease localized to one lung, such as pneumonia, pulmonary contusion, or single-lung transplant, body positioning, with the good lung dependent, may improve blood flow to a well-ventilated lung while increasing recruitment of the diseased lung. Care should be taken to avoid soiling the good lung when the infected lung is placed in the nondependent position. In this circumstance, placement of a double-lumen endotracheal tube may allow differential ventilation of the lungs (ie, simultaneous independent lung ventilation) to optimize recruitment of the diseased lung while protecting the healthy lung.

Extracorporeal membrane oxygenation (ECMO) is perhaps the most risky and labor-intensive technique for improving oxygenation in a patient with refractory hypoxemia. ECMO involves venovenous or venoarterial cannulation, a pump, and an oxygenator to allow oxygenation of the blood and CO_2 removal. This technique has become the standard in the neonatal population. In adults, using ECMO has become more common with improved systems and experience, most recently with outbreaks of H1N1 influenza. Given the complexity of managing patients on ECMO, this intervention is best reserved for institutions with sufficient experience.

Although these rescue therapies may improve oxygenation in many patients with refractory hypoxemia, no mortality benefit has been demonstrated. Still, these therapies may be appropriate in selected patients.

CARDIAC EVENTS

Hypotension is a common perioperative complication. Multiple causes of shock need to be considered, including hypovolemia, sepsis, pulmonary embolism, and an acute coronary syndrome.[6] While completing diagnostic studies to determine the cause, the initial management includes ensuring adequate plasma volume resuscitation, supporting cardiac function with inotropes as needed, and judicious use of vasopressors. Specific causes of hypotension may require specific rescue therapies when the initial management is insufficient.

If the patient is hypovolemic, the first concern is bleeding. In addition to fluid and blood resuscitation, this condition may necessitate surgical intervention or perhaps embolization by interventional radiology. Coagulopathy (warfarin anticoagulation) including therapeutically induced platelet dysfunction (aspirin, clopidrogel) should be concomitantly addressed. A massive transfusion protocol that is jointly developed with transfusion medicine may be lifesaving in those with massive gastrointestinal tract hemorrhage, postoperative hemorrhage, or iatrogenically induced blood loss (eg, torn iliac vein during sheath introducer insertion).

Septic patients often require initial plasma volume resuscitation. Vasopressors should be added only when the patient remains hypotensive despite fluid resuscitation. Adequate cardiac performance should be ensured. Controlling the source of sepsis is critical. Although there is plenty of controversy, there may be a role for steroids in patients with absolute or relative adrenal insufficiency.[7] Activated protein C has been recently withdrawn from the market because of lack of efficacy.

Surgical patients are at high risk of pulmonary embolism because of hypercoagulable states, immobility, and vessel trauma. Diagnosis of pulmonary embolism in an unstable patient may be difficult. Bedside echocardiography can be helpful in these circumstances if it demonstrates right ventricular hypokinesia, asymmetric dilatation of the right ventricle versus the left ventricle, or strain. In addition to standard anticoagulation, rescue therapies for patients who remain hypotensive due to massive pulmonary embolism include intravenous thrombolytic therapy (there is no evidence that catheter-directed therapy is more effective or safer), catheter embolectomy, or operative embolectomy.[8] These therapies carry significant risks but may be lifesaving.

Acute coronary syndrome occurs in the perioperative period because of stress and, possibly, hypercoagulable states. Often, the issue is demand ischemia (eg, from hypoxemia or hypotension) in a patient with fixed coronary atherosclerotic disease. Rapid correction of the underlying process, plus beta-blockade if possible, is the main strategy for management in such circumstances. Occasionally, however, acute coronary occlusion occurs in the perioperative period. Standard management for an acute myocardial infarction, including the administration of oxygen, aspirin, beta-blockade, and anticoagulation, is indicated unless there is a significant contraindication. Therapies aimed at rapid revascularization should also be used if possible. However, based on the perceived risk of hemorrhage in the perioperative period, the use of lytic therapy is too risky in the immediate perioperative period. Cardiac catheterization, although the patient may still require antiplatelet therapy after stent placement, may be indicated. In many hospitals, a system is in place for rapid mobilization of the cardiology team to minimize the event-to-balloon time.[9] If patients develop profound cardiac dysfunction despite maximum medical therapy, mechanical circulatory support with an intra-aortic balloon pump in the short term, or a ventricular assist device for long-term support, may be necessary.

Patients may also suffer a cardiac arrest in the perioperative period. Traditionally, code teams respond to these events. Although, intuitively, use of METs decreases the incidence of cardiac arrests and/or improves outcomes, this has been difficult to prove.[10] Sudden events leading to cardiac arrest include pulmonary embolism and myocardial infarction. In addition, cardiac arrest may be the end result of deterioration because of multiple organ dysfunction, sepsis, or hemorrhage and may not be reversible. When sudden cardiac arrest occurs, standard advanced cardiac life support therapies should be initiated. Frequently, spontaneous circulation cannot be restored. Those who regain a pulse, however, may not rapidly recover neurologic function.[11] Randomized clinical trials in comatose survivors of out-of-hospital cardiac arrest with initial rhythms of ventricular fibrillation (VF)/ventricular tachycardia (VT) demonstrated improved neurologic outcomes and survival with therapeutic hypothermia. The American Heart Association now recommends that comatose survivors of out-of-hospital VF/VT be cooled to 32°C to 34°C for 12 to 24 hours. Therapeutic hypothermia should be considered for patients who suffer a cardiac arrest in hospital and for patients with other initial rhythms. Unless there is a clear contraindication, surgical patients should be treated similarly.

Postcardiac arrest care has, until recently, received little direct attention. It seems clear, however, that optimizing management could readily affect outcomes. To this end, the primary cause of cardiac arrest should be addressed rapidly with, for example, cardiac catheterization for coronary occlusion or thrombolytic therapy for acute pulmonary embolism. In addition, appropriate blood pressure and glucose control are recommended. Neurologic evaluation and prognostication, as well as referral for rehabilitation, are needed. Some institutions have organized teams to assist in the management of patients after cardiac arrest.

NEUROLOGIC EVENTS

Critically ill surgical patients frequently develop delirium in the perioperative period. This may be associated with medications (new agents or failure to continue existing agents), alcohol withdrawal, sepsis, and exacerbation of underlying comorbidities.

Optimal therapy for the delirious patient remains unclear. Therefore, strategies to prevent delirium, such as judicious use of sedatives and analgesics in patients at risk, optimizing environmental factors, and rapidly treating perioperative complications, should have a greater impact. Without focal findings on examination, computed tomography (CT) or magnetic resonance imaging of the head is rarely helpful.

More severe neurologic events, particularly stroke, can occur in the perioperative period.[12] Any patient who has a new focal neurologic deficit should undergo a stat CT of the head. If an ischemic stroke is suspected, administration of tissue plasminogen activator (tPA) should be considered if standard criteria are met and tPA use is not contraindicated. Some institutions have a designated stroke service that is prepared to quickly evaluate such patients. Urgent angiographic evaluation with possible stent placement is a new therapy that is used in some situations, particularly in patients for whom thrombolytic therapy is contraindicated, although these therapies are not mutually exclusive in select patients. It is clear that the more rapidly tissue oxygen delivery is re-established, the better is the postevent neurologic outcome.

SUMMARY

Critical events are common in the perioperative period. Rapid identification of patient deterioration and rapid deployment of a team prepared to manage the patient's condition may affect morbidity and mortality. When necessary, rescue therapies should be used for airway management, ventilatory and cardiovascular support, and severe neurologic deficits. Use of these rescue therapies may improve patient outcomes.

REFERENCES

1. DeVita MA, Bellomo R, Hillman K, et al. Findings of the first consensus conference on medical emergency teams. Crit Care Med 2006;34:2463–78.
2. Chen J, Bellomo R, Flabouris A, et al. The relationship between early emergency team calls and serious adverse events. Crit Care Med 2009;37:148–53.
3. Lavery GG, McCloskey BV. The difficult airway in adult critical care. Crit Care Med 2008;36:2163–73.
4. Berkow LC, Greenberg RS, Kan KH, et al. Need for emergency surgical airway reduced by a comprehensive difficult airway program. Anesth Analg 2009; 109(6):1860–9.
5. Pipeling MR, Fan E. Therapies for refractory hypoxemia in acute respiratory distress syndrome. JAMA 2010;304(22):2521–7.
6. Cheatham ML, Block EF, Promes JT, et al. Shock: an overview. In: Irwin R, Rippe J, editors. Irwin and Rippe's intensive care medicine. 6th edition. Philadelphia: Lippincott Williams & Wilkins; 2008. p. 1831–42.
7. Bernard GR, Vincent JL, Laterre PF, et al. Recombinant Human Protein C Worldwide Evaluation in Severe Sepsis (PROWESS) Study Group. Efficacy and safety of recombinant human activated protein C for severe sepsis. N Engl J Med 2001; 344(10):699–709.
8. Jaff MR, McMurtry MS, Archer SL, et al. Management of massive and submassive pulmonary embolism, iliofemoral deep vein thrombosis, and chronic thromboembolic pulmonary hypertension: a scientific statement from the American Heart Association. Circulation 2011;123:1788–830.
9. Nallamothu BK, Bradley EH, Krumholz HM. Time to treatment in primary percutaneous coronary intervention. N Engl J Med 2007;357:1631–8.
10. Hillman K, Chen J, Cretikos M, et al. Introduction of the medical emergency team (MET) system: a cluster-randomised controlled trial. Lancet 2005;365:2091–7.

11. Peberdy MA, Callaway CW, Neumar RW, et al. Part 9: post-cardiac arrest care: 2010 American Heart Association Guidelines for Cardiopulmonary Resuscitation and Emergency Cardiovascular Care. Circulation 2010;122:S768–86.
12. Lukovits TG, Goddeau RP. Critical care of patients with acute ischemic and hemorrhagic stroke: update on recent evidence and international guidelines. Chest 2011;139(3):694–700.

The American College of Surgeons Trauma Quality Improvement Program

Avery B. Nathens, MD, PhD[a,b],*, H. Gill Cryer, MD[c],
John Fildes, MD[d,e]

KEYWORDS

• ACS TQIP • Benchmarking • TRISS

The American College of Surgeons Trauma Quality Improvement Program (ACS TQIP) is a recent addition to the many quality improvement collaboratives that have been established in surgery. On the background of a well-established trauma center and its performance improvement activities, ACS TQIP offers the potential to further advance trauma care and offers participating centers the opportunity to better understand their strengths and areas for improvement. The rationale for ACS TQIP's development, implementation challenges, and potential for advancing the quality of trauma care are described.

WHY EVOLVE? A HISTORY OF TRAUMA PERFORMANCE IMPROVEMENT AND A PLACE FOR ACS TQIP

Continuous quality improvement is an integral component of trauma center care. This striving for high-quality care is complex, given the nuances in defining quality. In 1966, Avedis Donabedian,[1] the renowned public health pioneer, described 3 distinct aspects of quality in health care: outcome, process, and structure. Outcome

---

[a] Department of Surgery, St. Michael's Hospital, University of Toronto, 30 Bond Street, Toronto M5B 1W8, Canada
[b] American College of Surgeons Trauma Quality Improvement Program, American College of Surgeons, ACS TQIP, 633 North St Clair Street 26th Floor, Chicago, IL 60611, USA
[c] Division of General Surgery, University of California-Los Angeles, UCLA Medical Center, 200 UCLA Medical Plaza, Suite 214 Los Angeles, CA 90095, USA
[d] Division of Trauma & Critical Care, Department of Surgery, University of Nevada School of Medicine, 2040 West Charleston Boulevard, Suite 301, Las Vegas, NV 89102, USA
[e] American College of Surgeons Committee on Trauma, American College of Surgeons, 633 North St Clair Street, Chicago, IL 60611, USA
* Corresponding author. American College of Surgeons, ACS TQIP, 633 North St Clair Street 26th Floor, Chicago, IL 60611.
E-mail address: abnathens@gmail.com

Surg Clin N Am 92 (2012) 441–454
doi:10.1016/j.suc.2012.01.003
0039-6109/12/$ – see front matter © 2012 Elsevier Inc. All rights reserved.

measures were challenging as a sole indicator of quality, given that in many cases outcomes might not be modifiable. Alternatively, "a particular outcome might be irrelevant, as when survival is chosen as a criterion of success in a situation which is not fatal but likely to produce suboptimal health,[1]" a challenge in reports from the Trauma Quality Improvement Program (TQIP) and in other literature pertaining to outcomes following severe traumatic brain injury.[2]

Donabedian[1] suggested that given the limitations associated with outcome assessment, it might be more meaningful to examine the process of care itself. He justified the use of process evaluation by the assumption that knowledge of whether medicine was properly practiced is important. If so, then quality care was delivered. He described a third approach to quality assessment, focusing on not the process, but the setting in which the care was provided or the structure.[1] The structure is concerned primarily with the adequacy of facilities and equipment; the qualifications of medical staff and their organization; the administrative structure and operations of programs and institutions providing care; and fiscal organization. The underlying assumption focusing on structure is that given the proper resources, good medical care will follow. Furthermore, structure is simple and deals with information that is relatively concrete and accessible. Unfortunately, this paradigm assumes that there is a relationship between structure, process, and outcome.

Structure, Process, and Outcome in the Context of Injury Care

In the context of injury care, measures of structure, process, and outcome are key elements of quality and have been recognized as such since the beginning of the trauma center verification process. In 1976, the ACS Committee on Trauma published "Optimal Hospital Resource for Care of the Seriously Injured," which described the general requirements for a trauma center.[3] By 1987, updates to this document outlined key structures required to provide high-quality care to the injured patient.[4] There was less focus on process and outcome. However, a multidisciplinary performance improvement process with a registry and a process for reviewing care delivery and outcomes were built into the structure. Appreciating the challenges in evaluating process and outcome, the Committee on Trauma provided assurances that the process and the outcome would be evaluated internally on an ongoing basis, while the integrity of this process was assured through the verification process.

The resultant trauma center performance improvement programs borne of these requirements served injured patients very well. Several processes of care believed to be important to outcome were evaluated routinely using a variety of audit filters that served to identify cases requiring review. More recent evidence suggested that these easily captured filters might not necessarily identify opportunities for improvement because outcomes among patients meeting filter criteria are not necessarily poor.[5,6] Reviews (both structured and unstructured) of sentinel events, mortality, and morbidity allowed centers to identify opportunities for improvement. The registry made it possible to routinely assess indicators that might call for a more focused review if the incidence of a particular event was greater than in previous years. This approach assured that a center's performance was consistent over time, but raised questions as to whether consistency is a high enough goal for which to strive.

Assessing outcomes objectively was challenging, but the introduction of the Trauma Score–Injury Severity Score (TRISS) allowed centers to identify patients with unexpected outcomes.[7] TRISS provides statistical comparisons of actual and expected numbers of survivors for each institution, and uses a regression model based on age ($\leq$54, >54), mechanism of injury (blunt vs penetrating), Injury Severity Score (ISS), and the Revised Trauma Score (comprising the Glasgow coma scale [GCS], systolic blood pressure, and respiratory rate). Regression coefficients for TRISS were widely disseminated and used. Although this is one method of evaluating performance, the regression coefficients, and thus the probabilities of survival, are those estimated from the Major Trauma Outcomes Study and so reflect expected outcomes over 1982 to 1987,[8] not the outcomes with contemporary trauma care. In addition, the injured population has changed significantly, with a greater number of comorbidities and a broader age distribution than in the 1980s. Clearly, a 55-year-old patient differs markedly from an 85-year-old patient with the same injuries. Using TRISS, these patients would have the same estimated probability of survival. If the quality of trauma care was to evolve, a higher bar than care provided in 1982 and a means of identifying centers that were not only consistent but also at the leading age of trauma care are needed.

External Benchmarking and Striving for Best in Class: the Next Stage of Trauma Performance Improvement

ACS TQIP, through the reports provided to participating centers, allows centers to compare their processes and outcomes to their peer centers. This external benchmarking provides an opportunity to advance the care of injured patients. Broadly defined, benchmarking is a systematic comparison of structure, processes, or outcomes of similar organizations, used to identify the best practices for the purposes of continuous quality improvement.[9] External benchmarking compares performance between organizations, provides more appropriate information about whether or how much of a performance issue an organization might have, and offers information about realistic goals for improving performance. If a peer organization can perform at a certain level, then that level is likely achievable in one's own institution.

External benchmarking takes quality improvement to a higher level. In most circumstances, we believe that our performance is equal to (or better than) our peer institutions. If a benchmarking exercise shows that this is not the case, it provides an opportunity to better focus performance improvement efforts. It also indicates how to improve, so long as the benchmarking exercise identifies who has achieved superior results. This second point is only advantageous if the exercise, whether it is a regional or national collaborative, enables networking between centers.

External benchmarking provides insights into the unwitting innovators. Centers' practices evolve over time in response to internal and external pressures and resources, case mix, and practitioners' interests. In time, practices might diverge from the average center. If the practice divergence provides an advantage, this advantage is likely to go unnoticed. The variability in outcomes (or processes) becomes evident through external benchmarking, leading to an exploration of the underlying practices that provide this advantage. External benchmarking capitalizes on the variability to identify best practices, only a fraction of which might be identified through other means. It provides opportunities to test ideas for further evaluation in the form of before-and-after studies or randomized controlled trials.

A CASE FOR ACS TQIP

The ACS TQIP was conceived in 2008 through a small working group assembled by the ACS Committee on Trauma. Its goal was to build on the foundations and infrastructure of trauma performance improvement as laid out in the ACS Optimal Resources Guide for Care of the Injured Patient and by the Committee on Trauma Subcommittees (Performance Improvement and Patient Safety, National Trauma Data Bank, Verification), local performance improvement activities, and national initiatives such as the Society of Trauma Nurses' Trauma Outcomes and Performance Improvement Course. The goal was to enable transformational change in trauma quality improvement.

The impetus for change came from the accruing evidence of the effectiveness of large national collaboratives that were based on (1) standardized data, (2) feedback to centers, and (3) a network that would allow for the sharing of challenges and best practices (**Fig. 1**). For example, prompted by a 1986 congressional mandate, the Veterans Health Administration (VHA) conducted the National Veterans Administration Surgical Risk Study (NVASRS), beginning in 1991, with the aim of developing and validating risk-adjustment models for the prediction of surgical outcome and the comparative assessment of the quality of surgical care among multiple facilities. NVASRS provided the critical tools necessary to monitor surgical outcomes and provide feedback to centers. Based on this foundation, the National Veterans Administration Surgical Quality Improvement Program (NSQIP) was established in 1994 with the goal of monitoring and improving the quality of surgical care in the VHA. The VA NSQIP was quite successful, with a reported 9% reduction in mortality and 30% reduction in morbidity over a 3-year period.[10]

Given the success of VA NSQIP, expansion began into the private sector as a pilot in 1998.[11] The ACS then received funding from the Agency for Healthcare Research and Quality (AHRQ) through a patient safety grant in 2001. This initiative supported the participation of 14 private sector hospitals funded by the AHRQ as well as 4

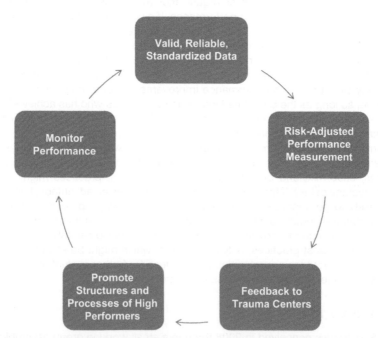

Fig. 1. The conceptual framework of continuous quality improvement underlying ACS TQIP and other quality collaboratives. High-quality data provide the opportunity to provide valid risk-adjusted performance measures back to centers. These institutions then review their performance in the context of their environment and seek areas to improve, if necessary relying on strategies used by high-performing centers. Performance is monitored and the loop continues.

community hospitals funded by the Partners Healthcare Corporation of Massachusetts.[12] Significant improvements in morbidity and mortality between 2001 and 2004 in this small program prompted the ACS to establish ACS NSQIP in 2004. A review of 3 years' experience with ACS NSQIP demonstrated that two-thirds of hospitals had significant improvements in mortality and 80% had improved their complication rates.[13] The greatest improvements were evident in the worst-performing hospitals, but high-performing centers also demonstrated improvement.

FROM ACS NSQIP TO TQIP

Simply incorporating trauma patients into NSQIP was not possible. ACS NSQIP had created a data infrastructure where none previously existed. In addition, it required a well-trained surgical clinical reviewer to collect and submit data. By contrast, each trauma center had a trauma registry, a team of registrars to collect the data, and a means of aggregating these data through the National Trauma Data Bank. To avoid creating a parallel data infrastructure and costly duplication, it was decided to use the existing infrastructure and work toward data standardization. This decision moved the process forward rapidly to allow the development of a 2-year pilot study involving 23 level 1 and level 2 trauma centers. This pilot study provided risk-adjusted outcomes for all patients with an ISS of 9 or more in the participating centers. To better understand opportunities for improvement, ACS TQIP also provided outcomes separately for patients injured through penetrating mechanisms, those with multisystem blunt trauma, and those with severe single-system injuries. This work confirmed that there was substantial variability across similarly designated centers, and a center that was high-performing for one patient population might very well have room for improvement for another patient population.[14,15]

CHALLENGES TO THE DEVELOPMENT AND IMPLEMENTATION OF ACS TQIP

To be successful, a large national collaborative requires interested participants. The success of ACS NSQIP and the long-standing interest in performance improvement in the trauma community assured that there was a place for ACS TQIP. However, the 2 fundamental challenges in moving forward related to data quality and risk adjustment to address differences in case mix across centers. Each of these challenges and solutions are now described.

Data Standardization and Quality

Trauma registries are critical structural components of trauma centers, and are essential to injury surveillance and performance improvement activities. The first hospital registry was developed in Chicago as early as 1969, which ultimately expanded as a statewide registry by 1971.[16] The use of registries expanded significantly over the next several years, and registries were often developed by interested local experts with some expertise in database design. The database fields incorporated into the registries were those that were thought to be important or of interest to a particular center. This approach addressed local performance improvement needs and served the injury community extremely well, with a proliferation of publications on injury and injury care in the wake of the recognition of injury as a disease worthy of study.[17] Over time, several registry vendors entered the market, all of whom offered user-friendly features related to data entry, injury coding, report writing, and customizable fields. Each registry evolved based on local needs and served a unique role in the trauma center, becoming a registry that other surgical (or medical) services often looked on with curiosity and envy.

By 2006, with each registry evolving based on local needs, the extent of variation across registries was extraordinary.[18] Inclusion criteria were inconsistent, with states variably requiring inclusion of drowning victims, differing minimum length of hospital stay, deaths in the emergency department (ED) (or deaths on arrival), and same-level falls. There was even variation in the definition of inclusion criteria, with 13 different definitions across states for same-level falls. This variability in case ascertainment posed problems in comparing outcomes across centers. For example, centers including elderly patients with isolated hip fractures tended to have lower risk-adjusted mortality than centers that did not include such patients.[19] This lower risk-adjusted mortality was no longer evident if this patient population was excluded from the analysis, which shows the challenge in risk adjustment when there is no overlap in selected patient populations across centers.

Different definitions and guidelines for coding also posed challenges. For example, across states there were 11 different coding conventions for recording of injury time when it was unavailable, and many variations on what constituted the ED GCS score, with 15 states requiring the initial score, 8 states requiring the initial and the last, 1 state the worst, 1 state the best, and another state the initial and worst. Injury coding in the context of a vignette also varied across registrars. Together, this lack of standardization limited any assurance that comparisons across centers were valid.

A means of responding to these challenges came with the development of the National Trauma Data Standard (NTDS). The NTDS version 1.0 was disseminated in 2006, after stakeholders representing physician professional organizations, state trauma program managers, trauma registry vendors, and others in the trauma community sought to identify the most critical core elements for a trauma registry. The NTDS also provided uniform field definitions, a source hierarchy outlining where the elements of the field should be found in the medical record, and the extensible markup language for each field, assuring a standard means of structuring, storing, and transporting information across platforms. Data submission from each center also required each record to pass through a validator with different error levels. This validator provided edit and logic checks to limit the potential for missing and out-of-range data. The introduction of the NTDS was the enabler, providing the first opportunity to compare data across centers.

There remain some challenges to data quality despite the NTDS. For example, the authors explored how deaths in the ED were classified among participating TQIP centers in 2009 using the NTDS field "ED death." Options in NTDS version 1 included declared dead on arrival (DOA) with minimal or no resuscitation attempt (no invasive procedures attempted), death after failed resuscitation attempt (failure to respond within 15 minutes), or died in ED (other than failed resuscitation attempt). In this analysis, more than 6% of patients labeled DOA had time to death in excess of 30 minutes from arrival, with some centers having more than 40% of their DOAs pronounced dead after 30 minutes. More than 10% of patients categorized as DOA were either intubated, had chest tubes inserted, or other procedures performed, and a similar number had documented blood pressure or respiratory rates. These findings varied considerably across centers. In their early reports, the authors excluded patients identified as DOA, but now appreciate the possibility that excluded patients might very well not be dead on arrival. The authors have now evolved to report risk-adjusted mortality both inclusive and exclusive of patients who die in the ED, and have defined a "signs of life" field on arrival to the ED to better capture unsalvageable patients. Subsequent work has demonstrated that this degree of misclassification has negligible effects on the risk-adjusted mortality.[20]

The evolution of TQIP has also allowed identification of other areas in which aggregated data quality can be improved. With the introduction of NTDS, many registrars had to map their existing fields to NTDS fields. An example of this mapping process might occur with the field called "primary method of payment," where there are 10 options. However, local registries might be far more granular with a greater number of options. The mapping process requires the vendor and client to identify which fields would map to the 10 existing fields in NTDS. If this mapping is not done correctly, there is the potential for misclassification or, more frequently, missing data. This particular issue is most relevant for complications and comorbidities. These 2 fields are a particular focus of attention, as both are important for risk adjustment and outcome assessment.

Ongoing registrar training and data quality assessments are a part of ACS TQIP. Each month, TQIP provides the registrars from participating centers with educational opportunities focused on the problem areas identified through assessments of data quality. In addition to education, TQIP provides the centers with data quality reports, and in 2012 will begin external validation of the data. This external validation process will require expert abstractors to review medical records at participating centers and compare these data with those submitted to TQIP. These site visits will be geared toward identifying areas where additional education or standardization is required.

The focus on data quality has been critical for TQIP. The authors think that these approaches lead to greater confidence in the validity of the reports, which in turn leads to a greater follow-through once the areas for improvement have been identified. Furthermore, the lessons learned in standardizing data and data quality will extend beyond the TQIP centers to include all centers contributing data to the National Trauma Databank.

Risk Adjustment in ACS TQIP

Once the data quality and standardization concerns were addressed, risk adjustment was a lesser challenge. There are a large number of published risk-adjustment methodologies in trauma care. Although most methodologies have been used to predict mortality and are useful at the center level, many can be modified to provide valid interfacility comparisons by assuring comparison of "apples to apples." There are wide variations in case mix across centers as a result of several factors. A trauma center located in the core of a large city might receive patients with very short prehospital times in comparison with a center that might serve a wide geographic area and receive many patients through transfer from a nontrauma center. The degree of physiologic derangement at the time of arrival to the trauma center depends on the interval between arrival and definitive care as well as the quality of preliminary care. Local rates of violent crime and penetrating injury, recreational opportunities, local industry, and proximity to major highways also affect the types of injuries cared for in trauma centers. Registry inclusion criteria and differing policies or philosophy related to pronouncing death in the field or in the ED might result in patients at some centers never receiving care in others. All of these factors and more must be considered in developing risk-adjustment models that balance risk of death and complications across centers.

Although there are a large number of published approaches to mortality risk-adjustment models, they all have their limitations. Risk-adjustment models should account for systematic differences in patients' characteristics across centers, but most modeling approaches are dependent on the centers having comparable risk profiles.[21] Regression modeling assumes that there is an overlap of risk distribution. If a group of centers systematically excludes a population of patients included at other centers, then this overlap cannot occur. In the case of TQIP participating centers, this is most evident in the inclusion of elderly patients with isolated hip fractures. Some centers routinely include these patients in their registries and thus need benchmarking data, whereas others do not. Ignoring the lack of overlap in this patient population leads to biased mortality estimates.[19] As a result, TQIP excludes this population from most analyses and provides a specific detailed report focusing only on these patients for those who require this information. Similarly, there are limitations with overlap across centers in patients who either present DOA or who die shortly after ED arrival. To overcome this limitation, data with and without these very early deaths are presented.

Although very complex risk-adjustment models are necessary to account for differences in case mix, it seems that ISS, age, the first ED systolic blood pressure, head Abbreviated Injury Scale (AIS) score, mechanism of injury, gender, and abdominal AIS are the most important factors considered in mortality modeling. TQIP models consider these factors along with the first ED GCS motor score,[22] ED pulse rate, transfer status, and the worst AIS in each body region. Modeling also brings in the *International Classification of Diseases, Ninth Revision* (ICD-9) injury codes using the ICD-9–based ISS.[23–25] The resultant mortality models have an excellent ability to discriminate between survivors and deaths (c-statistic of 0.93) and excellent calibration, the ability of the model to accurately predict expected rates of death across all levels of risk. Separate risk-adjustment models with their own coefficients are produced annually and for each subpopulation, so that centers are compared with the contemporary performance of their peer centers for each patient group.

The mortality models are used to predict the number of deaths expected given a particular institution's case mix. This estimate of expected (E) number of deaths is compared with the observed (O) number of deaths in that institution, creating an O/E ratio, which is presented in a graphical format. If the O/E ratio exceeds 1 and the confidence interval around the O/E ratio excludes 1, then the center has statistically more deaths than expected. If the O/E ratio is less than 1 (and the confidence interval excludes 1), then the center has fewer deaths than expected. While the authors' approach to date has used caterpillar graphs to demonstrate the O/E ratios (**Fig. 2**), they are tending toward the use of funnel plots, which are more intuitive and are becoming the standard for comparing institutional performance (**Fig. 3**).[26] Funnel plots are simply scatter plots with the O/E plotted by hospital volume, with the confidence intervals placed directly on the graph. Although the caterpillar graphs give the appearance of centers being ranked, this is spurious, with centers in the middle all being average. This perception is obviated using funnel plots.

Length of stay (LOS) is modeled in a manner similar to mortality, with the inclusion of payer type as a covariate, given how this factor plays a large role in determining the ease of disposition. In presenting LOS, the length of stay for each patient is estimated and if the patient's LOS exceeds this by 25%, then they are considered to have an excess length of stay (ELOS). The proportion of patients who have ELOS at each center is then presented after adjustment for case mix. The development of risk-adjustment models for selected complications is under way and is likely to be presented in 2012 reports.

CURRENT STATE OF ACS TQIP

Now entering its third year, ACS TQIP has more than 120 participating centers. The components of ACS TQIP have evolved considerably through lessons learned in the pilot and the authors' early experiences (**Fig. 4**). The authors have standardized inclusion criteria to ensure that case ascertainment is similar across the centers to include all adults (age ≥16 years) with an ISS of 9 or more, exclusive of patients with advanced

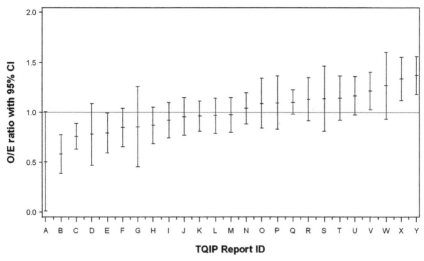

Fig. 2. A sample caterpillar graph demonstrating observed to expected (O/E) ratios for mortality. Expected number of deaths is estimated from the risk-adjustment models. Each center has a unique identifier as shown on the x-axis. In this example, centers B and C are high performers, with their O/E ratios and their confidence intervals all below 1. V, X, and Y are low performers, with their O/E ratios and their confidence intervals (CI) all below 1. It seems the remaining centers are ranked but statistically, each of the centers whose CIs touch unity have similar levels of performance.

directives to withhold life-sustaining interventions. Elderly patients with isolated hip fractures are captured (and reported on) separately, given the variability in the capture of this population across registries and the implications to risk adjustment.[19] Aggregate outcomes by center are reported as well as outcomes in 2 distinct subsets of patients: multisystem blunt trauma and penetrating trauma. In addition to this all-patient report, the authors also provide quarterly reports that focus separately on patients with traumatic brain injury (TBI), shock, or the elderly population. Realizing that performance is not necessarily consistent across patient populations, these diverse reports allow centers to identify their strengths and the areas with opportunities for improvement.[15,19,27] The need for focused reports on selected patient populations was evident, as each of these populations challenges expertise and resources differently. For example, the elderly require a different approach to care than the young. This phenomenon was highlighted by the poor correlation and concordance when assessing the performance within a center for the young compared with a center for the older patients.[27] In addition, reports to date have also provided information regarding the processes of care. For example, the authors have reported on the use of intracranial pressure monitors for patients with TBI (**Fig. 5**), and the use and timing of angiography for patients presenting in shock.

These reports will be expanded as additional data fields to capture processes of care are added. Over 2012 to 2013, the authors will be adding specific fields that will better identify patients with severe TBI and capture the use of intracranial monitoring in this patient population, which provides more granularity than is possible through the current fields in the NTDS. Data on the timing of fracture fixation, the use of pharmacologic venous thromboembolism prophylaxis, the time to hemorrhage control, and transfusion practices will also be captured. There has been tremendous interest in understanding the end-of-life practices, which reflect both quality and

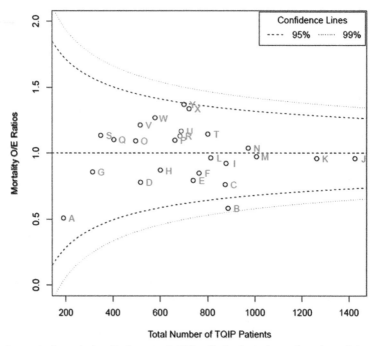

Fig. 3. A sample funnel plot. Each center's O/E ratio is plotted as a function of the center's volume. If a center is outside the 95% confidence interval, it is an outlier. A center below the lower line (eg, B) is a high performer, whereas center Y is just at the limit of average performance. Unlike the caterpillar graph, there is no perception of ranks.

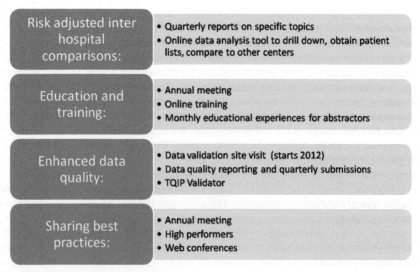

Fig. 4. The key components of ACS TQIP.

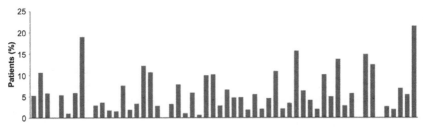

Fig. 5. The variability in use of cerebral monitoring across centers as an example of a process measure. Each vertical bar represents a center and the y-axis represents the proportion of intubated patients with isolated traumatic brain injury who have a cerebral monitor for either intracranial pressure or cerebral oximetry. These data were derived from ICD-9 procedure codes 01.10 (intracranial pressure monitoring), 01.16 (intracranial oxygen monitoring), 01.17 (brain temperature monitoring), and 02.20 (ventriculostomy). A new data field specific to intracranial monitoring along with education on its use will lead to a more consistent data capture and a likely increase in the use of cerebral monitoring for patients with severe traumatic brain injury.

perceptions of salvageability. To address this issue, data on withdrawal of life-sustaining therapy will be captured.

The intermittent nature of the reports provides an opportunity for the engagement of participants throughout the year. In addition, ACS TQIP has created an online tool that allows centers to obtain a probability of survival for each of their patients. This opportunity to drill down on selected patients allows centers to incorporate ACS TQIP into their performance improvement programs in real time, and provides objective assessments of whether an outcome could have been different.

FUTURE INITIATIVES IN ACS TQIP

The development and successful implementation of ACS TQIP has paved the way for several initiatives, including the identification and promulgation of best practices, and the creation of regional collaboratives.

Best Practices

External benchmarking of performance allows for the identification of centers that have particularly good outcomes or processes of care. The practices that result in these outcomes need to be identified for all participants to benefit. Some of these processes, as complex as they may be, might result from institutional culture and might not be easily translatable to other environments. To evaluate this possibility, the authors have explored the feasibility of semistructured interviews with institutional stakeholders to better understand the cultural elements of a high-performing center. Other factors that might lead to better outcomes include practices or structures that have been adopted for any variety of reasons. These factors will need to be identified through a process that requires a close relationship between ACS TQIP and participating centers. Stakeholders at consistently high-performing centers need to be interviewed to understand precisely how care is different at these centers. This challenge is probably one of the most significant of ACS TQIP and will be enabled, in part, through the development of smaller, regional collaboratives.

Regional Collaboratives

Collaboratives represent clusters of centers that share data and exchange information. In organizational theory, these are best referred to as communities of practice.

These communities are groups of people who "share a concern, set of problems, and who deepen their knowledge and expertise by interacting on an ongoing basis.[28]" In theory, both TQIP and NSQIP are collaboratives, but there might be an additional benefit to smaller, regional collaboratives. Historical connections, better networking, and preexisting relationships might lead to a greater trust, and thus better information transfer across centers. In addition, smaller, more frequent in-person meetings focusing on local initiatives or challenges might offer a greater opportunity for an effective change. These regional collaboratives are effective in altering processes and outcomes of care in oncologic surgery, major general surgery, and cardiovascular surgery.[28] Limited evidence suggests that these regional collaboratives might even be more effective than larger, national initiatives such as NSQIP. For example, the Michigan Surgical Quality Collaborative is a group of 34 Michigan hospitals that use ACS NSQIP quality reporting infrastructure. In one study, this collaborative reported its performance relative to ACS NSQIP and demonstrated a significant improvement in the rates of postoperative complications that were not evident in the larger ACS NSQIP collaborative.[29]

It Is plausible that larger initiatives do not facilitate the exchange of details that might be very important for translation of knowledge into practice, and the wide array of institutions might provide a limited opportunity to evaluate relationships between processes and outcomes of care. Regional, customized processes that allow for sharing of best practices and implementation of effective strategies might very well be more successful. Several states are working with ACS TQIP to leverage the existing data and reporting infrastructure, analytic resources, and expertise to develop regional collaboratives. These states will be receiving reports that show their centers' risk-adjusted outcomes in comparison with each other and with the entire TQIP participant base, and might extend to include system-level data as well (eg, interfacility transfer times).

The State of Michigan is farthest ahead, in large part because of the relationship between its trauma centers and Blue Cross Blue Shield of Michigan/Blue Care Network (BCBSM/BCN). The Michigan Trauma Quality Improvement Program (MTQIP) was formalized as a BCBSM/BCN statewide collaborative quality initiative (CQI) in 2011. Since 1997, BCBSM/BCN have partnered with Michigan hospitals and providers in creating statewide CQI, aimed at improving safety and quality of specific procedures and clinical practices across a diverse spectrum of specialties. There are now 12 CQI programs existing as components of a "Value Partnerships" effort, whereby BCBSM/BCN supports hospitals' participation in both national and regional quality initiatives such as TQIP/MTQIP in a pay-for-participation approach, rather than pay-for-performance approach. A pay-for-performance approach might lead to competitiveness and limited willingness to share best practices (or poor performance) with others, whereas a pay-for-participation approach involves minimal risk. CQI programs, such as MTQIP, are focused on participation and engagement of hospitals at a regional level. MTQIP leverages the learning and the resource infrastructure offered by ACS TQIP.[30] In return, the Collaborative has offered its lessons learned in developing a collaborative and in piloting new ideas back to ACS TQIP for others to benefit.

Pediatric TQIP

There has been an extraordinary amount of interest in developing TQIP for the pediatric population and creating a pilot study involving a small number of pediatric trauma centers. This population is particularly difficult to study, as populations are relatively small in number and outcomes such as mortality are rare. There might very well be a greater focus on the processes of care and morbidity, rather than mortality. At present, pediatric stakeholders are working on identifying pediatric indicators of quality that are evaluable across institutions.

SUMMARY

ACS TQIP provides participating centers with risk-adjusted benchmarking data. The information received through quarterly reports is focused and directed, and thus actionable. The collaborative nature of the program allows for the sharing of best practices and the identification of novel approaches to care for the injured. Smaller, regional collaboratives will further enable the sharing of implementation strategies that are practical and translatable to the local environment.

REFERENCES

1. Donabedian A. Evaluating the quality of medical care. 1966. Milbank Q 2005;83: 691–729.
2. Turgeon AF, Lauzier F, Simard JF, et al. Mortality associated with withdrawal of life-sustaining therapy for patients with severe traumatic brain injury: a Canadian multicentre cohort study. CMAJ 2011;183:1581–8.
3. Optimal hospital resources for care of the seriously injured. Bull Am Coll Surg 1976;61:15–22.
4. Hospital and prehospital resources for optimal care of the injured patient. Committee on trauma of the American College of Surgeons. Bull Am Coll Surg 1986;71:4–23.
5. Copes WS, Staz CF, Konvolinka CW, et al. American College of Surgeons audit filters: associations with patient outcome and resource utilization. J Trauma 1995;38:432–8.
6. Cryer HG, Hiatt JR, Fleming AW, et al. Continuous use of standard process audit filters has limited value in an established trauma system. J Trauma 1996;41: 389–94.
7. Boyd CR, Tolson MA, Copes WS. Evaluating trauma care: the TRISS method. J Trauma 1987;27:370–8.
8. Champion HR, Copes WS, Sacco WJ, et al. The Major Trauma Outcome Study: establishing national norms for trauma care. J Trauma 1990;30:1356–65.
9. Camp RC. Benchmarking: the search for industry best practices that lead to superior performance. Milwaukee (WI): Quality Press; 1989.
10. Khuri SF, Daley J, Henderson W, et al. The Department of Veterans Affairs' NSQIP: the first national, validated, outcome-based, risk-adjusted, and peer-controlled program for the measurement and enhancement of the quality of surgical care. National VA Surgical Quality Improvement Program. Ann Surg 1998;228:491–507.
11. Fink AS, Campbell DA Jr, Mentzer RM Jr, et al. The National Surgical Quality Improvement Program in non-veterans administration hospitals: initial demonstration of feasibility. Ann Surg 2002;236:344–53.
12. Khuri SF, Henderson WG, Daley J, et al. The patient safety in surgery study: background, study design, and patient populations. J Am Coll Surg 2007;204: 1089–102.
13. Hall BL, Hamilton BH, Richards K, et al. Does surgical quality improve in the American College of Surgeons National Surgical Quality Improvement Program: an evaluation of all participating hospitals. Ann Surg 2009;250:363–76.
14. Shafi S, Stewart RM, Nathens AB, et al. Significant variations in mortality occur at similarly designated trauma centers. Arch Surg 2009;144:64–8.

15. Hemmila MR, Nathens AB, Shafi S, et al. The Trauma Quality Improvement Program: pilot study and initial demonstration of feasibility. J Trauma 2010;68: 253–62.
16. Goldberg J, Levy PS, Gelfand HM, et al. Factors affecting trauma center utilization in Illinois. Med Care 1981;19:547–66.
17. National Academy of Sciences/National Research Council, Division of Medical Sciences. Accidental death and disability: the neglected disease of modern society. Washington, DC: National Academy of Sciences/National Research Council; 1968.
18. Mann NC, Guice K, Cassidy L, et al. Are statewide trauma registries comparable? Reaching for a national trauma dataset. Acad Emerg Med 2006;13:946–53.
19. Gomez D, Haas B, Hemmila M, et al. Hips can lie: impact of excluding isolated hip fractures on external benchmarking of trauma center performance. J Trauma 2010;69:1037–41.
20. Gomez D, Xiong W, Haas B, et al. The missing dead: the problem of case ascertainment in the assessment of trauma center performance. J Trauma 2009;66: 1218–24.
21. Shahian DM, Normand SL. Comparison of "risk-adjusted" hospital outcomes. Circulation 2008;117:1955–63.
22. Healey C, Osler TM, Rogers FB, et al. Improving the Glasgow Coma Scale score: motor score alone is a better predictor. J Trauma 2003;54:671–8.
23. Osler T, Rutledge R, Deis J, et al. An international classification of disease-9 based injury severity score. J Trauma 1996;41:380–6.
24. Meredith JW, Kilgo PD, Osler TM. Independently derived survival risk ratios yield better estimates of survival than traditional survival risk ratios when using the ICISS. J Trauma 2003;55:933–8.
25. Clarke JR, Ragone AV, Greenwald L. Comparisons of survival predictions using survival risk ratios based on International Classification of Diseases, Ninth Revision and Abbreviated Injury Scale trauma diagnosis codes. J Trauma 2005;59: 563–7.
26. Spiegelhalter DJ. Funnel plots for comparing institutional performance. Stat Med 2005;24:1185–202.
27. Haas B, Gomez D, Xiong W, et al. External benchmarking of trauma center performance: have we forgotten our elders? Ann Surg 2011;253:144–50.
28. Fung-Kee-Fung M, Watters J, Crossley C, et al. Regional collaborations as a tool for quality improvements in surgery: a systematic review of the literature. Ann Surg 2009;249:565–72.
29. Campbell DA Jr, Englesbe MJ, Kubus JJ, et al. Accelerating the pace of surgical quality improvement: the power of hospital collaboration. Arch Surg 2010;145: 985–91.
30. Michigan Trauma Surgery Collaborative. Michigan trauma quality improvement program. 2011. Available at: http://www.mtqip.org. Accessed November 1, 2011.

Index

Note: Page numbers of article titles are in **boldface** type.

A

Abdominal compartment syndrome (ACS). *See also* Intra-abdominal hypertension (IAH)/
    abdominal compartment syndrome (ACS)
    defined, 207
    IAP measurement in, 208
    treatment of, 215–216
Abdominal sepsis
    damage-control sequence for, 244–248
Acetaminophen
    in chronic pain management after surgical nerve injury, 398–399
Acinetobacter calcoaceticus–baumannii complex
    antibiotic resistance by, 360–361
ACS. *See* Abdominal compartment syndrome (ACS)
ACS TQIP. *See* American College of Surgeons Trauma Quality Improvement Program
    (ACS TQIP)
Acute colonic pseudo-obstruction
    POI *vs.,* 264–265
Acute lung injury
    transfusion-related
        in surgical patient, 227–229
Acute pain
    after surgical nerve injury
        management of, 395–398
Acute respiratory failure
    postoperative, 337–339
Afterload
    increased
        in IAH, 210
Aging
    delirium related to, 415
Albumin
    for surgical patients, 193
Alcohol withdrawal
    POD related to, 418–419
Alpha-2 adrenoreceptor agonists
    in POD management, 423–424
Alvimopan
    for POI, 266
American College of Surgeons Trauma Quality Improvement Program (ACS TQIP),
    441–454
    case for, 443–445

Surg Clin N Am 92 (2012) 455–470
doi:10.1016/S0039-6109(12)00039-4
surgical.theclinics.com
0039-6109/12/$ – see front matter © 2012 Elsevier Inc. All rights reserved.

Printed and bound by CPI Group (UK) Ltd, Croydon, CR0 4YY
030502024
0840416003

Moving?

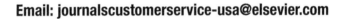

Make sure your subscription moves with you!

To notify us of your new address, find your **Clinics Account Number** (located on your mailing label above your name), and contact customer service at:

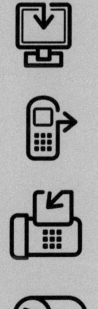

Email: journalscustomerservice-usa@elsevier.com

800-654-2452 (subscribers in the U.S. & Canada)
314-447-8871 (subscribers outside of the U.S. & Canada)

Fax number: 314-447-8029

Elsevier Health Sciences Division
Subscription Customer Service
3251 Riverport Lane
Maryland Heights, MO 63043